The Neurological Patient in History

Rochester Studies in Medical History

Senior Editor: Theodore M. Brown
Professor of History and Preventive Medicine
University of Rochester

ISSN 1526-2715

The Neurological
Patient in History

EDITED BY
L. STEPHEN JACYNA
AND
STEPHEN T. CASPER

UNIVERSITY OF ROCHESTER PRESS

First published 2012
Transferred to digital printing and reprinted in paperback 2014

University of Rochester Press
668 Mt. Hope Avenue, Rochester, NY 14620, USA
www.urpress.com
and Boydell & Brewer Limited
PO Box 9, Woodbridge, Suffolk IP12 3DF, UK
www.boydellandbrewer.com

ISSN: 1526-2715
hardcover ISBN-13: 978-1-58046-412-3
paperback ISBN-13: 978-1-58046-475-8

Library of Congress Cataloging-in-Publication Data

The neurological patient in history / edited by L. Stephen Jacyna and
Stephen T. Casper.
      p. ; cm. — (Rochester studies in medical history, ISSN 1526-2715 ; v. 20)
   Includes bibliographical references and index.
   ISBN 978-1-58046-412-3 (hardcover : alk. paper)
   I. Jacyna, L. S. II. Casper, Stephen T. III. Series: Rochester studies in medical
history. 1526-2715
   [DNLM: 1. Nervous System Diseases—history. 2. Patients—history. 3. History,
19th Century. 4. History, 20th Century. 5. Neurology—history. WL 11.1]
   616.8—dc23

                                                              2011047390

A catalogue record for this title is available from the British Library.

This publication is printed on acid-free paper.

Contents

Part Four: The Patient Constructs the "Neurological Patient"

Part Five: Historians Construct the "Neurological Patient"

Preface

It is now a quarter of a century since Roy Porter began examining the place of the patient in the history of medicine and health. It thus appears an appropriate moment to revisit the historical development of the patient-doctor relationship and the privileging of the patient's perspective—themes that have animated historians of medicine since the mid-1980s. While this volume is concerned with the history of a specific patient, the neurological patient, its essays reveal that many interesting lacunae and unquestioned assumptions about the patient proper remain poorly examined. Among these, the most striking is that historians have too readily employed an essentialist and ahistorical conception of the patient in their historical analysis. In other words, the question of how the patient has been constituted in the era of modern medicine has too often been ignored.

All of the essays assembled in this volume begin the work of addressing that problem. The authors first gathered together for a workshop entitled *The Neurological Patient in History*, sponsored by the Wellcome Trust Centre for the History of Medicine at University College London in the winter of 2008. Although the historical approaches and perspectives of the authors varied, all the attendees agreed that the workshop had facilitated an unusually coherent attempt to study a complex skein of issues raised by the history of the patient proper and the neurological patient in particular. A number of the contributors made strong claims for the potential of historical research to enhance contemporary attitudes and approaches to neurological conditions and enact health policy reforms. Others noted that these essays could serve to revise historical consideration of the patient's place in the history of medicine. This volume consequently derives from those initial discussions.

It has become practically cliché to say that edited volumes are notoriously difficult to organize around unifying themes. To address this challenge, we have attempted wherever possible in each individual essay to draw out parallels or contrasting lines of reasoning among our authors, to whom we otherwise gave no instructions. In addition, we divided the volume into four sections. It was a happy coincidence that our chapters organized rather neatly into the couplets listed in the table of contents, but it is clear that in the various constructions of the patient we identify there were thematically significant and dominant means of viewing patients. In addition, in our historiographic introduction we have described ways that other scholars have examined the patient in history, with an eye toward both explaining areas our volume addresses and neglects, and to providing a richer, theoretically informed structure to the overall work. Finally, while we do not suppose, as many popular authors have done, that the neurological patient is unique among patients, the authors of this volume do hold firmly to the view that the neurological patient as a category of historical analysis uniquely illustrates the peculiar and historically rich circumstances of the patient proper. We thus offer this volume as a history of the patient first and only secondarily as a history of neurology.

—The Editors

Acknowledgments

We wish to express our gratitude to our colleagues—historians and clinicians—who have contributed to our many discussions. In particular, we wish to thank Professor John C. Burnham for attending the workshop that led to this volume and sharing his notes and observations from that day, and for his extensive comments on the introduction of this volume. Clarkson University provided generous support for this project. We would also like to thank the librarians and archivists at the Wellcome Library and at Clarkson University for their assistance.

Finally, we wish to acknowledge the generous support of the Wellcome Trust Centre for the History of Medicine at University College London. Through its support of academic workshops, colloquia, and conferences, the centre provided an unusual, wholly unique, and essential venue for historians of medicine from across the globe to analyze the history and philosophy of medicine, science, and technology. Thoughtful historians should regret the loss of the centre and the resources it provided for historical research, as well as the circumstances that led to its closure.

Introduction

L. Stephen Jacyna and Stephen T. Casper

The essays in this volume deal with the construction of the "neurological patient" as a category in Western medicine. They therefore touch upon how doctors have constructed categories of nervous disease over the past two centuries, and on how medicine has viewed and treated those it has diagnosed as suffering from these complaints. This volume is therefore concerned with one particular version of the clinical gaze. These essays proceed from the premise that neurological disease is not an essence waiting to be discovered but rather a construct with a discernible historicity. But this collection is also concerned with the experience of nervous disease: with what it was to be a neurological patient. One major contention appearing throughout these contributions is that the neurological patient cannot be viewed from a purely clinical perspective. The experience of nervous disease can affect all aspects of an individual's persona, and can permeate the social nexus within which he or she lives. In this respect the neurological patient shares much in common with those who suffer from other kinds of illness. But neurological disease has a peculiar capacity to strike at the core of what in Western culture is taken to constitute personal identity, social status, and competence—indeed even what it is to be human.

"The Patient" in Medical History

For much of the twentieth century historians of medicine were chiefly concerned with changes in medical knowledge, discoveries, and hagiography.[1] From the 1960s onward, however, a generation of social historians of medicine who had been inspired by new trends in sociology, philosophy of science, and general history began to gravitate toward topics that would come to dominate the new historiography of medicine, namely, the professions of medicine, the institutions of medicine, and the social transformations wrought by endemic and epidemic diseases in modern society.[2]

In the 1960s and 1970s as these new patterns were taking hold, many historians of medicine distanced themselves from the conventional narrative of triumphant progress that had been recorded in medical history since the time of the French Revolution. Much of their new suspicion arose in a context in which authority of all kinds—not simply medical authority— was being challenged,[3] but for medicine the challenges seemed especially trenchant. On the one hand, there were intellectual critiques by the likes of Michel Foucault, Erving Goffman, Thomas Szasz, and Ivan Illich.[4] On the other hand, a number of what became infamous medical scandals and treatments—for example, thalidomide and Tuskegee—came to the public's attention and called into question physicians' much-touted humanist ideals.[5] Culturally it became increasingly common to place all scientific and medical conclusions under a critical eye. The confusing data produced by the placebo effect, the mass availability of alternative medicine, the increased prominence of Chinese medicine, and the widespread availability of vitamins further encouraged individuals to question the unchallenged authority of Western scientific medicine.[6] The best doctors might have their patients' interests at heart, but even the best doctors were fallible. Personal health, many came to believe, had become the individual's responsibility.

Much scholarship in the history of medicine from the Vietnam era and after appears to have sought a middle ground in these widespread critiques of the authority of medicine. Partially, of course, this resistance was due to the dispassionate tendencies of the academy. But there were other reasons. Many former physicians had turned medical historians, and not a few of the more respected professional historians of medicine had come originally from a biomedical background. For most historians, it was challenging tradition enough to turn away from the biographies that had dominated the scholarship and focus on public health movements, nutrition, the construction of disease, technology, and (for the more politically inclined) to argue for the equitable distribution of medical resources. If the public fell ever more under the sway of the claim that health was an individual responsibility, then historians of medicine, so it seems, argued against this view and in favor of a social understanding of medicine and for medical policies informed by social perspectives.

Medical power and authority remained very much in the foreground in both public antipathy and in historians' sweeping surveys and narrower case studies, in which they relied upon sources produced by doctors or in medical institutions. From both viewpoints the relationship between the patient and the practitioner was presented in terms of a stark opposition. On the one hand, the doctor was endowed with all the power and authority that his profession and expertise conferred, while on the other, the patient assumed the role of passive object entirely bereft of agency. The British sociologist N. D. Jewson provided a schematized historical account of how this polarization had occurred, when in a much-cited 1976 paper he sketched the "disappearance of the sick man" in Western scientific medicine.[7] While the simplicity of this monochromatic view had some appeal, its limitations soon became apparent.

In what quickly became a classic article in the history of medicine, Roy Porter drew attention to patient agency and called for a realignment of the history of medicine around the patient's perspective.[8] At first glance, Porter appeared to be writing in 1985 from a vaguely leftist perspective. His paper could be read as an attempt to give a voice to a constituency that had been effectively silenced through the tyranny of medical power. The concept of the "patient" was thus configured as akin to other repressed groups, such as women and the working classes, that had been effectively marginalized in conventional historiography.

But ironically, by proposing inter alia a history from below, Porter articulated a program for medical history that sat comfortably alongside the company of the contemporaneous new liberalism propounded in the era of Ronald Reagan and Margaret Thatcher. In the United Kingdom in particular, during the 1980s the healthcare system underwent a substantial reconfiguration as an extension of the marketplace. Within this newly imagined space, the patient occupied the central and privileged role of consumer— a role endowed with the attributes of agency and choice. While this new role elevated the status of the patient, the new liberalism reviled the medical profession as a reactionary bastion of corporate privilege.[9] Porter's later writings, in which the unfettered early modern marketplace for medical services became an object of implicit celebration, served only to strengthen this unlikely alliance with the new Right.

The Porter program, insofar as there was one, challenged historians to move beyond histories that aggrandized bedside acumen and thus reduced the patient "to something akin to the corpse in the detective story."[10] Against the likes of Foucault, Goffman, Szasz, and Illich, Porter argued that patients became patients when they finally decided to seek healing.[11] Beyond this claim, which was perhaps inadvertently calculated toward interests in choice, consumption, commerce, and tastes in the same way that the new cultural history of medicine was, little more explanation of how the patient's perspective could be developed was forthcoming.[12] Porter appears to have almost desired a hagiography of patients, and as other historians have commented, his work fixated often upon patients of wealth and reputation. Porter's penchant for charting the sickness careers of persons of means may be contrasted with Mary Fissell's deliberate choice to focus on poor and disadvantaged patients in her writings on eighteenth-century England.[13]

In one sense, Porter's aim to make the patient an object of medical history was successful—although in another sense the patient's place in the social history of medicine was all but assured anyway; not simply because of the political commitments of historians or the wide array of sources about them, but also because the patient could never really be absent from medicine.

The number of articles in journals devoted to patients rapidly increased.[14] Many studies dating from the 1990s, especially for the medieval and early modern period, recounted the wide varieties of medical practice on offer, the relationships between practitioners and their patients, the disparate experiences of wealthy and poor patients, and the strategies that people used to avoid illnesses.[15] It became clear as well that early modern lay people possessed their own frames for understanding disease and its treatment, and that sometimes medical knowledge was actually the stuff of common lore. As Jewson would put it, the barriers between lay and professional knowledge were more permeable than they later became, a view that implied that the patient became a more unequal partner in the modern clinical encounter as a result of the growing gulf between lay and professional discourses.[16]

There is a superficial similarity between Jewson's analysis and that found in the work of Michel Foucault. In *The Birth of the Clinic* Foucault argued that a new clinical gaze emerged in early nineteenth-century Western medicine. Within this new regime the patient was reduced to a congeries of organs to be scrutinized through techniques of objective examination in order to discern the anatomical lesions that might account for symptoms. The era of Paris medicine also saw the emergence of statistical modes of analysis that reduced the patient to a mere numerical value within a diseased aggregate, further depriving the sufferer of individuality and agency.[17]

In his later work, Foucault developed the notion that modernity was characterized by new modes of exercising power over the body. Central to these disciplinary systems was the notion of "normalization." This presumed a human physiological norm from which various forms of deviance and disorder could be seen as departures. Medicine, conceived as both a body of knowledge and a set of practices, played a central role in establishing and policing these criteria of health and pathology. The protocols established by this disciplinary system determined when and whether an individual or collection of individuals was to be classified as abnormal and therefore to assume the aspect of a patient. Thus arose what Jacqueline Duffin describes as the "tyranny of the normal," the view that the patient no longer needed to feel sick to be sick.[18] In other words, it was the clinical gaze that established illness.

Many historians came to regard Foucault's claims as overwrought and empirically suspect.[19] At first glance a neat separation between early modern and modern patients does appear somewhat exaggerated. Porter's refrain that the patient's agency should not be disputed seemingly applied for all periods. This is, however, to overlook significant features of medicine in the modern era.

First, there was an authoritarian streak to modern medicine. The involuntary commitment of women and men into insane asylums was one especially obvious example, but there were others. Physicians had frequently denied the legitimacy of patient self-reports for which they had no patho-physiological explanation, or alternatively, they had often classified deviance from accepted norms as evidence of illness, as in, for instance, implicitly comparing drapetomania (a supposed mental illness that led North American slaves to flee captivity) or homosexuality to a palsy. Second, there were pressures in modern society pushing individuals toward a model of health that was youthful, strong, and energetic. While reflective individuals in all epochs might have spotted these fountains of youth for what they were, the mass commodity culture and the magic bullet mentality that accompanied these desires was at least partially spring fed by medicine and its tributaries in pharmacy (the latter was often aligned with the cosmetics market). The notion of patient agency in the modern era, in its most base rendering, seemingly implied that patients might choose to die. Yet there were confusing limits. Parents who, for example, opted to remove their children from medical treatments risked social condemnation and even legal sanctions, and few individuals were allowed to avoid the medical progress stipulated by voluntary vaccinations. Modern medicine simply had a depersonalizing effect; the social good trumped individual expectations and agency.

This depersonalization of the patient was not lost on medical practitioners, many of whom, as Christopher Lawrence has shown,[20] worried about the replacement of bedside acumen with laboratory knowledge. Yet the tendency by the mid-nineteenth century was for physicians to view their patients not only as problems for therapeutic intervention but also as statistical points and experimental subjects. While in the early nineteenth century physicians could discover a new condition with reference to only a few similar cases, by the mid-twentieth century standards had so shifted that usually a large number of patients were required to pass muster.[21] Statistical thinking and awareness of differences within populations had become dominant modes of thought in medicine. Not surprisingly, histories of modern medicine that relied upon case records tended to adopt a similar statistical methodology. The sheer quantity of case records meant that mapping large transformations in hospital practice became problems for computer-aided analysis.[22] Few historians followed the early model of Stanley Reiser and examined the actual practices involved in producing the case records that implicitly reduced the patient to the status of standardized description.[23] Still fewer followed Elizabeth Lunbeck's technique in using patient records as the foundational sources for historical narrative.[24]

One of the central issues represented by the modern patient, of course, was precisely the question of the significance of the sources about them. Lunbeck's study had come under criticism by Jack Pressman—an historian with interests in case notes—for its effort to extrapolate from the limited case of one hospital to a larger narrative about medicine in twentieth-century America.[25] But how many case notes would be representative of that larger narrative? The problems did not stop there. Another problem was that historians writing narratives about patients using patient records nevertheless continued to orient around the standard themes of medical history—doctor-patient relations, hospitals, and disease (or madness). Despite Porter's desire for a history from below, everything below was pretty thin on top.

Historians of medicine had too readily employed an essentialist and ahistorical conception of the "patient" in their historical analysis. Theoretically informed histories were few, and much of the most interesting work being done on patients and their experiences occurred in science and medicine studies and focused on the increasing standardization of medical practices,[26] or alternatively in contestations with that scholarship.[27] A few historians, among them Roger Cooter and John Pickstone, had made a substantive effort to use the history of the body as a means of fragmenting the patient into a postmodern subject,[28] but that important point was largely lost upon historians most comfortable in the so-called new (by the twenty-first century it was old) social history of medicine, whose techniques, concepts, and devices, even if they were dead, continued to haunt the whole of the field.[29] Few, moreover, were the studies that were able to break with the patient-practitioner model and examine other roles for the sick person. Historians failed in particular to consider the impact of illness upon the patient's economic, familial, legal, and civic status.

The caregiver was also an absent entity. Moreover, the patient tended to be viewed exclusively as an individual—or as at most a loose aggregate of individuals. Patient organizations received little attention. The legal status of patients was regarded as topic of sociological interest chiefly for the light it might cast on jurisdiction disputes between the professions of law and medicine. The doctor as a patient appeared mostly as a topic of antiquarian interest. Even such an obvious question as how physicians or scientists had derived knowledge from patient's bodies was often ignored.

More than twenty years after Porter's putative gestalt shift, the history of the patient remains therefore curiously underwritten. As Flurin Condrau has noted:

> The patient's point of view remains enigmatic. On the one hand, there is a call to consider the patient in the history of medicine as an important partner, voice, subject, object, or whatever you like to name it with the ultimate aim of rewriting the history of medicine according to the patient's view. On the other hand, we have statements that the patient has actually disappeared from the medical narrative or is merely a by-product of medicine. A full debate between these two positions—that the patient's view can be unearthed from the sources against the statement that the patient is a construct of the medical gaze—has to my knowledge never taken place.[30]

The Neurological Patient in History

The Neurological Patient, in contrast with the patient of medical history, has enjoyed a somewhat different status in the historiography of medicine, being at once a much used subject and at the same time a curiously neglected figure. On the one hand, historians of medicine routinely use patients with neurological diseases or deficits to illustrate their surveys and case studies and to put *the patient* back into medical history.[31] On the other hand, few have commented upon, analyzed, or even recognized the preponderance and variety of sources on neurological patients.

Warwick Anderson's study of kuru is a case in point. Anderson uses the kuru patient to show the ways in which biomedical scientists in the modern era colonized primitive bodies even as they acquired fame for their scientific discoveries. Yet the subject matter of Anderson's study lends itself in grisly ways to making the point stick. The brain of kuru patients was embedded within traditional aboriginal discourses and prized in the practice of ritualistic cannibalism of the dead. It was also a highly sought after commodity by Western scientists, who emerge in Anderson's narrative almost as clinical zombies with unsavory proclivities.[32]

Yet why is the kuru patient especially suited for the making of this argument? Like Walter B. Cannon's studies of voodoo death so diligently described by Otniel Dror,[33] the harnessing of the customs and traditions of aboriginal peoples to Western scientific discourse is the gripping feature of Anderson's study. But as in the case of Dror's work on the emotions, it is the brain (and thereby implicitly the mind) that holds Anderson's narrative together. In other words, it is contemporary fascination with what Fernando Vidal calls the "cerebral subject" that makes the work so engrossing.[34] It is the brain of the kuru patient that ultimately reveals colonizing forces or biomedical prospecting. In Anderson's work, and many others, the neurological patient functions as a totem that forges the physical and metaphysical worlds together into a comprehensible, coherent order.

If this claim about the status of the neurological patient holds, then the obvious question becomes, why? The answer is complicated. One reason is that often neurological patients presented to their physicians and caregivers as already determined subjects, fixed entities, and incurables. For those patients with genetically determined disorders of the nervous system, discussions à la Porter of patient agency, for example, would have to be contrasted with the certainty of their conditions' outcomes.[35] Many authors, among them neurologists, consequently succumbed to temptations to imbue these patients with special social and cultural significance, and as the example of Anderson's work illustrates, this is an especially attractive viewpoint in terms of public consumption.[36] Yet for our purposes here, the more important point about neurological patients is not that they are or should be treated as exemplary figures, which is their typical representation in the literature, but rather that they make manifest in an exemplary way features that all patients share in common.

In that sense the neurological patient has had few experiences differing from other patients in history, but for the reasons outlined above, substantial source material about neurological patients abounds. As in other fields of medicine, physicians approached the patient with mental and nervous disorders as a diagnostic challenge and as an object from which new physiological, pathological, psychological, and even philosophical knowledge might be obtained. Nerve doctors, however, adopted a broadly physiological view of their patients earlier than other areas of medicine, and they routinely made their physiological claims comprehensible by described their patients in exhausting detail.[37]

Nineteenth-century British neurologist John Hughlings Jackson was typical of this strategy. Jackson made many of his classical observations about the nervous system and its physiology through careful clinical examination of his epileptic patients (and others), and he was not alone.[38] Henry Head, trained by physiologist Michael Foster, literally *made* himself a patient when he famously and intentionally sectioned part of his own radial nerve in the course of his scientific investigations of the sensory nervous system. (Head, interestingly, *became* a neurological patient as the result of Parkinson's disease that caused him to retire from professional life.)[39]

Although such episodes of self-experimentation were atypical, the use of patients as subjects for experimentation, contemplation, teaching, and heroic medicine had been the pattern in medicine since the birth of the Paris clinic. Perhaps the most notorious case was the woman in whom the American physician, Roberts Bartholow, demonstrated localization in the brain.[40] From the mid-nineteenth century, whole generations of physicians had used their patients as instructional devices for training clinical students in teaching hospitals. Doctors often displayed their most typical or difficult patients as specimens at meetings of societies, especially those devoted to the investigation of the science and medicine of the nervous system, which began forming in the 1870s and had become increasingly common across the Western world by the close of the first decade of the twentieth century.[41]

From a purely instructional or illustrative point of view, the neurological patient was little different from other patients. For doctors concerned with patients as instructive resources, the new patient and the ideal patient became sought after commodities. The new patient, that is, a new disease incidental to the patient, represented potential discovery and eponymous fame that could consequently establish a physician's reputation in day-to-day practice and likely medical history.[42] An ideal patient, by contrast, could be offered as an exemplary illustration of a specific condition against which less exemplary patients harboring the same condition might be measured. The ideal neurological patient functioned practically as an archetype, and often these patients achieved a measure of fame within neurological circles.

As physicians began investigating patients with nervous diseases, seeking both the new and ideal cases, reports on individual patients appearing in the medical literature changed in tone and perspective. Alongside this new literature was another curious cultural product—the case history or story that captured public attention. This genre, often of a more literary nature, concerned itself with extraordinary cases or extraordinary interpretations of cases, many of which were neurological. Sometimes the literary imagination and the clinical gaze thoroughly fused together, resulting in the widespread fame of the patient, as in the case of Phineas Gage, who in 1848 survived the direct entry of an iron rod up and through the left side of his head and frontal part of his brain.[43] But the literary case note perhaps first fully emerged in psychoanalytical circles and through the wide and growing readership of the works of Sigmund Freud in the 1890s and 1900s. Sometimes the works were even fictional, as, for instance, were Charlotte Perkins Gilman's *The Yellow Wallpaper* and Dalton Trumbo's *Johnny Got His Gun*. But increasingly the genre operated to popularize neurological science, and the doctor-authors who penned these popular medical narratives, such figures as Aleksandr Romanovich Luria and Oliver Sacks, acquired celebrity status.[44]

Many of these case histories focused on the experiences of the neurological patient and usually with an eye toward questions of being and human nature. The neurological patient, of course, was not alone in such depictions. Transplantation patients, for example, received special attention as well and from a similar perspective that raised questions about whether they shared experiences with their donors. But while the transplantation patient might carry some of the significances of the neurological patient, the neurological patient was a decidedly more ambiguous figure.[45]

That ambiguity marked the neurological patient: their status as a neurological patient had to be assumed. The distance, for example, between insanity and neurology was not so very great. Contrary to the view that there were sharp divides between alienism, psychiatry, and neurology, physicians with interests in nervous and mental diseases, at least in the nineteenth century, made few distinctions, save to classify some disorders as functional and others as organic. The functional disorders increasingly fell less clearly within the neurologist's province, for these disorders, in distinction to organic conditions, had no obvious etiological markers. Yet most physicians conflated nervous and mental disorders. Organic conditions often included derangement of higher mental functions. Furthermore, many doctors assumed that the structural pathology of individual mental disorders would eventually be discovered, and thus the classification of a functional disorder was an invitation for investigation.[46]

But the problems did not stop there. There was also the troubling issue caused by conditions that were generally disseminated across the body even as they wrought havoc upon the nervous system. Tertiary syphilis, for one, was a condition many neurologists claimed fell within their purview, but that was a claim held in low regard by more generally minded physicians. The same was true of cases of stroke, cancer, orthopedic injuries, schizophrenia, rheumatoid arthritis, encephalitis lethargica, and poliomyelitis.[47]

There was a corollary to this problem as well. For just as there were patients who appeared to neurologists to be neurological but somehow were not, there were other patients whom general practitioners, psychiatrists, and psychologists regarded as neurological cases, even in the absence of etiological knowledge and demonstrated involvement of the nervous system. The hysteric and the neurasthenic, at times welcomed and at other times vilified by neurologists, were two such patients, but the depressed patient, the psychosomatic patient, the obsessive patient, the malingerer, and the shell-shocked patient were also counted among their numbers.[48]

The neurological patient's ambiguous status, contrary perhaps to expectations, actually justifies the claim that these patients can be understood as being highly representative of all medical patients. It is no easy task to understand how economic, social, cultural, and political discourses defined any patient in the era of modern medicine, but the contributions in this volume suggest that neurological disorders and diagnoses provide highly illustrative case studies. Neurological conditions include acute, chronic, and hereditary diseases. Some neurological conditions such as dystonia, myasthenia gravis, and amyotrophic lateral sclerosis are rare and have come to the public's attention chiefly through their appearance among famous figures or whole professional groups, such as focal dystonia among musicians.[49] Coma has been routinely featured in films, often inaccurately functioning through a Cinderella-like conceit in which the patient awakes to find love or seek revenge.[50] Other conditions like Parkinson's and Alzheimer's disease, migraine, multiple sclerosis, spinal injuries, and stroke, by contrast, occur frequently. The neurological diagnosis of brain death, necessary for organ donation, and management decisions regarding treatment of patients in persistent vegetative states routinely stirs public controversy.[51] Most neurological patients have mental and physical symptoms, and many of those suffering from these often-degenerative conditions remain without treatment options and therefore exist as continuing reminders of the limits and aspirations of modern medical workers and patients alike.

Beyond these reasons, there are still further motivations for examining the neurological patient. For even if the neurological patient is representative of the experiences of all medical patients, the neurological patient has also served an important role in a wider cultural shift that has placed ever increasing value on neuroscientific knowledge. Since the so-called

Decade of the Brain, there has been a growing scholarly appreciation of the prevalence and potency in contemporary society of what some term "neuroculture," a culture in which human nature is ever more to be explained, modified, and controlled through concepts and techniques drawn from the neurosciences.[52] Given the emerging centrality of the nervous system to the conception of selfhood that has become ever more prevalent over the past century, any affliction that affects these organs strikes at the core of the contemporary sense of personal identity.[53]

For the physician, primary caregiver, or even the passive observer, neurological conditions testify to cognitive processes and states often beyond imaginable experience. When confronted with such calamities, the sufferer can strain to find words adequate to characterize the experience. One stroke sufferer described her condition in a best-selling self-help book as akin to that of "a wounded animal," but also compared the state of her consciousness to "a fluid of cells at peace and one with nature."[54] The construction of this neurological patient was not, however, an occurrence merely mediated by the interaction of patients with doctors or through the remarkable variety of public portrayals of patients. Instead, something more significant occurred over the last century to the neurological patient. The neurological patient became a thing through which humans fashioned their sense of identity.[55]

Overview of the Volume

The essays in this volume cannot help but reflect upon these observations, revealing as they do the growing contemporary purchase of these views of the neurological patient. Yet these essays also use the neurological patient to identify the various lacunae that remain underexamined or even absent in the fuller discussion of the patient in medical history. Additionally, they make clear that the patient, neurological or otherwise, can be reconstructed through a wide variety of sources, many of which have been underutilized in patient studies. These sources range from medical writing by doctors and scientists; materials from patient advocacy groups; laboratory records; hospital case notes; cultural sources like magazine articles, newspapers, and films; and sources produced by the patients themselves. Indeed, one interesting observation about the essays in this volume is that even as many of them seek to preserve patients' rights, autonomy, dignity, and humanity, their authors, nevertheless, often infer the patient's perspective through sources of authority other than those generated by the patients themselves. Put differently, one irony in this volume is that the patient continues to be described through the discourses that originally produced him or her as an object first for medicine and then only secondarily for the historical record.

But that irony, banal as it might first appear, tells a story too: the historians contributing to this volume were given no explicit instructions about how to focus their essays, creativity, or narratives, and in consequence their strategies for examining the history of their patients were various. In one sense, then, the patient appears in these essays, as Roger Cooter reflects in his essay in this volume, as "the hole in the middle of the donut." Yet in another way, the patient emerges from these essays as a collage that showcases the variety of ways that historians can approach the patient, even as the essays tell stories and make arguments about patients. Indeed, the essays even reveal the ways in which the patients and the historians have become embedded in the same changes.

We consider this point to be one of the wider justifications for this volume. For the patient in this volume is both absent and present throughout it. In a modernist sense, the patient appears in all of these essays in a commonplace fashion: The patient seeks knowledge of his or her own neuroses. The caregiver copes with the expectations of a debilitated spouse. The courts navigate the murky waters that separate individual autonomy from patient senescence. The doctor names the illness and thus treats the condition. Laboratory knowledge turns the experimental subject into a therapeutic means. In other words, the authors of this volume gravitate toward themes commonplace in modernist understanding, especially in their focus on scientific method, process, categorization, standardization, rule making, institutions, and even in the disciplining of the body.

Yet at some point within this volume, the collage acquires a new order. The patient ceases to be the patient—the patient disappears. Diseases and syndromes become questionable and contingent. Notions of self become a matter of choice, design, and taste. The legitimacy and value of medical authority becomes a matter for debate. The authors become preoccupied with narrative and performance, themes that increasingly seem to link the arguments within the essays together. Some authors resist this interest more than others, seeking to hold steadily to the fixed, dispassionate, scientific, and humanistic strategies of modernity; others shift from those colonizing discourses of modernity toward, as Jesse Ballenger writes in his essay, "a radical reconsideration of what we think it means to be a human being." The patient, the hole in the donut, arises as a new postmodern subject—what Paul Forman describes as the subject defined by a "self-aggrandizing character, undiluted, unmoderated, unmodulated by a sense of obligation, subordination, or subservience of the individual to some other, any other, entities—be they, again, persons, or social, natural, or supernatural entities."[56]

This transformation, of course, occurs not in the primary sources that determine the narratives of this volume, but rather in the imaginations and arguments of the volume's authors. The tension examined implicitly and explicitly throughout this volume is between selfhood and medicine. No technology, means of diagnosis, categorization, or even treatment thoroughly overrides individual experience and agency, a point with which certainly Roy Porter would have agreed. Indeed, this point reveals an underlying cruelty of the turn away from modernity, for several of the essays in this volume record how individuals experiencing the extremes of disease, disorders, or syndromes have been literally whitewashed out of existence in the contemporary moment. Sufferers of Tourette's or Alzheimer's that take forms closer to modern medical discourses' classical typologies of these conditions became problems for their contemporary advocacy groups. The classical cases revealed the awkwardness and the natural ontology of the extreme cases, and thus made manifest the simultaneous limits of narratives of cure, diversity, science, solidarity, entrepreneurship, and technology.

Finally, a number of common themes can be discerned in these essays that merit further attention. A number of the contributions reinforce the received view of a contrast, even an antagonism, between patient and practitioner. Stephen Casper's essay, for example, addresses the limits that patients' bodies imposed upon the neurological examination, showing that even as medical practices that made patient reflexes "speak" were developed, patient bodies proved highly resistant to medical understanding. Similarly, Marjorie Lorch's account of the impact of the new discipline of aphasiology on legal discourse in nineteenth-century England provides evidence of conflicts between the patient's narrative and medical opinion. Lorch makes clear that the notion of a simple binary relationship between doctor and patient overlooks the role of other parties—in this case witnesses—in defining the status of the sufferer. Ellen Dwyer's paper also provides support for the view that modern medicine is characterized by a shift of power away from the patient toward the medical professional. In her case study, the patient does indeed figure as the hapless object of a clinical gaze that seeks to objectify. Indeed the doctors in her study seem determined to reduce their patients to the status of experimental subjects and have a remarkable lack of empathy for these individuals. Moreover, Dwyer shows how governmental and sociological, as well as clinical, discourses sought to define these cases and pathologies. Jesse Ballenger, on the other hand, presents a picture of a far more proactive and empowered set of patients. Sufferers from Alzheimer's disease have, he shows, sought to take control of their destiny despite suffering from what might be deemed the most hopeless of conditions. Ballenger also provides an insightful analysis of why dementia in particular and neurological disease in general so profoundly drive conceptions of the self that are at the heart of modern Western culture. Howard Kushner similarly describes how the construction of the modern Tourette's patient was very much a collaborative effort between doctors and sufferers, and how current preconception and stereotypes contributed to this process.

The history of Tourette's syndrome moreover exemplifies the instability of the distinction made by neurology between functional and organic disorders—a second theme that is also evident in Paul Foley's and Stephen Jacyna's papers. Katrina Gatley provides a more intimate account of the experience of one sufferer and the impact of a chronic neurological condition upon those around him, in particular upon his wife who was obliged to take on the role of caregiver. While in this case the patient himself appears as bereft of agency, Gatley shows that his partner took an active role in seeking and judging medical opinions and support. Finally, the afterword of this volume includes two short commentaries analyzing all of the chapters. Roger Cooter's and Max Stadler's commentaries provide very different estimations of the content of this volume; Cooter argues forcefully that the patient remains as elusive as ever, and Stadler counters that the essays in this volume individually reflect facets of patient identity that allow the patient as a category of historical contemplation to emerge rather more fully formed than has hitherto been the case.

Notes

1. Susan Reverby and David Rosner, eds., *Health Care in America: Essays in Social History* (Philadelphia: Temple University Press, 1979). An early and important work on patients, however, appeared in L. J. Henderson, "Physician and Patient as a Social System," *New England Journal of Medicine* 212 (1935): 819–23.

2. John Harley Warner and Janet A Tighe, eds., *Major Problems in the History of American Medicine and Public Health: Documents and Essays* (Boston: Houghton Mifflin, 2001), 1–23; and John C. Burnham, *How the Idea of Profession Changed the Writing of Medical History* (London: Wellcome Institute for the History of Medicine, 1998). Two works that were especially important for establishing these new trends were Thomas S. Kuhn, *The Structure of Scientific Revolutions* (Chicago: University of Chicago Press, 1970) and E. P. Thomas, *The Making of the English Working Class* (New York: Vintage Books, 1966).

3. Jean-François Lyotard, *The Postmodern Condition: A Report on Knowledge* (Minneapolis: University of Minnesota Press, 1984).

4. See, for instance, Erving Goffman, *The Presentation of Self in Everyday Life* (New York: Anchor, 1959); Thomas Szasz, *The Myth of Mental Illness: Foundations of a Theory of Personal Conduct* (New York: Harper & Row, 1974); Paul Rabinow, ed., *The Foucault Reader* (New York: Pantheon, 1984); and Ivan Illich, *Limits to Medicine: Medical Nemesis, the Expropriate of Health* (London: Marion Boyars, 2000).

5. On the thalidomide tragedy, see "The Thalidomide File," *London Times*, May 10, 1968, 49–52. On Tuskegee, see Susan M. Reverby, *Examining Tuskegee: The Infamous Syphilis Study and Its Legacy* (Chapel Hill: University of North Carolina Press, 2009).

6. Anne Harrington, *The Cure Within: A History of Mind-Body Medicine* (New York: W. W. Norton, 2008).

7. Nicholas Jewson, "The Disappearance of the Sick Man from Medical Cosmology, 1770–1870," *Sociology* 10 (1976): 225–44.

8. Roy Porter, "The Patient's View: Doing Medical History from Below," *Theory and Society* 14 (1985): 175–98. A parallel and important work that appeared at about the same time and is thus of interest here is Edward Shorter, *Bedside Manners: The Troubled History of Doctors and Patients* (Simon & Schuster, 1985).

9. Nancy Tomes, "Patients or Health-Care Consumers?: Why the History of Contested Terms Matters," in *History and Health Policy in the United States: Putting the Past Back In*, ed. Rosemary A. Stevens, Charles E. Rosenberg, and Lawton R. Burns (New Brunswick: Rutgers University Press, 2006), 83–110; and Nancy Tomes, "Merchants of Health: Medicine and Consumer Culture in the United States, 1900–1940," *Journal of American History* 88 (2001): 519–47.

10. Dorothy Porter and Roy Porter, *Patient's Progress: Doctors and Doctoring in Eighteenth-Century England* (Stanford: Stanford University Press, 1989), 13.

11. Ibid., 15.

12. See, for example, Mark S. R. Jenner and Patrick Wallis, eds., *Medicine and the Market in England and Its Colonies, c. 1450–c. 1850* (Basingstoke: Palgrave Macmillan, 2007); and Roberta Bivins and John V. Pickstone eds., *Medicine, Madness, and Social History: Essays in Honour of Roy Porter* (Basingstoke: Palgrave Macmillan, 2007).

13. Mary E. Fissell, *Patients, Power, and the Poor in Eighteenth-Century Bristol* (Cambridge: Cambridge University Press, 1991); see also Guenter B. Risse, *Hospital Life in Enlightenment Scotland: Care and Teaching at the Royal Infirmary of Edinburgh* (Cambridge: Cambridge University Press, 1986).

14. John C. Burnham, *What is Medical History?* (Cambridge: Polity Press, 2005), 135–36.

15. Much of the impetus to the interest in the history of the patient derives from the work of Michel Foucault, above all from *The Birth of the Clinic: An Archaeology of Medical Perception*, trans. A. M. Sheridan (London: Tavistock, 1973). In Foucault's work the patient is the product of a clinical gaze that first attained its modern form in the early nineteenth-century Parisian clinic. For an application of Foucault's work, see L. Stephen Jacyna, *Lost Words: Narratives of Language and the Brain, 1825–1926* (Princeton: Princeton University Press, 2000), especially chap. 3. For the patient more generally, see Andrew Wear, ed., *Medicine in Society: Historical Essays* (Cambridge: Cambridge University Press, 1992).

16. Jewson, "Disappearance of the Sick Man," 225–44.

17. Foucault, *Birth of the Clinic*, 5, 9, 11, 16, 191, and 198.

18. Jacalyn Duffin, *History of Medicine: A Scandalously Short Introduction*, 2nd ed. (Toronto: University of Toronto Press, 2010), 242.

19. For a critical discussion of the impact of Foucault upon medical history, and thus the Paris clinic, see Colin Jones and Roy Porter, eds, *Reassessing Foucault: Power, Medicine, and the Body* (London: Routledge, 1994).

20. "Incommunicable Knowledge: Science, Technology, and the Clinical Art in Britain, 1850–1914," *Journal of Contemporary History* 20 (1985): 503–20.

21. This is a point made in Douwe Draaisma, *Disturbances of the Mind*, trans. Barbara Fasting (Cambridge: Cambridge University Press, 2009).

22. John Harley Warner, "The Use of Patient Records by Historians: Patterns, Possibilities, and Perplexities," *Health and History* 1 (1999): 101–11.

23. Stanley Joel Reiser, *Medicine and the Reign of Technology* (Cambridge: Cambridge University Press, 1978).

24. Elizabeth Lunbeck, *The Psychiatric Persuasion: Knowledge, Gender, and Power in Modern America* (Princeton: Princeton University Press, 1994).

25. Jack Pressman, "Psychiatry and Its Origins," *Bulletin of the History of Medicine* 71, no. 1 (1997): 129–39.

26. Marc Berg and Annemarie Mol, *Differences in Medicine: Unraveling Practices, Techniques, and Bodies* (Durham: Duke University Press, 1998).

27. See, for example, Ilana Löwy, *Preventative Strikes: Women, Precancer, and Prophylactic Surgery* (Baltimore: Johns Hopkins University Press, 2010).

28. Roger Cooter and John V. Pickstone, *Companion to Medicine in the Twentieth Century* (London: Routledge, 2003).

29. It is striking that no essay in Frank Huisman and John Harley Warner, eds., *Locating Medical History: The Stories and Their Meanings* (Baltimore: Johns Hopkins University Press, 2006) deals with *the patient* as a conceptual problem in the history of medicine.

30. Flurin Condrau, "The Patient's View Meets the Clinical Gaze," *Social History of Medicine* 20 (2007): 529.

31. For example, Roy Porter, *The Greatest Benefit of Mankind: A Medical History of Humanity from Antiquity to the Present* (New York: HarperCollins, 1997), 534–50.

32. Warwick Anderson, *The Collectors of Lost Souls: Turning Kuru Scientists into Whitemen* (Baltimore: Johns Hopkins University Press, 2008).

33. Otniel E. Dror, "'Voodoo Death': Fantasy, Excitement, and the Untenable Boundaries of Biomedical Science," in *The Politics of Healing: Essays in the Twentieth-Century History of North American Alternative Medicine*, ed. Robert D. Johnston (London: Routledge 2004), 71–81.

34. Fernando Vidal, "Brainhood, Anthropological Figure of Modernity," *History of the Human Sciences* 22 (2009): 5–36.

35. Alice Wexler, *The Woman Who Walked into the Sea: Huntington's and the Making of a Genetic Disease* (New Haven: Yale University Press, 2008).

36. The obvious examples are Oliver Sacks and Aleksandr Romanovich Luria, discussed below. But many authors have picked up on this theme. See, for instance, J. Bogousslavsky and F. Bollwer, eds., *Neurological Disorders in Famous Artists* (Basel: Karger, 2005).

37. Roger Smith, *Inhibition: History and Meaning in the Sciences of the Brain and Mind* (London: Free Association, 1992).

38. George K. York and D. Steinberg, *An Introduction to the Life and Work of John Hughlings Jackson with a Catalogue and Raisonné of his Writings* (London: Wellcome Trust Centre for the History of Medicine, 2006).

39. L. Stephen Jacyna, *Medicine and Modernism: A Biography of Sir Henry Head* (London: Pickering & Chatto, 2008), chap. 6.

40. J. P. Morgan, "The First Reported Case of Electrical Stimulation of the Human Brain," *Journal of the History of Medicine and Allied Sciences* 37 (1982): 51–64.

41. Stephen T. Casper, "The Idioms of Practice: British Neurology, 1880–1960" (PhD diss., University College London, 2007), chap. 3.

42. Draaisma, *Disturbances of the Mind*, 1–10; and Peter J. Koehler, G. W. Bruyn, and John M. S. Pearce, *Neurological Eponyms* (Oxford: Oxford University Press, 2000), 266–366.

43. Malcolm Macmillan, "Phineas Gage: A Case for All Reasons," in *Classic Cases in Neuropsychology*, ed. Chris Code, Claus-W. Wallesch, Yves Joanette, and André Roch Lecours (Erlbaum: Psychology Press, 1996), 243–62.

44. A. R. Luria, *The Man with a Shattered World: The History of a Brain Wound*, trans. Lynn Solotaroff (London: Cape, 1973). Oliver Sacks, *The Man Who Mistook His Wife for a Hat* (London: Duckworth, 1985); and Oliver Sacks, *An Anthropologist on Mars: Seven Paradoxical Tales* (London: Picador, 1995). On Luria, see also Anne Hunsaker Hawkins, "A. R. Luria and the Art of Clinical Biography," *Literature and Medicine* 5 (1986): 1–15.

45. For a broader discussion of transplant patients, see Margaret Lock, *Twice Dead: Organ Transplants and the Reinvention of Death* (Berkley: University of California Press, 2001).

46. One important discussion of the broad integrative definition of neurology can be found in Andrew Abbott, *The System of Professions: An Essay on the Division of Expert Labor* (Chicago: University of Chicago Press, 1988), chap. 10.

47. Anne Hardy, "Poliomyelitis and the Neurologists: The View From England, 1896–1966," *Bulletin of the History of Medicine* 71 (1997): 249–72; and Kenton Kroker, "Epidemic Encephalitis and American Neurology, 1919–1940," *Bulletin of the History of Medicine* 78 (2004): 108–47.

48. Janet Oppenheim, *Shattered Nerves: Doctors, Patients, and Depression in Victorian England* (Oxford: Oxford University Press, 1991); and Cooter, *Companion to Medicine.*

49. See for example, S. E. Brown, "Focal Dystonia in Musicians," *Western Journal of Medicine* 157, no. 6 (1992): 666. For further examples, see the essays in Bougousslavsky, *Neurological Disorders*; and Barron Lerner, *When Illness Goes Public: Celebrity Physicians and How We Look at Medicine* (Baltimore: Johns Hopkins University Press, 2006).

50. Eelco F. M. Wijdicks and Coen A. Wijdicks, "The Portrayal of Coma in Contemporary Motion Pictures," *Neurology* 66 (2006): 1300–1303.

51. James L. Bernat, "Theresa Schiavo's Tragedy and Ours, Too," *Neurology* 71 (2008): 964–65.

52. Vidal, "Brainhood," 5–36.

53. Roger Smith, *Being Human: Historical Knowledge and the Creation of Human Nature* (New York: Columbia University Press, 2007); Susanne Antonetta, *A Mind Apart: Travels in a Neurodiverse World* (New York: Jeremy P. Tarcher, 2007); and Polly Morrice, "Otherwise Minded," *New York Times*, January 29, 2006, review of *A Mind Apart*, http://www.nytimes.com/2006/01/29/books/review/29morrice.html?_r=1.

54. Jill Bolte Taylor, *My Stroke of Insight: A Brain Scientist's Personal Journey* (New York: Viking, 2008), 64, 70.

55. Lorraine Daston, ed., *Things That Talk: Object Lessons from Art and Science* (New York: Zone, 2004).

56. Paul Forman, "(Re)cognizing Postmodernity: Help for Historians—Of Science Especially," *Berichte zur Wissenschaftsgeschichte* 33 (2010): 165.

Part One

Medicine Constructs the "Neurological Patient"

Chapter One

The Patient's Pitch

The Neurologist, the Tuning Fork, and Textbook Knowledge

Stephen T. Casper

In 1946, British neurologist and clinical neurophysiologist Gordon Holmes wrote in his *Introduction to Clinical Neurology*:

> There is perhaps no branch in practical medicine in which the help and co-operation of the patient is so essential as in the approach to a neurological disorder. For, in the first place, it is on the patient we must mainly rely for an accurate history of the development of his illness, and such a history is often extremely valuable in determining its nature.... In the second place, many neurological symptoms are purely subjective; they are abnormalities experienced by the patient, and may be accompanied by no ... visible sign of disease.[1]

A long discussion of how a neurologist should examine a neurological patient followed this passage. Holmes, drawing upon his past practical and clinical experiences, described lessons that had reinforced his ability to determine primary, and when necessary, differential diagnoses. At the end of his volume he appended a procedural scheme that a student of neurology might employ for fact-finding on the patient's body.[2] Intentionally or not, Holmes was addressing the challenge of translating a tacit knowledge learned through years of practice into logical, comprehensible prose for students.[3] The appendix of his volume provided little more to the reader than the outlines of rules that structured patient-neurologist relations (fig. 1.1 and fig. 1.2). The outline was a tool; the examination of the patient, by contrast, was a practice with historically determined scientific and clinical logics. It was impossible, therefore, for Holmes to express clearly in prose the relations between the neurologist and the patient and their meaning. In a world before high-definition X-rays, computer-aided analyses, and PET, CAT, and MRI imaging, the living body, normal and pathological, and the dead body determined the neurologist's practices.[4] Life was the formal barrier preventing absolute neurological knowledge.

APPENDIX

A Scheme for the Clinical Investigation of the Functions of the Nervous System

THE advantage of employing a standard method or scheme in the examination of a patient who presents, or may present, signs of disorder in the functions of the nervous system is that it assures an adequate investigation in the shortest possible time, reduces the risk of oversight or omission of symptoms and enables the clinician to arrange his observations in a concise and logical manner. Frequently such a scheme can serve only as a preliminary or general survey of a case; facts brought to light by it, or special disorders, may require fuller investigation or the use of additional methods.

The aim of any scheme or plan of operation should be to ensure a methodical investigation of the separate functions of the nervous system; the use of the simplest methods that can furnish reliable results or observations, and the arrangement of tests so that the analysis or interpretation of each observation should be, as far as possible, independent of facts revealed by subsequent tests should be adopted, though a final conclusion can be reached only by correlation of all available evidence.

Many schemes are in use: the following will prove adequate for a preliminary examination of most cases. It may, however, be necessary or advisable to vary the sequence of tests, or modify them according to the state of the patient or the nature of his illness.

Special Senses

Smell.—Exclude local conditions as rhinitis, catarrh, etc. Use standard set of common odours, as camphor, cloves, peppermint, asafœtida.

Taste.—Apply sugar, salt, quinine, citric acid in powder to the anterior and posterior parts of the tongue.

Vision.—*Acuity of Central Vision* after errors of refraction have been corrected and opacities and other abnormalities of the media have been allowed for. Extent of *visual fields* for white and colours, first by confrontation methods and later, if necessary, by use of a perimeter. Presence or absence of *scotomata*, or areas of defective vision within the fields, first by confrontation and later by use of a perimeter or a Bjerrum's screen. *Ophthalmoscopic examination*, noting the edges and central pit of each optic disc, the colour of each disc, the condition of the retinæ, particularly of the macular regions, and the state of the retinal vessels.

Hearing.—Response to whispered voice, to a watch or tuning-fork. Conduction of sound of a vibrating tuning-fork through air and through

Figure 1.1. One example of a scheme for examining the patient in Gordon Holmes, *Introduction to Clinical Neurology* (Edinburgh: E & S Livingstone, 1946), 184. Courtesy of Elsevier.

bone. Lateralisation of sound of tuning-fork placed on middle line of skull. Presence of tinnitus.

CRANIAL NERVES

Third, Fourth and Sixth Nerves.—Range of movements of each eye and of conjugate movements. Presence or absence of squint, diplopia or nystagmus. Size, symmetry and regularity of pupils. Direct and consensual reaction of the pupils to light and on convergence. Posture and movement of the lids.

Fifth Nerve.—Size of the masseter and temporal muscles when contracted. Deviation of lower jaw on opening and closing the mouth, preferably against resistance. Sensibility of the face to touch, pin-prick and temperature. Corneal reflexes.

Seventh Nerve.—Expression and symmetry of face at rest. Voluntary and expressional movements of the upper and lower portions of the face.

Ninth and Tenth Nerves.—Position and movement of the soft palate. Palatal and pharyngeal reflexes. Position and movements of the vocal cords as seen by the laryngoscope. Articulation, phonation and swallowing.

Twelfth Nerve.—Presence or absence of wasting, fibrillation and tremor of the tongue. Movements of the tongue.

MOTOR SYSTEM

Presence of atrophy or fibrillation of muscles. Tone of muscles; nature of increase of tone if present. Power of contraction of individual muscles (in peripheral lesions) and strength of movement of each segment of the limbs and of the trunk. Automatic movements, as swinging the arms in walking. Co-ordination of movement, testing first simple, later more complicated movements, as gait and the use of tools. Influence of excluding vision on accuracy of movement. Alternating movements. Presence or absence of involuntary movements.

REFLEXES

Note presence, absence or modification of the following:—

Proprioceptive or Deep Reflexes.—Flexion and extension reflexes of the forearm and finger-jerks. Knee and ankle jerks.

Superficial or Cutaneous Reflexes.—Abdominal, cremasteric and plantar reflexes.

SENSATION

Spontaneous Sensations.—Presence or absence of pain and abnormal sensations. Their nature, distribution and the factors that influence them if present.

Cutaneous Sensibility.—Response to tactile, painful and thermal stimuli. Localisation of stimuli and discrimination of compass points.

Figure 1.2. Another page from the same scheme for examining the patient in Gordon Holmes, *Introduction to Clinical Neurology* (Edinburgh: E & S Livingstone, 1946), 185. Courtesy of Elsevier.

Scholars as various in their approaches to the history of medicine as Erwin Ackerknecht and Michel Foucault have noted that the project of modern Western medicine began in the Paris clinic with the realization that death allowed a knowledge of life.[5] So-called Paris medicine, in contrast with the humoral medicine of the early modern period, placed the corpse at the center of its system of knowledge.[6] Unlike the medicine of the early modern period, physicians ceased to see the patient as an individual. Instead, physicians categorized patient symptoms in terms of an inner, imagined pathology that ultimately referred to their experiences in the morgue and thus constituted a statistical body. Physicians increasingly correlated the visible lesions of the dead with the discernible symptoms of disease in the living patient. Throughout the nineteenth century, new means of revealing hidden pathology became part of medicine's practices—the laying on of the hand preceding the revealing capacities of the stethoscope, thermometer, ophthalmoscope, laryngoscope, and in the twentieth century, the X-ray, ventriculogram, and electroencephalograph.[7] As historian Stanley Reiser describes, tools like the stethoscope "could, in a sense, autopsy the patient while still alive."[8]

For nineteenth-century physicians with an interest in nervous diseases, such technological innovations did little to facilitate a complete break with medicine's early modern modes of practice. Aspects of constitutional medicine remained part of medical understanding well into the twentieth century. The pathology of many nervous diseases was simply hidden from postmortem inspection. In his textbook *A System of Clinical Medicine,* Thomas Dixon Savill captured the essential challenge and thus technique of the neurological exam. He wrote: "The method of examining a nerve case differs somewhat from that in other departments of medicine, partly on account of the inaccessibility of the nervous system to direct examination, and partly owing to the widespread effects of its diseases. It is, however, not difficult provided the beginner adopts a fixed order of examination."[9] As this chapter will show, part of that fixed order was a throwback to early modern medicine's observational techniques and interest in patient narratives. Each became part of neurology's productive discourses and made invisible pathologies suddenly perceptible.

This chapter focuses on the history of the neurological examination, that is, the means by which physicians with an interest in the nervous system diagnosed patients with nervous and mental disorders. In other words, it calls attention to a little-examined area of medicine, what historian John Harley Warner has described as the means with which "protean signs and symptoms" came to be deemed important by clinicians in the making of diagnoses.[10] In particular, the emphasis here is upon the internal logic of this exam, especially the ways early modern medical understanding combined with approaches pioneered in the Paris clinic in order to constitute the modern neurological exam and thus also the neurological patient. It also examines the means by which practitioners transmitted and interpreted the modern neurological exam between generations, and the ways patients were consequently conceived of by their doctors, and accordingly how patients experienced and participated in the exam's performance. This approach is in contrast to other scholarship, which has tended to exhaustively delineate the origins of each individual test, while paying less attention to the production and reproduction of the practices underlying the exam. It was those practices that eventually fused together a knowledge of signs and their corresponding lesions with a knowledge of the significance of the patient's narrative.[11]

The focus of this essay is limited mainly to Britain. In addition, the sources—primary and secondary—for such a study are limited and tend toward brief but germane vignettes on the neurological exam.[12] Yet this paper claims to follow representative threads. It begins by examining some of the origins and influences on British neurology, and then considers how early physicians with an interest in nervous diseases began to conceive of their patients and how these doctors transmitted that new and often tacit knowledge to their students. The processes by which the medical student received this knowledge of the patient were not merely dependent upon neurological training. The student also had to acquire a special way of viewing and judging the patient's body before he or she could fully appreciate the view the neurological window provided of pathology.[13] In the nineteenth century, the tools framing that window were often improvised or made. By the 1940s, as government administrators formally institutionalized neurology in Britain's hospitals, the tools of the neurological exam had become more standardized. The patient's experience of the rituals of the exam thus became increasingly routine.

Body and Constitution: Origins and Influences on the Science and Medicine of the Nervous System

If medicine in the nineteenth century was different in many ways from the medicine of the early modern period, then modern medicine nevertheless kept alive many of the older traditions of medical practice as well, especially in the way that physicians observed their patients. In his *Handbook of Physical Diagnosis*, which appeared in 1880, Paul Guttman, noted that while auscultation, percussion, palpation, spirometry, and pneumatometry, as well as tests of the blood and excretions, comprised the physician's diagnostic armamentarium, none of these tests could proceed without a general inspection of the patient's body, for "a practiced eye often discovers ... a multitude of signs, which not merely declare which of the organs is at fault, but frequently reveal the nature and stage of the disease with absolute accuracy."[14]

In the subsequent twenty-one pages, Guttman described the implications of fever, accelerated pulse, blanching, jaundice, cyanosis, swelling, and emphysema in diagnosis. Although he made only subtle reference to the patient's constitution, he left unacknowledged obvious aspects of patient individuality such as occupation, class, gender, race, or creed. Yet the individuality of the patient, so important to the early moderns, had not become obsolete in the nineteenth century.[15] An interest in the patient's narrative instead became tacitly incorporated into modern medicine's new practices of revealing illness. Modern medicine thus demanded knowledge of the patient's individuality, later to be termed lifestyle. At the same time, it harnessed that knowledge to an objective discourse of postmortem pathology, a language especially necessary for neurology.

By the mid-nineteenth century, physicians and scientists had established many of the concepts central to the sciences of the nervous system, yet the formation of such knowledge had not yet led to any specific pattern of academic or clinical institutionalization.[16] Many histories of neurology note that institutionalization of neurology coincided with wars in the nineteenth and twentieth century.[17] Although historians have noted the limitations to ascribing too much causal import to wartime events, it seems evident that the injuries caused by shrapnel or bullets during, for example, the American Civil War extended the Paris approach to the nervous system in a way novel for the medicine of the nervous system but in keeping with the new practices of nineteenth-century medicine. Shrapnel and bullet wounds made visible what were normally hidden lesions in the peripheral and central nervous system. These wounds also made manifest behavioral and physiological symptoms. American physicians like Silas Weir Mitchell and William Hammond were able to use the diversity of injuries appearing in their wounded patients to observe and categorize a range of hitherto unknown functions of the nervous system.[18] By the end of World War I, research reports of this kind had become commonplace in studies of the nervous system.[19]

In Europe, the impulse toward specialization in medicine lent itself increasingly to the creation of specialist institutions and clinics for nervous diseases.[20] Most famously, the Salpêtrière in Paris contained numerous patients with nervous conditions.[21] Medical students from Europe and North American flocked there to train under the celebrity-physician Jean-Martin Charcot (1825–93).[22] Charcot had been appointed to the Salpêtrière in 1862 and by 1892 held a clinical chair of diseases of the nervous system in the Paris Faculty of Medicine.[23] In his lectures, published in English by the Sydenham Society in 1889, Charcot exhorted his students to make themselves "anatomists for today" so that "examination of the *living* subject" could continue tomorrow.[24] Without a broad knowledge of anatomy, physiology, and pathology, Charcot's remarks implied, the accurate diagnosis of nervous conditions would be impossible.

Circumstances in Britain were similar to those in contemporary France. Though less famous than Charcot, James Crichton Brown, John Hughlings Jackson, David Ferrier, and other physicians with interests in the pathophysiology of the nervous system increasingly placed physiology at the center of the diagnosis of nervous conditions.[25] Initially, these physicians had used patients housed in the West Riding Lunatic Asylum for research. In articles appearing in the *Medical Reports* of that institution, these physicians began delineating the relations between nervous and mental symptoms and postmortem pathology by utilizing the "valuable information hitherto buried in case-books and diaries."[26] Some of these younger physicians were able to take advantage of the new hospitals for epilepsy and paralysis that began appearing in London from the 1860s onward.[27] As historian Chandak Sengoopta has observed, following the formation of the hospitals, these physicians focused increasingly on the localization of neurological functions to specific anatomical structures within the brain. As a corollary, these physicians and their students increasingly lost interest in conditions for which they could find no physioanatomical correlate, mainly functional nerve disorders.[28] By the 1920s, the distinctions between psychopathology, psychiatry, psychology, and neurology, if still blurred in practice, were becoming delimited.

The neurologists' decreasing interest in so-called functional disorders did not indicate failing interest in the patient's constitution. Charcot, for one, was interested, and he has traditionally captured scholarly attention with his emphasis on hypnosis and classification of the nervous diseases of women. Yet many—perhaps most—Victorian and Edwardian physicians believed that the constitution of the patient could prove determinative in nervous disease.

Women, for example, were especially vulnerable to specific nervous and mental disorders.[29] William Gull, a consultant physician at Guy's Hospital, and the Fullerian Professor of Physiology from 1847 to 1849, had unified observations of eating disorders in young women into a coherent disease classification, anorexia nervosa, which linked weakened nervous organization with physiological principles.[30] Today the language that informed much of this constitutionalism rings with misogynistic undercurrents that feminist scholars like Elaine Showlter have been quick to note.[31] And indeed when James Purves-Stewart described his barking, grunting, and snorting hysterical patients in his textbook *Diagnoses of Nervous Diseases*, he noted perhaps too drolly that in the case of one "her bark made her society a mixed pleasure."[32]

Women were not the only victims of this late-nineteenth-century medical constitutionalism. Henry Head, a German-trained physician-neurologist, remarked that "the world . . . is singularly like my East End Jew patients" of whom, Head's biographer Stephen Jacyna remarks, he made scapegoats for his own "growing sense of angst with the realities of professional life."[33] If we see now that Head's comment reflected commonly held anti-Semitic attitudes, then it is necessary to note that they were also part of profounder assertions about the threat of degeneration and the nervous system (this issue of cultural stereotypes and diagnosis is addressed in many of the papers in this volume, and most prominently in Howard Kushner's examination of Tourette's syndrome).

From this, the logics of the neurological exam begin to become obvious. The neurologist it seems could read two pathologies: the inner anatomical pathologies of lesions and the outer pathologies caused by everyday life that weakened or worked upon an already genetically weak body. Putting it differently, the logic of the neurological examination assumed that lifestyle and hereditary predispositions were productive of nerve lesions and thus were proximate causes of symptoms observed in practice. Frederick Mott, physician-neurologist at the central pathological laboratories at the Maudsley Hospital, articulated this attitude when during the course of his 1911 Presidential Lecture before the neurological section of the Royal Society of Medicine he asserted that "every neurologist recognises the importance of the inborn factor in the production of neuroses and psychoses; and in certain degenerative conditions of the nervous system." It was due to these inborn factors, and their degenerative effects upon the patient's constitution, that Mott could claim that "Jews were, on account of their neurotic temperament, more liable to insanity than Christians."[34]

Textbooks and Tacit Knowledge

Textbooks are one source that can make the logics of the patient's examination clearer to us.[35] They show the ideal ways that physicians were instructed to observe their patients. Textbooks reveal, moreover, one way that a conception of the patient could be transmitted from one generation of physicians to the next.[36] In any case, they make especially manifest for us the special and novel way that neurologists forged the patient's illness narrative with a diagnostic reading of the patient's body.

Until the 1850s, there were few textbooks, manuals, or book-length works devoted completely to the subject of nervous diseases, the nervous system, or neurology. As early as 1855, John Russell Reynolds noted that the essential task in diagnosis of diseases of the brain, spinal cord, and nerves was to identify "locality, nature, and lesion" in the patient.[37] But how? It was in the 1880s that the first major textbooks began to appear that possessed a detailed nomenclature of the conditions encountered in patients with nervous and mental diseases and a means of diagnosing them. William R. Gowers's *Manual of Nervous Diseases* and the translation of Charcot's clinical lectures arrived shortly after Thomas Buzzard's *Clinical Lectures on Diseases of the Nervous System*. The 1890s saw the publication of Charles Beevor's handbook for students and practitioners on diseases of the nervous system, and by the first decade of the twentieth century, the publication of James Purves-Stewart's *The Diagnosis of Nervous Diseases*. By then works by North American authors were in circulation in Britain as well; so too were other translated works from the European continent.[38]

Such texts were always wide-ranging and expansive in their conception of the neurological patient. They tended to systemize clinical practices while simultaneously advertising to a wider public the author's expertise in treating nervous conditions.[39] In their general features, Victorian and Edwardian manuals and textbooks mirrored one another in layout and content. They opened with general discussions exploring the anatomy and physiology of the nervous system, and then usually considered diagnosis. Most of these texts contained either a full chapter or appendix wholly devoted to describing the methods a physician should follow for taking case histories and for conducting detailed neurological examinations.[40] Consequently these sections articulated and ordered the textbook author's bedside experiences. At the same time, as will be shown below, the authors linked these methods of history taking and examination with further discussion of the anatomical and physiological principles underlying their methods for understanding the patient's illness.[41]

The first textbook on the subject in English appeared in 1886. Titled the *Manual of Nervous Diseases*, it had been written by William Gowers, Professor of clinical medicine at University College London. His was a first attempt to systematize knowledge of nervous and mental diseases into a comprehensive scheme (in two volumes). His book was intended for medical students and young physicians. It was, moreover, among the first texts discussing ways of making visible those nervous conditions that could only otherwise be diagnosed in patients with any certainty through postmortem inspection. In a section titled "Symptoms and their Investigation," Gowers remarked that the "nervous system is almost entirely inaccessible to direct observation" save for the eyes, a point worth noting because Gowers had published an earlier work on that new technology of revealing, the ophthalmoscope.[42] Yet because "morbid states reveal their presence by the derangement of function which they cause," Gowers argued that it was possible to link the most frequent symptoms with the actual process of their elucidation, and from both—the symptoms and system of examination—to proceed to a diagnosis.[43] Gowers furthermore divided patient symptoms into their mental, motor, and sensory states. Although he noted that some patients would have diseases of unknown pathology, he guessed that in time researchers would discover lesions caused by malnutrition or a degenerative constitution.[44]

Gowers's textbook seems to have become the model for subsequent works. While his book was extraordinarily comprehensive, his competitors in the 1890s and 1900s attended mainly to the commoner nervous diseases or diseases of a part of the nervous system like the spinal cord or brain.[45]

It seems that the most commonly used of the textbooks was James Purves-Stewart's *The Diagnosis of Nervous Diseases*. First published in 1906, translated and later described by neurologist Edwin Bramwell as "the best book of the kind in the English language," it subsequently appeared in many languages; its ninth and final edition appeared in 1945.[46] Purves-Stewart's stated goal in his textbook was to avoid "abstruse details of theoretical interest" and to focus on the diagnosis of patients alone.[47] His book, like Gowers's, began with lectures outlining the anatomical and physiological knowledge required for accurate diagnosis. He wrote, "there is no department of medicine where an accurate knowledge of anatomy is of greater importance."[48] Though clinical practice in nervous diseases required scientific knowledge, a particular value system nevertheless distinguished his system. He wrote, for example that "the examination of a nervous case should not be confined to the nervous system alone. All the systems of the body should be investigated. An accomplished neurologist must be in the first place a sound physician."[49] He cautioned as well against the risks of spot diagnosis of patients, a tendency prevalent among the elite consultants, which when correct marveled an ill-advised and incautious audience, but when wrong put the patient's life in jeopardy.

Like Gowers, Purves-Stewart also held that discrimination between organic and functional disorders was complicated. The changes in the nervous system were so minute, he thought, that they could go unrecognized, even with the aid of a microscope in postmortem examination. He thus observed: "The term 'functional' then, is a confession of our etiological ignorance."[50] On the other hand, if a patient's lesion could be detected, then the nerve doctor's task was to determine its location (its anatomy) and its nature (its pathophysiology). Crucially, the answer to the question of where the lesion was located could only be constituted through both the physician's knowledge of signs, that is, through examination of the patient's body, and the physician's reconstruction of the history of symptoms, or the patient's narrative. The answer to the nature of the lesion could only be obtained through the patient's narrative—the patient's self-reporting of the chronology and sequence in which the symptoms had begun to appear. According to Purves-Stewart, a proper neurological examination required that the physician combine the patient's narrative with the physician's diagnostic reading of the patient's body.

Both Gowers's and Purves-Stewart's textbooks were representative of those that appeared between 1880 and 1950. Gowers's textbook, and others like it, aimed for encyclopediclike coverage. Purves-Stewart's sought a balance between comprehensiveness and instructional quality; in other words, where Gowers focused on facts, Purves-Stewart was prescriptive. Unlike Gowers's book, then, Purves-Stewart's book included numerous drawings and photographs, perhaps explaining its popularity. Both books had their competitors.

H. Campbell Thomson's *Diseases of the Nervous System*, which appeared in 1908, was reprinted in 1915, 1921, and 1925, and mirrored Gowers's overall organization while updating, if limiting, its content. Donald Core's *The Examination of the Central Nervous System* and Frederick Nattrass's *The Commoner Nervous Diseases for General Practitioners and Students*, in contrast, were written for a nonspecialist market, and they sought audiences among clinicians working far from regional metropolitan centers. Their works might have competed with Purves-Stewart's, but they notably had few illustrations and neither went to a second edition.

Further encyclopedic tomes appeared: in 1933 the first edition of Walter Russell Brain's *Diseases of the Nervous System*, and in 1940 the posthumous publication of Samuel Alexander Kinnier Wilson's three-volume *Neurology*. All of these works began with discussions of the nervous system's anatomy and physiology. With the exception of Brain's textbook, they all also utilized their author's vast clinical experiences and thus most provided some account of the techniques and skills required for elucidating signs and recording and interpreting the patient's history. In hindsight, the textbook that appears the most unique in this period was Gordon Holmes's *Introduction to Clinical Neurology*. At 183 pages, it was the smallest of the textbooks and the only one to contain barely a word on psychiatric conditions.[51] At its heart, however, Holmes's textbook provided the most detailed discussion of diagnosis because it focused entirely on the meaning of signs and symptoms.

Revealing Practices: The Plantar Reflex as an Illustration

Little is known about the process by which students learned to examine their patients.[52] Historians of medicine have largely avoided examination of the work and rituals involved in patient diagnosis. Although Koehler, Bruyn, and Pearce have made a significant effort to trace the history of some neurological tests, it is not certain that most of the neurological tests described in recent works are remotely equivalent to those appearing in earlier textbooks.[53] Most students would likely have learned how to examine their patients by observing and mimicking their teachers. Films of neurological patients from the interwar period and after, some of which are housed at the Queen Square Library, provide little insight into the transmission of this tacit knowledge.

Yet it is significant that the earliest textbooks on nervous diseases contained a section or chapter devoted to the patient examination and the process of recording the patient's narrative.[54] Indeed, by the 1950s and 1960s whole monographs were devoted to the subject.[55] At almost eight hundred pages, Russell DeJong's *The Neurological Examination* (the fourth edition appeared in 1979), was the most comprehensive work on the subject.[56] The existence of such full-length works raise many questions, not least of which is how, historically, did the practices described in them become a part of the neurological repertoire? The answer to this question can be established through analysis of the logics underlying the examination. In all cases, the goal was to make the patient's lesion and constitution qua hereditary weaknesses and lifestyle influences simultaneously visible for medical inspection.

By far the most familiar neurological tests are the knee jerk and plantar reflex tests.[57] The neurological examination, however, became over time extraordinarily comprehensive; similar tests involved pins, tuning forks, vials of liquids smelling of camphor, mint, or other odors, von Frey hairs, dynamometers, spinal taps, temperature tests, as well as close observation of the patient's habits and state of mind. Each of the tests employing these various technologies of revealing would be worthy of exploration. However, for brevity this chapter shall explore the plantar reflex only, a test that Francis Walshe, neurologist at University College London, described as the perhaps most "important single physical sign in clinical neurology," and one that now seems highly representative of the logic underlying the other tests used to diagnose the neurological patient.[58]

In 1896 Joseph Babinski described his sign and its neurological implications.[59] In his 1906 textbook, Purves-Stewart described the procedure: in an upward motion, the physician gently stroked the sole of the patient's foot with a hard object. Normally all of the toes would flex. When abnormal, however, the big toe extended slowly while the other toes would curl toward the sole. In his book, Purves-Stewart noted that this sign was "practically always pathology . . . and if constantly present it indicates an organic lesion, and one which implicates the pyramidal tract," an area of the brain involved in movement.[60]

Papers assessing the relative diagnostic value of the plantar reflex in patient diagnosis had begun appearing as early as 1899.[61] Yet it was a 1904 paper in the *Review of Neurology and Psychiatry* by a young Birmingham physician, Arthur Stanley Barnes, that most fully established the reflex's utility. Barnes had been a house physician at the National Hospital for Epilepsy and Paralysis, Queen Square, between 1900 and 1902, and had spent another year in practice at Queen's Hospital in Birmingham. In total, his paper reviewed 2,500 instances in which the plantar reflex had been used as a part of patient diagnosis. His study included evidence from 150 postmortem findings as well.[62] Barnes described his technique:

> I found that the most constant and delicate results were produced by stimulation of the outer part of the sole, that is, the edge of the sole corresponding roughly to the outer and lower surfaces of the fifth metatarsal and adjacent tarsal bones. The sole here is not quite so sensitive as at the inner side, so that frequently a stronger stimulus is necessary to evoke the reflex from the outer side of the sole than from the inner side; but in all cases when patients are "ticklish," it is far easier to obtain from this position a constant result.[63]

After describing the patient's reflex under normal conditions, Barnes offered a picture of the various neurological conditions that might bring on the sign. Any damage to the pyramidal area of the patient's brain brought about derangement, but Barnes's clinical experience suggested that the strength of the sign in the patient depended upon whether it was a progressive neurological condition or one caused by immediate trauma. Thus a stroke affecting that region of the brain would almost certainly lead to the pathological response, whereas progressive conditions like cancer, tabes, meningitis, and increased intercranial pressure gave a more ambiguous picture.[64] Sydenham's chorea never showed the extensor form of the reflex; diplegia, on the other hand, usually did. The complete absence of the sign in a patient could be significant, and usually indicated the destruction of the nerves involved in the pathway; therefore, the physician could suspect conditions like neuritis, disseminated sclerosis, and even severe hysteria, although Barnes was quick to caution that fatigue could sometimes lead to the sign's absence altogether.[65]

None of these observations mattered greatly without reference to other signs, and it was in combination with the other components of the exam that the diagnostic value of the reflex became clear. Unlike the knee reflex, Barnes demonstrated that one of the advantages of the plantar reflex was that there seemed to be no cases where the sign could be present without pathology. The knee reflex, by contrast, was a far less certain indicator; an exaggerated or diminished kick was always a measure of qualitative sensibility. Yet in the case of the plantar reflex, extension of the big toe consistently indicated the presence of a lesion in the central nervous system. An absent knee reflex but the presence of a normal plantar reflex likely indicated a disease of the spinal cord. If both knee reflexes were absent, then an abnormal plantar reflex indicated the side of the brain in which a stroke had occurred. The distinction between disseminated sclerosis and hysteria tended to be tricky, but the presence of the extending toe immediately suggested the degeneration of the brain, a point Barnes ultimately demonstrated for one case through postmortem examination.[66]

The neurological examination required many more tests than the plantar reflex, but the way in which Barnes described its presence in relation to the other reflexes and the patient's history and connected these facts to anatomical and physiological principles makes explicit to us the logic of the patient's examination. The neurological exam literally turned the patient's body into a machine of its own revealing. A simple test of the toe revealed a localized pathology of the brain; in the absence of a technology of revealing like the stethoscope or X-ray, the reflex became a substitute. Other examples abound: a prick of a pin, when sensed only after an interval of time, was one sign that the patient suffered from locomotor ataxy; his or her inability to sense the vibrations of a tuning fork was likely a sign of syphilitic infection.[67]

If the body as a machine allowed the patient's invisible lesions to become visible to the physician, then the practices of the everyday life of the patient allowed the physician to read a constitutional pathology through observations of habits. In *Introduction to Clinical Neurology*, Gordon Holmes recommended observing the patient's normal activities. "The manner in which he uses his hands in dressing or undressing himself, in arranging his bed-clothes, and even in gestures during conversation" could provide important clues to the patient's underlying condition.[68]

The occupation of the patient proved crucial as well. In his original paper on the plantar reflex, Stanley Barnes constantly noted the occupations of his patients.[69] The "exact details of his occupation" Walter Russell Brain insisted in his 1933 textbook, offered an important clue to the possible "exposure to injury or to toxic substances."[70] Alternatively, the occupation of the patient could also reveal the time and sequence of the appearance of new symptoms; a musician might lose fine motor skills in the hand long before simpler skills like grasping diminished.[71]

How precisely patients understood the rituals of the examination is almost impossible to tell. An anecdote like that recorded by Jacyna must surely have indicated some amusement on the part of the patient. According to Jacyna, the naturalist Bruce Frederick Cummings reported that Henry Head had chased him "round his consulting room with a drum-stick, tapping my nerves and cunningly working my reflexes. Then he tickled the soles of my feet and pricked me with a pin—all of which I took like a man."[72] All of the authors of textbooks reminded their readers that the neurological exam, if done comprehensively, was exhausting to the patient. For his part, Francis Walshe noted that the patient had an irritating habit of describing his or her symptoms in "terms of what he thinks them due to." Walshe admonished his reader that "it is facts rather than amateur interpretations that are needed in diagnosis."[73] Gordon Holmes noted too that it was best to advise the patient to report facts rather than interpretations. Unlike Walshe, Holmes nevertheless urged the physician to engage the patient's interest in the examination in order to insure cooperation, attention, and willingness to express fatigue.[74] In this sense, the patient's narrative was simply another form of information to be extracted: words and reflexes. The body spoke; so did the reflexes.

In any case, for the patient there must have been an element of theater to the examination, at least in the performance of James Purves-Stewart.[75] Purves-Stewart had worked at Westminster Hospital, and one of his colleagues recalled the persona he fashioned for students, patients, and staff:

> Purves-Stewart's demonstration of neurology drew visitors from all over the world. He possessed that curious trick, almost showmanship, found in many great teachers, which employs a slight exaggeration of a normal gesture to ram

home a point. To see him take the patient's pulse or elucidate the Babinski reflexes left no doubt in the audience's mind of the essential importance of these fundamental acts. His retinue, too, was impressive: the House Physician carried his gold patella hammer; his secretary attended to take notes and his chauffeur carried a bag containing other instruments. When he entered a ward followed by these functionaries, the Sister and her nurses and the students and visitors, and the patients could not fail to be impressed.[76]

If such a spectacle impressed the neurological patient, then it is less clear that medical students and junior doctors found equally impressive the idiosyncrasies of the neurological examination or deemed helpful their instruction in the technique. In his autobiography, neurologist John Walton described, for example, how Francis Walshe, the ever-caustic vituperative at the National Hospital, had with "consummate showmanship" publicly conducted a superficial neurological exam and made a wholly inaccurate diagnosis before a gathering of medical students. A young registrar perhaps too impetuously tickled the patient's toes, thus disproving through the ease of the plantar response his chief's diagnosis, for which he received the honest rebuke that "a young man with his eye on the future would never have done that." Walton also recalled that the most obsessive physician at the National Hospital was Michael McArdle, a technically brilliant and diagnostically unparalleled physician, who spent "interminable hours studying and examining a single patient." Walton remembered that by the time McArdle had arrived at a diagnosis, "clerks and house-officers alike had often lost interest, not so much from boredom . . . but simply through exhaustion."[77]

The practice of revealing, the rigorous and exacting methods, and the tacit knowledge it entailed acquiring, ultimately demanded the persistence of student and patient alike and their collaboration. The student needed to study the textbooks and to try to distill from the description of the practice these methods of revealing lesion and constitution. In the end, however, the practice of revealing could only be learned through participation. The young student, budding neurologist, had to practice his or her way into the tacit knowledge of neurological disease; the neurological patient was every bit as much a teacher as the clinical professors.

Institutionalizing Tacit Logics:
The Patient Exam Becomes Routine

As the specialty of clinical neurology emerged, its practices and areas of diagnosis became more focused. The neurological exam, in fact, had become amenable to government standardization, inviting the hypothesis that patient diagnosis had become routine as well. Some Ministry of Health documents offer important clues. In 1948, the British government took over the hospitals and medical schools, establishing the country's National Health Service.[78] Part of this process entailed the creation of healthcare regions supported by teaching centers and ancillary clinics and hospitals. Prior to 1948, many of these areas would not have had neurologists or neurological departments. Neurologists had been located chiefly in London, Oxbridge, Newcastle, Edinburgh, and Glasgow. The creation of the NHS entailed not only the improvement of rural medical services but also made parity in patient access a priority. Hence, areas long underserved by either specialists or special departments were to be modernized; throughout the late 1940s and 1950s the government hired neurologists and, where necessary, created new departments.[79]

Among the fascinating sources documenting this transformation of clinical neurology are minutes from the National Hospital Service Medical Supplies Working Party. The government charged this committee to standardize the supplies provided in each NHS hospital for the various specialties.[80] This committee co-opted representatives from each medical specialty and asked them to draft a list of equipment necessary to their practice. The list for neurology is particularly instructive. The Working Party had asked two neurologists from the National Hospital, Macdonald Critchley and Denis Williams, to become official representatives for the subgroup on neurology and neuropsychiatry. In early 1948, the committee asked Critchley and Williams to "furnish lists of apparatus required for a neurological unit in a special hospital and for a similar unit in a general hospital."[81] By May, Williams and Critchley had supplied their list.[82] Unlike other specialists, their list not only discussed the needs of a neurological department, but it also identified items required for departments of histology, clinical pathology, biochemistry, and psychology—all were departments that supplied their own lists.[83] Critchley and Williams thus identified items required for insulin therapy, electronarcosis, electroconvulsive therapy, and electroencephalography. The diagnostic equipment for the department was equipment that had basically been deemed necessary in the latest textbooks: a dynamometer, tuning forks, patella hammers, bottles filled with substances for testing taste and odors, skin pencils, special mattresses, and a set of von Frey hairs. Critchley and Williams even considered it necessary to explain which toys were appropriate for entertaining child inpatients. Male dolls with detachable clothing that could make them a father or policeman and female dolls with clothing that could make them a mother, nurse, or teacher were apparently necessary for play.[84]

Hence, alongside the neurological diagnostic equipment necessary for the actual examination of the patient, the neurologists attempted to create a microuniverse for eliciting normal behavior for children. It was perhaps not coincidental that beneath the list of children's toys necessary for playtime was yet one additional list of psychological tests deemed necessary for neurological examination—these ranged from the Rorschach to the Minnesota Pre-School Scales. Between the tools of the psychological tests and the toys of play, neurology defined and delimited a space of the normal and the pathological—the pathologies of anatomy, psychology, genetics, and ultimately constitution. Even in this list of standard equipment required by all British neurological departments—as far as known, the only record of its kind—the constitution of the normal individual and the pathologies of the body and constitution became unified in language and practice.

Conclusion

This discussion of the organization of the neurological exam, its logics, transmission, and implications for the neurological patient, tells a broader, well-known story of medicine since the birth of the clinic. Yet that story would not be complete for neurology without an enhanced means of perceiving invisible pathologies. In other words, the science and medicine of the nervous system had to acquire modern medicine's special relation with the body in ways distinctive from other areas of medicine. The neurological patient was surely a special case, one that other chapters in this volume describe by focusing specifically on the problem of diagnosis or efforts to define an emblematic patient. In fact, Tourette's syndrome, encephalitis lethargica, multiple sclerosis, and Alzheimer's disease, conditions that are all discussed in this volume, were illnesses of unknown etiology. They still remain so today. The diagnosis of patients with these conditions depended upon practices that were fashioned from both knowledge of patient individuality and postmortem observation.

For much of the twentieth century, there was no technological means of peering into the internal workings of the nervous system, save in those few special instances when the ophthalmoscope could be used. Even during an autopsy the nervous system could conceal the causes of its illnesses. In the living patient, the physician could only infer a lesion from actions produced by the patient's body. In concert, the tuning fork, the pin, and the reflex hammer were tools that made the body's behavior—normal and pathological—evident. The links between anatomical structure and physiological function remained tenuous at best, and in any case difficult to reveal confidently in the diseased state. The textbooks of diseases of the nervous system were thus predicated upon morbid relations, yet the logic of the neurological examination entailed turning the body into the technology of its revealing and in recognizing the individuality of each patient. The authors of the works routinely exhorted their readers to remember that the absence of a sign in the patient was as important as the presence of another. They also cautioned that ignorance of the patient's habits, occupation, or customs could prove detrimental in the diagnosis of disease. Thus, even as these practices were institutionalized within the new bureaucratic structures of modern medicine, they carried along with them the essences of these ambiguities, ambiguities that arose from practices established for medicine in an earlier epoch. At its heart, then, neurology collapsed together earlier modes of diagnosis with newer ones. These ambiguities were far from being an insufficient break from the antiquated notions of the past. Instead, they were the ultimate justification for neurology's continued preoccupation with the philosophical status of man, a preoccupation wholly dependent upon the neurological patient.[85]

Notes

1. Gordon Holmes, *Introduction to Clinical Neurology* (Edinburgh: E & S Livingstone, 1946), 10.

2. Ibid., 185–86.

3. Michel de Certeau, *The Practices of Everyday Life* (Berkley: University of California Press, 1988), 45–60; and Pierre Bourdieu, *The Logic of Practice* (Cambridge: Polity Press, 2003).

4. A number of works led me to this particular argument. Of particular importance were studies of the body, disability, and power—the motives of which I am attempting to collapse together in this paper into a coherent model for understanding clinical knowledge. Jean Starobinski, "The Natural and Literary History of Bodily Sensation," in *Fragments for a History of the Human Body*, ed. Michel Feher, Ramona Naddaf, and Nadia Tazi (New York: Zone, 1989), 2:351–405; Susan Wendell, *The Rejected Body: Feminist Philosophical Reflections on Disability* (London: Routledge, 1996), 117–38; Roger Cooter and John Pickstone, eds., *Companion to Medicine in the Twentieth Century* (London: Routledge, 2003), 187–486; and Michel Foucault, *Madness and Civilization: A History of Insanity in the Age of Reason* (New York: Vintage, 1988), 375–422.

5. Michel Foucault, *The Birth of the Clinic: An Archeology of Medical Perception* (London: Routledge, 1986), 149; and Erwin H. Ackerknecht, *Medicine at the Paris Hospital, 1794–1848* (Baltimore: Johns Hopkins University Press, 1967), 3–12.

6. L. Stephen Jacyna, "Medicine in Transformation, 1800–1849," in *The Western Medical Tradition, 1800–2000*, ed. William F. Bynum, Anne Hardy, L. Stephen Jacyna, Christopher Lawrence, and E. M. Tansey (Cambridge: Cambridge University Press, 2006), 11–101; esp. 41–47.

7. Bynum, *Western Medical Tradition*, 2006; and Jack Pressman, *Last Resort: Psychosurgery and the Limits of Medicine* (Cambridge: Cambridge University Press, 1998). For a critique of these developments relevant to neuroscience, see M. R. Bennett and P. M. S. Hacker, *Philosophical Foundations of Neuroscience* (London: Blackwell, 2003).

8. Stanley J. Reiser, *Medicine and the Reign of Technology* (Cambridge: Cambridge University Press, 1981), 36.

9. Thomas Savill, *A System of Clinical Medicine Dealing with the Diagnosis, Prognosis, and Treatment of Disease for Students and Practitioners*, 3rd ed. (New York: William Wood, 1912), 711.

10. John Harley Warner, "The Use of Patient Records by Historians: Patterns, Possibilities, and Perplexities," *Health and History* 1 (1999): 106.

11. Stephen T. Casper, "The Idioms of Practice: British Neurology, 1880–1960" (PhD diss., University College London, 2007).

12. Peter Koehler, G. W. Bruyn, and John M. S. Pearce, *Neurological Eponyms* (Oxford: Oxford University Press, 2000).

13. Thomas Osborn, "On Anti-Medicine and Clinical Reason," in *Reassessing Foucault: Power, Medicine, and the Body*, ed. Colin Jones and Roy Porter (London: Routledge, 1994), 34–35.

14. Paul Guttmann, *A Handbook of Physical Diagnosis Comprising the Throat, Thorax, and Abdomen*, trans. A. Napier (New York: William Wood, 1880), 2.

15. Andrew Wear, "Medical Practice in Late Seventeenth and Early Eighteenth-Century England: Continuity and Union," in *The Medical Revolution of the Seventeenth Century*, ed. R. K. French and Andrew Wear (Cambridge: Cambridge University Press, 1989), 301–2.

16. Edwin Clarke and L. Stephen Jacyna, *Nineteenth-Century Origins of Neuroscientific Concepts* (Berkeley: University of California Press, 1987); Daniel Kevles and Gerald Geison, "The Experimental Life Sciences in the Twentieth Century," *Osiris* 10 (1995): 97–121; and Casper, *Idioms of Practice.*

17. A. Oliff, "History and Development of Neurology as a Distinct Specialty in America," *Journal of Civil War Medicine* 3 (1999): 33–41.

18. Silas Weir Mitchell, G. R. Morehouse, and W. W. Keen, *Gunshot Wounds and Other Injuries of the Nerves* (Philadelphia: Lippincott, 1864); William A. Hammond, ed., *Military Medical and Surgical Essays: Prepared for the United States Sanitary Commission* (Philadelphia: Lippincott, 1864); William A. Hammond, *A Treatise on Diseases of the Nervous System* (New York: Appleton, 1871); Silas Weir Mitchell, *Some Personal Recollections of the Civil War* (Philadelphia, 1905; repr. Transactions of the College of Physicians of Philadelphia, 1905); Silas Weir Mitchell, *The Medical Department in the Civil War* (Chicago: American Medical Association, 1914); Silas Weir Mitchell, *Injuries of Nerves and Their Consequences* (New York: Dover, 1965); Bonnie Ellen Blustein, "New York Neurologists and the Specialization of American Medicine," *Bulletin of the History of Medicine* 53 no. 2 (1979): 170–83; Bonnie Ellen Blustein, *Preserve Your Love for Science: Life of William Hammond, American Neurologist* (Cambridge: Cambridge University Press, 1991); Roger Cooter, Mark Harrison, and Steve Sturdy, eds., *War, Medicine, and Modernity* (Stroud: Sutton, 1998); and Roger Cooter, Mark Harrison, and Steve Sturdy, eds., *Medicine and Modern Warfare* (Amsterdam: Rodopi, 1999).

19. For example, Gordon Holmes, "Disturbances of Vision from Cerebral Lesions, with Special Reference to the Cortical Representations of the Macula," *Brain* 46 (1917): 34–73; see also Casper, *Idioms of Practice*, 156–99.

20. George Rosen, *The Specialization of Medicine with Particular Reference to Ophthalmology* (New York: Froben Press, 1944); Rosemary Stevens, *Medical Practice in Modern England: The Impact of Specialization on State Medicine* (New Haven: Yale University Press, 1966); and George Weisz, *Divide and Conquer: A Comparative History of Medical Specialization* (Oxford: Oxford University Press, 2006).

21. Lawrence McHenry, *Garrison's History of Neurology* (Springfield, IL: Charles C. Thomas, 1969), 254–57.

22. Roger Smith, *History of the Human Sciences* (New York: W. W. Norton, 1997), 710–13.

23. Christopher Goetz, M. Bonduelle, and Toby Gelfand, *Charcot: Constructing Neurology* (New York: Oxford University Press, 1995), 222–31.

24. Jean-Martin Charcot, *Lectures on the Diseases of the Nervous System*, trans. G. Sigerson (London: The New Sydenham Society, 1881), 21–22.

25. The value of physiology for general clinical practice was not self-evident; see Gerald Geison, *Michael Foster and the Cambridge School of Physiology: The Scientific Enterprise in Late Victorian Society* (Princeton: Princeton University Press, 1978); Christopher Lawrence, "Incommunicable Knowledge: Science, Technology, and the Clinical Art in Britain, 1850–1914," *Journal of Contemporary History* 20 (1985): 503–20; and Gerald Geison, "Divided We Stand: Physiologists and Clinicians in the American Context," in *The Therapeutic Revolution: Essays in the Social History of American Medicine*, ed. M. J. Vogel and Charles Rosenberg (Philadelphia: University of Pennsylvania Press, 1979), 115–29.

26. James Crichton-Browne, "Preface," *Medical Reports of the West Riding Lunatic Asylum* 1 (1871): iv.

27. Gordon Holmes, *The National Hospital, Queen Square* (Edinburgh: E & S Livingstone, 1954); and Anthony Feiling, *A History of Maida Vale Hospital for Nervous Diseases* (London: Butterworth, 1958).

28. Chandak Sengoopta, "'A Mob of Incoherent Symptoms'?: Neurasthenia in Medical Discourse, 1860–1920," in *Cultures of Neurasthenia: From Beard to the First World War*, ed. Marijke Gijswijt-Hofstra and Roy Porter (Amsterdam: Rodopi, 2001), 107.

29. Jesse F. Ballenger, *Self, Senility, and Alzheimer's Disease in Modern America* (Baltimore: Johns Hopkins University Press, 2006), 11–35; Anne Hardy, *Health and Medicine in Britain Since 1860* (New York: Palgrave, 2001), 1–58; and Janet Oppenheim, *"Shattered Nerves": Doctors, Patients, and Depression in Victorian England* (New York: Oxford University Press, 1991), 181–232.

30. Joan J. Brumberg, *Fasting Girls: The History of Anorexia Nervosa* (New York: Vintage, 1989), 104–23.

31. Elaine Showalter, *The Female Malady: Women, Madness, and English Culture* (London: Virago Press, 1985).

32. James Purves-Stewart, *The Diagnosis of Nervous Diseases* (London: Edward Arnold, 1906), 311–12.

33. L. Stephen Jacyna, *Medicine and Modernism: A Biography of Sir Henry Head* (London: Pickering & Chatto, 2008), 76.

34. F. Mott, "Presidential Address: The Inborn Factors of Nervous and Mental Disease," *Proceedings of the Royal Society of Medicine* 5, no. 2 (1911): 1, 2.

35. A hint appears in Henry Miller, "Textbooks for Pleasure," *Journal of the American Medical Association* 192, no. 2 (1965): 145–48.

36. As a primary source, medical and scientific textbooks and manuals are rather unpopular. It seems a widespread view—if one not often acknowledged by historians—that few people utilized them and that textbooks were generally inaccurate and in no way reflected the work of practitioners or scientists. Such views make little sense. In the first place, the commitment required by such a project alone suggests that someone thought that the works had contemporary purchase. Second, people, and not just students, actually spent money on them, while publishers produced

multiple editions of the same volume. Finally, the transience of the knowledge communicated in the textbooks suggests that their most important role was to summarize the state of knowledge. They consequently also held out the promise of the future refinement of that knowledge. In no way, of course, am I suggesting that we can reconstruct a community's entire past from textbooks. I am, however, claiming that we can sense the development and transmission of tacit knowledge between generations through examination, a view very much in accordance with an older Kuhnian tradition in the history of science. On textbooks, see R. G. Collingwood, *Essays in the Philosophy of History* (Austin: University of Texas Press, 1965), 30; Thomas Kuhn, *The Structure of Scientific Revolutions* (Chicago: University of Chicago Press, 1996), 136–38; and M. Smyth, "Certainty and Uncertainty Science: Marking the Boundaries of Psychology in Introductory Textbooks," *Social Studies of Science* 31 (2001): 389–416.

37. James R. Reynolds, *The Diagnosis of Diseases of the Brain, Spinal Cord, Nerves, and Other Appendages* (London: John Churchill, 1855), 50.

38. Julius Althaus, *Diseases of the Nervous System: Their Prevalence and Pathology* (London: Smith Elder, 1877); Charles Edward Beevor, *Diseases of the Nervous System* (London: H. K. Lewis, 1898); Silas Weir Mitchell, *Lectures on Diseases of the Nervous System: Especially in Women* (Philadelphia: Lea Brothers, 1885); Samuel Wilks, *Lectures on the Diseases of the Nervous System* (London: Churchill, 1878); William A. Gowers, *A Manual of Diseases of the Nervous System* (London: Churchill, 1892); Thomas Buzzard, *Clinical Lectures on Diseases of the Nervous System* (Philadelphia: Blakiston, 1882); H. Oppenheim, *Diseases of the Nervous System: A Textbook for Students and Practitioners of Medicine* (London: Lippincot, 1904); Judson S. Bury, *Diseases of the Nervous System* (Manchester: Manchester University Press, 1912); Smith E. Jelliffe and W. A. White, *Diseases of the Nervous System: A Textbook of Neurology and Psychiatry* (Philadelphia: Lea & Febiger, 1917); and A. Gordon, *Diseases of the Nervous System: For the General Practitioner and Student* (London: H. K. Lewis, 1908).

39. Henry Miller, "Personal Book List: Neurology," *The Lancet* 2 (1968): 972; and McHenry, *Garrison's History*, 269–341.

40. For example, Purves-Stewart, *Diagnosis of Nervous Diseases*, 39–41; Donald Core, *The Examination of the Central Nervous System* (Edinburgh: E & S Livingstone, 1928), viii; and Frederick J. Nattrass, *The Commoner Nervous Diseases* (London: Oxford University, 1931), 28–29.

41. Casper, *Idioms of Practice*, 73–82.

42. William A. Gowers, *Manual and Atlas of Medical Ophthalmoscopy* (London: Churchill, 1879).

43. Gowers, *Manual of Diseases*, 7–8.

44. Ibid., 1; and McHenry, *Garrison's History*, 345.

45. Byrom Bramwell, *The Diseases of the Spinal Cord* (Edinburgh: Clay, 1895); F. S. Pearce, *A Practical Treatise on Nervous Diseases for the Medical Student and General Practitioner* (London: Appleton, 1904); J. Collins, *The Treatment of Diseases of the Nervous System: A Manual for Practitioners* (New York: William Wood, 1900); Gordon, *Diseases of the Nervous System*; and R. T. Williamson, *Diseases of the Spinal Cord* (London: Hodder and Stoughton, 1908).

46. Edwin Bramwell, *Rough Notes and Recollections, 1945*, section titled "Sir James Purves Stewart KCMG CB MD FRCP," private collection.

47. Purves-Stewart, *Diagnosis of Nervous Diseases*, iii–iv.

48. Ibid., 1.

49. Ibid., 38.

50. Ibid., 39.

51. Holmes, *Introduction to Clinical Neurology*.

52. Mark W. Weatherall, *Gentlemen, Scientists, and Doctors: Medicine at Cambridge, 1800–1940* (Woodbridge, UK: Boydell Press, 2000).

53. Koehler, *Neurological Eponyms*. Consider, for instance, the Heel-Toe-Shin test for ataxia. It is now a standard test, but its appearance is mysterious. Who discovered it? How did it propagate in training?

54. The earliest discussion I have found is C. W. Suckling, *On the Diagnosis of Diseases of the Brain, Spinal Cord, and Nerves* (London: H. K. Lewis, 1887), 53–92.

55. Derek Denny-Brown, *Handbook of Neurological Examination and Case Recording* (Cambridge: Harvard University Press, 1957); E. R. Bickerstaff, *Neurological Examination in Clinical Practice* (Oxford: Blackwell, 1963); and R. S. Paine and T. E. Oppe, *Neurological Examination of Children* (London: Spastics Society of Medical Education and Information Unit, 1966).

56. Russell DeJong, *The Neurological Examination: Incorporating the Fundamentals of Neuroanatomy and Neurophysiology*, 4th ed. (New York: Harper & Row, 1979).

57. Suckling, *Diagnosis of Diseases*, 175a.

58. F. M. R. Walshe, *Diseases of the Nervous System Described for Practitioners and Students* (Edinburgh: E & S Livingstone, 1940), 22.

59. J. van Gijn, *The Babinski Sign: A Centenary* (Utrecht: Universiteit Utrecht, 1996); J. van Gijn, "The Babinski Sign," *Practical Neurology* 2 (2002): 42–44.

60. Purves-Stewart, *Diagnosis of Nervous Diseases*, 270–71.

61. James Collier, "An Investigation Upon the Plantar Reflex, with Reference to the Significance of Its Variations Under Pathological Conditions, Including an Enquiry into the Aetiology of Acquired Pes Cavus," *Brain* 22, no. 1 (1899): 71–97; and Wilfred Harris, "The Diagnostic Value of the Plantar Reflex," *Review of Neurology and Psychiatry* 1 (1903): 320–28.

62. Arthur Stanley Barnes, "The Diagnostic Value of the Plantar Reflex," *Review of Neurology and Psychiatry* 2 (1904): 345–46.

63. Ibid., 347.

64. Ibid., 349–51.

65. Ibid., 353–57.

66. Ibid., 375–76.

67. Bury, *Diagnosis of Nervous Diseases*, 68.

68. Holmes, *Introduction to Clinical Neurology*, 14.

69. Barnes, "Diagnostic Value," 371–76.

70. Walter Russell Brain, *Diseases of the Nervous System* (Oxford: Oxford University Press, 1933), 135.

71. Walshe, *Diseases of the Nervous System*, 7.

72. Jacyna, *Medicine and Modernism*, 63.

73. Walshe, *Diseases of the Nervous System*, 4.

74. Holmes, *Introduction to Clinical Neurology*, 11.

75. The performance of neurology and neurosurgery has been discussed at length by Delia Garvis. See "Men of Dreams and Men of Action: Neurologists, Neurosurgeons, and the Performance of Professional Identity, 1925–1950," *Bulletin of the History of Medicine* (forthcoming).

76. J. G. Humble and P. Hansell, *The Westminster Hospital, 1716–1966* (London: Pitman Medical, 1966), 98–99.

77. John Walton, *The Spice of Life: From Northumbria to World Neurology* (London: Royal Society of Medicine, 1993), 165.

78. Hardy, *Health and Medicine in Britain*, 139–79.

79. The Organization of Neurology in London After the War [undated, ca. 1945–52], MS 3226/99 Walter Russell Brain Papers, Royal College of Physicians, London; and Casper, *Idioms of Practice*, 97–105.

80. Medical Supplies Working Party 1948, PRO MH 77/141, Public Record Office, London.

81. Working Party to Critchley and Williams, March 5, 1948, PRO MH 77/141.

82. Williams to Coppin, May 7, 1948, PRO MH 77/141.

83. Attached List, Williams to Coppin, May 7, 1948, 1–5, PRO MH 77/141.

84. Ibid., 2–3.

85. Foucault, *Birth of the Clinic*, 197–98.

Chapter Two

Neurological Patients as Experimental Subjects

Epilepsy Studies in the United States

Ellen Dwyer

For almost one hundred years in the United States and elsewhere, researchers, regulatory agencies, and the public have argued about what constitutes the ethical use of human subjects in biomedical experiments. Yet despite its continuing importance, much of this discussion has been forgotten. Few histories reach back further than the Nuremberg Code of 1946. In neglecting the lively early debate, truncated accounts limit our understanding of the development of research ethics in the United States.

According to Susan Lederer, during the first three decades of the twentieth century, and thus well before the horrors of Nazi Germany, biomedical researchers began to design large-scale clinical experiments for the first time. The resulting need for human subjects generated an intense public discussion that appeared in newspapers, medical journals, and even popular fiction. Many Americans did not like the idea of being used as research guinea pigs. Angry exposés of abuse appeared in pamphlets with lurid titles like "Foundlings Cheaper Than Animals." As early as 1900, one legislator introduced a bill for the regulation of scientific experiments upon human beings in the District of Columbia to the United States Senate, albeit to no effect. In 1916, a number of concerned doctors proposed that the American Medical Association adopt a formal code of ethics.[1]

Although no formal regulatory policy emerged, the intensity of the public outcry pushed biomedical researchers toward a form of limited self-regulation. Some began to ask clinical patients for permission to involve them in an experiment. A few tried out new serums on themselves and their families before using them in clinical trials. There was an occasional discussion of the need to avoid excessive risk.[2] In *Subjected to Science*, a pathbreaking study of this early period, Lederer argues that contrary to popular wisdom, "ethical guidelines influenced the conduct of research with both human and animal subjects" well before World War II.[3]

Historian Harry Marks makes a complementary argument. In the first half of *The Progress of Experiment: Science and Therapeutic Reform in the United States, 1900–1990*, Marks describes early twentieth-century reformers' efforts to make direct clinical therapeutic practice more scientific, largely by involving the laboratory sciences.[4] Their hope was that rational therapeutic agents could be discovered and tested in laboratories before being introduced into clinical practice.[5] The benefits would be twofold. Biomedical research would become more scientific and those in need of new therapies better protected. The best way to achieve these ambitious goals, reformers felt, was through cooperative studies involving researchers at several institutions. Unfortunately, although cooperative studies had obvious advantages, in practice they proved difficult to organize. Most researchers proved reluctant to sacrifice their intellectual autonomy for the sake of advancing research.[6] During the 1920s and 1930s, however, they were increasingly willing to reach across departmental and divisional lines within their own universities in order to locate research partners and facilities.[7]

Inspired by the work of Lederer and Marks, this chapter tackles a more specialized history: the changing attitudes toward and the use of neurological patients in experimental research, particularly having to do with epilepsy. In the 1920s and 1930s, unlike many of their colleagues, neurological researchers were relatively protected from public scrutiny, even though they targeted that seemingly most human of organs, the brain. Especially in the case of convulsive disorders, much about the brain remained mysterious. Research groups at medical schools like Harvard, Yale, Johns Hopkins, and the Montreal Institute were determined to learn more. With funding from the Rockefeller Foundation, the Josiah Macy Foundation, and others, they devised a number of ambitious research experiments that involved not just neurologists and neurosurgeons but also pathologists, physiologists, anatomists, and chemists. (Unlike the researcher studied by Lederer, the neurologists proudly proclaimed their desire to conduct experiments.) Their goal was to replace anecdotal evidence about convulsive disorders, often gathered in a haphazard way, with scientific data collected under carefully controlled conditions.

According to William Lennox and Stanley Cobb, there were multiple puzzles confronting epileptologists in the late 1920s, including the neurological mechanisms of convulsions, the pathology of the nervous tissue, and abnormalities outside of the nervous system including circulatory problems, glandular abnormalities, and carbohydrate and fat metabolism. In earlier decades, the path to the understanding of seizure disorders had wound through the experiences of individuals with epilepsy. By 1928, neurologists' interests had moved on to "the cause of the seizure . . . what pulled the trigger rather than what happened after the trigger was pulled."[8] In the course of this move, despite their increasing reliance on human subjects, neurologists seldom mentioned individuals with epilepsy in published accounts of their experiments. To invert a later comment by William Lennox, in the late 1920s he and his colleagues viewed epileptics as patients, not as persons.[9] The shift went largely unnoticed by them.

Testing the expansive list of theories of epilepsy proposed by Lennox and Cobb proved to be a major challenge for neurologists. The enterprise also raised a number of ethical issues, only some of which were addressed. In order to explore this situation, this chapter relies heavily on a 1936 research report published by Northwestern University Medical School. While other research groups also engaged in extended neurological research projects, they generally published their findings in medical journals. The Northwestern researchers did the same, but in addition they compiled a comprehensive 537-page *Report on the Assistance of Indigent Epileptics*. In this volume, they laid out their experimental protocols and experimental results in unusual detail.[10]

The report describes first the goals and then the results of what was called The Northwestern Plan, an experimental epilepsy project funded by the Minnie Frances Kleman Fund. Set up to test multiple hypotheses in a relatively short period of time (initially, three months), The Northwestern Plan suggested (often inadvertently) the ways in which neurological patients were viewed as research subjects in a situation in which the etiology of their disorder was but poorly understood and the demand for efficacious treatments strong.

The Northwestern Plan

The Northwestern Plan for studying epilepsy was developed by two Northwestern Medical School faculty members, Loyal Davis and Lewis J. Pollack, and carried out under their supervision. In 1934, Davis was a young but already well-respected neurosurgeon who had trained with Harvey Cushing at Yale. He had been chair of the Department of Surgery at Northwestern since 1932. His collaborator, Lewis J. Pollack, was slightly older. He had served as chair of the Department of Nervous and Mental Disease since 1926. Like Davis, Pollock had a long and illustrious career, the high point of which (his election to the presidency of the American Neurological Association in 1942) had yet to come. Why Davis and Pollack got involved in epilepsy research is not clear. They had worked together on earlier, very different projects, most notably anemic cerebration in cats,[11] but up to this point had done little work with epileptics. Nonetheless, when the Minnie

Frances Kleman Memorial Foundation announced the availability of funds for epilepsy research that used indigent patients as subjects, Davis and Pollack were quick to apply. The location of the foundation in Chicago may have spurred their proposal, but given the relative scarcity of epilepsy research monies it is curious that none of the other major neurological centers applied for this funding.[12]

According to their application, Davis and Pollack intended to use the rich resources of Northwestern University: its many labs, large medical staff, and full complement of social services, to reach conclusions about the origins of epilepsy and the efficacy of specific treatments quickly and economically.[13] In addition to the existing neurological clinic at Northwestern Medical School, the project also would use the facilities of Passavant Memorial Hospital, located next door. (Several months into the experiment, Northwestern set up a special Montgomery Ward Clinic for epileptics.) Thus, Davis and Pollock could offer cost-effective medical care to indigent epileptics that would replace the existing wasteful and futile direct assistance programs. Further, they hoped, the promise of high-quality medical care would attract the large numbers of research subjects needed to carry on experimental research.[14]

Early in their proposal, Davis and Pollock justified their project in somewhat unconventional terms, those perhaps most pleasing to the Kleman Foundation. They began with an eloquent description of the unmet social needs of those with epilepsy. Too often, Davis and Pollock observed, misconceptions about the connection between, on the one hand, heredity and mental retardation, and, on the other, epilepsy, had led many to hide their disorder and neglect treatment. Seizures often deprived them of education; misconceptions about the hereditary nature of epilepsy led parents to outlaw friends with epileptic children. Reared in an abnormal atmosphere, epileptics were likely to become maladjusted. Unable to pursue schooling or a career, many ultimately became dependent on a variety of relief organizations or ended up in state-funded institutions. The Northwestern Plan promised to stop this downward social drift by offering epileptics and their families help and support.

Having demonstrated the social utility of their project, Davis and Pollock turned to their major interest, medical research. The mechanics of convulsive disorders, they observed, remained controversial. Some researchers focused on brain anatomy; others looked for chemical abnormalities; a third group was interested in physiological processes. Much work already had been published on these issues. However, Davis and Pollock justified their plans on the grounds that earlier research had not involved careful science. In a burst of what seems now exuberant hyperbole, Davis and Pollack proclaimed that "nowhere else in America is there opportunity for the study of epilepsy comparable to this."[15]

Evidently, the Kleman Foundation agreed. Initially, its directors awarded Northwestern University Medical School $2,500 to realize The Northwestern Plan. For various reasons, the grant was extended twice: first for an additional two months and then for another four. By the end of the project, the Kleman Fund had provided a total of $8,333.31. This money was supplemented by $2,700 from Passavant Hospital and an additional $2,600 from Northwestern Medical School itself.

From the beginning of their work, the Northwestern researchers confronted the difficulties of attracting nondeteriorated extramural patients to their experiments. As Davis and Pollock frankly acknowledged, indigent clinic patients, especially when enrolled in experiments, needed incentives if they were to return regularly and hence provide long-term data. To entice such experimental subjects, who were free to leave the clinic at any time, Davis and Pollock promised a range of services, both medical and social. As a result, The Northwestern Plan, in its initial formulation at least, was extraordinarily ambitious. Fourteen doctors were to be involved in the project, along with as an unspecified number of residents, interns, clinical clerks, nurses, social service workers, X-ray technicians, psychologists, and lab technicians. Almost fifty experiments were planned.

The project also was expensive. For example, when patients first became part of the experiment, they were given complete and free medical and neurological examinations. Female patients got gynecological examinations as well. Then there were a number of routine X-rays of the skull and laboratory tests. Within and without the clinic, social workers played a vital role. They took detailed patient social histories. They also helped patients with their diets, housing, schooling, employment, and provided money for carfare. Finally, the clinic planned to offer a number of educational programs for families in order to sustain their faith in the Northwestern experiments and to improve their supervision of epileptics at home.[16]

Initially, those patients in need of special tests were admitted to Passavant Memorial Hospital rather than the clinic. If surgery was required, they were then transferred from the Department of Clinical Neurology to the Department of Clinical Neurosurgery. Following this period of hospital study, most patients went back to the clinic for outpatient treatment. There, the medical staff asked patients to keep diaries of their medications, attacks, bowel movements, and any special circumstances, such as a menstrual period, fatigue, or lack of sleep, and to submit them to their clinician upon each visit.[17] These diaries were intended to complement patients' more detailed hospital records, but few patients complied—to the doctors' regret.

This rich array of services almost immediately proved too expensive and had to be curtailed. In place of offering psychological and social support, social workers found themselves struggling with more mundane tasks. They spent hours taking patient histories. In addition, they were asked to ensure that patients took their prescribed medications and returned for follow-up care—two impossible assignments. In addition, certain studies were assigned to a nearby state hospital as a way of further cutting costs. In return, Northwestern promised to make any new methods of treatment that emerged out of the project available to state hospital patients.[18] Despite these problems, Davis and Pollack did not lose faith. The Northwestern Plan was still a success, they asserted, because even a short involvement in the research project benefitted both subjects and researchers. Especially important here was the discovery of a number of other complicating physical diseases (such as Bright's disease and a toxic goiter) in the course of the lengthy physical examinations and multiple laboratory tests. Davis and Pollock eagerly called attention to this inadvertent outcome, in part because the Northwestern doctors generally found the newly identified problems easier to manage than patients' convulsive disorders.

The Subjects

Drawing on case histories collected by social workers, the Northwestern report described the patients enrolled in the Kleman-funded project in great detail. Between February 1935 and January 1936, the Northwestern researchers recruited fifty-eight males and thirty-eight females as experimental subjects. Two of the women were diagnosed with hysteria, not epilepsy, but were allowed to continue in the experiments. Most were between the ages of fifteen and thirty-five. They all were labeled indigent whites, although Northwestern never developed criteria for indigence. There also were several young children who had been born with multiple physical problems. In general, these epileptics were poorly educated and unemployed. About one-quarter had held jobs in the past but lost them when head traumas produced adult-onset epilepsy.[19]

According to the Northwestern social workers, the stigma against epileptics had produced a very narrowed existence for most of their patients. Over the course of eleven months of the Northwestern experiment, social welfare agencies, most notably the Illinois Emergency Relief Fund, referred some 150 patients to Northwestern. Only 97 were chosen to become research subjects. The report failed to specify whether those not included had refused to take part or been rejected as unsuitable. Initially, Davis and Pollock hoped to focus on cases of idiopathic epilepsy. However, to get a sufficient number of experimental subjects, they had to accept many whose seizures were rooted in organic deficiencies or trauma. Whatever the cause of their seizures, for the purposes of the Northwestern experiment every subject was the same.

The Experiments

Over the course of eleven months, the Northwestern researchers conducted forty-eight different experiments and tests on ninety-seven of the indigent epileptics who came to the Montgomery Ward Clinic for assistance. In the literature reviews that opened their individual experiments, the Northwestern researchers made clear that none of the work was particularly innovative, despite occasional allegations to the contrary. Repetition of the research of others was justified on the grounds that the Northwestern experiments were more carefully controlled than those that had preceded them. Most of the experiments were relatively unobtrusive—and also unrewarding. For example, blood morphology tests, urinalyses, and blood pressure tests revealed few if any differences between those with convulsive disorders and those without. Hyperventilation increased muscular irritability but did not produce seizures. Even heredity tests failed to support conventional wisdom. For example, Harry Paskind reported that the seizure records of thirty-three patients with evidence of hereditary neuropathic complaints looked much the same as those of thirty-three with no negative family history. Finally, ocular and dental examinations uncovered multiple problems that could be corrected fairly easily but little else of significance.

Even Loyal Davis's neurosurgical procedures, while hardly unobtrusive, produced few new insights. Davis was notably cautious, and for the most part he removed only intracranial tumors that had been identified clearly through encephalography. These surgeries generally decreased the frequency and severity of attacks—at least for the present, Davis was quick to add.[20] According to him, an "astonishingly large" number of patients at the Montgomery Ward Clinic had attacks that suggested cortical lesions. However, the clinical evidence remained too "inadequate and inconclusive" to justify surgical removal. If patients objected to the prospect of surgery, Davis did not operate, even when he was fairly certain of success. Others, Davis and Pollock make clear in the report, were not so careful. "It is striking," they observed, "that during each decade one or more [new] forms of treatment have been proposed," only to be later discarded. Among the procedures they mentioned were ovarectomies, the removal of the colon to prevent the reabsorption of putrefactive bodies from the intestines, the resection of crooked septa, circumcisions, adrenalectomies, and cervical sympathectomies. Several years later, Davis explained that he operated only with great caution, when doing so could be justified in terms of the results of experimental laboratory work done by others.[21]

While other surgeons were less careful than Davis, they too agreed that surgical interventions required justification. In looking back over the four hundred craniotomies he had performed over a period of nineteen years, the result of which he used to support the theory of cerebral localization,

Wilder Penfield said: "These surgical procedures are not experiments, for we are dealing with human beings."[22] Neither Davis or for that matter Penfield, however, felt a need to justify or even discuss the negative side effects of the encephalographies they frequently ordered. Encephalography involved the replacement of some of the cerebrospinal fluid with air or another gas for the purpose of obtaining an X-ray record of the ventricles, cisternae, and subarachnoid spaces of the central nervous system. They thus helped surgeons determine which cases of epilepsy would benefit from surgery. Electroencephalography also was used as a diagnostic procedure, albeit one that revealed relatively little of use in a number of nonsurgical experiments. Patients strongly disliked lumbar punctures, fraught with the potential for infection and medical error, which frequently left them nauseous and with headaches that sometimes lasted for a week or more. Yet during the 1930s in particular, lumbar punctures were performed ever more frequently (some patients endured eight or ten spinal taps in a short period of days) and for increasingly novel reasons.[23] In 1934, a researcher suggested that repeated lumbar punctures not only relieved these symptoms in cases of traumatic epilepsy but that they allegedly reduced antisocial behavior in children as well.[24] The year before, at the Infant and Children's Hospital in Boston, a Harvard researcher had used encephalography to determine which children were suitable for a special high-fat diet.[25] Finally, in a startling piece, researchers at Kings Park State Hospital characterized encephalography as a "safe and simple procedure" that could be done by "any well-grounded physician" who had time, X-ray equipment, and a hospital bed.[26] Fortunately for their patients, by the late 1930s many neurologists had abandoned encephalography for the less invasive but more revealing electroencephalogram. In addition to Davis's surgeries, there were three notable experimental areas at Northwestern that demanded much of human subjects: an experiment with anoxia, studies of water and carbohydrate metabolism, and the testing of a serum prepared from moccasin poison. The researchers who ran each of the experiments described them in great detail. Little if any evidence of a concern for human subjects appeared in their reports. While presumably patients agreed to take part, several of the research protocols involved serious threats to health.

Perhaps the most extreme Northwestern experiment grew out of a widely shared interest in the relationship between oxygen levels in the blood and seizures. After a relatively innocuous experiment involving changes in barometric pressure, two Northwestern researchers decided to test systematically the impact of lowering oxygen levels on seizures. To do so, they confined thirteen patients (eleven males and two females) in a double oxygen chamber. There were two rooms within the chamber, so that the occupants were free to walk about, talk with one another, and play cards. (The intent here was to minimize the apprehension that typically emerged during what were called rebreathing experiments.) They then gradually reduced the oxygen content of the air by pumping in nitrogen. Ten of the patients stayed in the chamber for at least thirty-six hours. (Two asked for early release and a third stayed for four days.) On multiple occasions, the researchers or their assistants observed but did not respond to signs of acute distress, ranging from incidents of unconsciousness and confusion to "several short attempts to tear off the handle" of the chamber door in an effort to escape. By the fourth day, the medical staff had difficulty in drawing blood specimens because of the collapsed condition of the single remaining patient's arteries. The twenty-four-year-old man had fallen unconscious and only artificial respiration revived him. With this event, they ended the human experiment.[27]

During the same few days, the researchers also conducted a similar experiment on six dogs, which were confined in a miniature oxygen chamber. The rationale for the parallel experiments was not explained but clearly the use of canine subjects freed the researchers to induce more intense levels of anoxia than they did with humans. After they lowered the oxygen content of the air to "asphyxial levels," three of the six dogs died. With this exception, there were no major differences in canine and human responses to anoxia. The researchers concluded in a matter-of-fact fashion, with no acknowledgment of the hardships their subjects had endured, that anoxia per se did not seem to be a factor in the production of epileptic seizures in either humans or dogs.[28]

There seemed to be no public protests against anoxia research at the time of the Northwestern experiment. Further, in their lengthy literature review, the Northwestern researchers made clear that their project followed the example of others. In particular, they pointed to the work of William J. Lennox and Stanley Cobb at Harvard Medical School during the same years.[29] Given the stressful nature of anoxia experiments, it is striking that not until 1960 did Lennox fully disavow his multiple experiments involving the deprivation of oxygen to human subjects. By that point he was scathingly critical. Once the experiments ended, the brain was expected to resume its normal functioning, but it did not always do so. As a result, he noted, "anoxia not only stops the machine but wrecks the machinery." The physiologic processes of the body have established safety zones, he went on, from which the body strays at its own risk.[30]

Like the anoxia experiments, the experiments with water metabolism that produced first overhydration and then dehydration entailed risks for human subjects. Once again, the Northwestern experimenters justified their plans by pointing to similar earlier research. That research allegedly proved that epileptics suffered a disturbance of the normal water-balance regulating mechanism and, as a result, had seizures. To retest this hypothesis, hopefully in a more rigorous fashion, the Northwestern experiments chose eighteen patients and discontinued all of their medication for the duration of the experiment.[31]

The experiment had three parts. During the first, patients were allowed a normal diet and unrestricted water. A variety of chemical tests was then used to determine their levels of bodily fluids. Next, the experimenters gave the subjects (reduced to thirteen) large quantities of water, along with pitressin, an antidiuretic, so as to produce a state of superhydration. Finally, during the third period, so to produce dehydration, the experimenters limited patients to the water contained in their food.[32]

The results of this taxing experiment were inconclusive. There was neither a positive correlation nor a negative correlation between water levels and seizures. Although measuring water balances in the body had proven nearly impossible, epileptics seemed to metabolize water at the same rate and in the same way as nonepileptics. Despite these minimal findings, once again the experimenters expressed no regret for the hardships they had inflicted on their subjects. Perhaps they, like William Lennox and Stanley Cobb, were attracted to the echoes of humoral theory in their work, echoes noted in other chapters in this volume. Translated into modern language, Lennox and Cobb claimed, Hippocrates had predicted that "whoever is acquainted with physiology and can render a man acidotic, dehydrated, and fully oxygenated could also repress this disease [of epilepsy]."[33]

For the most part, the Kleman Fund experiments took place in the clinics and hospitals of Northwestern University. In two instances, however, they were run at the nearby Elgin State Hospital. The first such experiment involved the administration of diacetone alcohol to eleven institutionalized epileptics in order to determine whether acetone bodies developed in the course of the ketogenic diet (a severely restricted diet intended to produce a state of acidosis) inhibited epileptic convulsions. Six drams of the diacetone alcohol were given daily to each of the subjects during two periods of treatment, the first of which lasted from 40 to 50 days, and the second, after an intervening period of 25 days, for 50 days. During these 125 days, patients were deprived of their usual medications, a move that risked incidents of status epilepticus. The alcohol raised blood sugar but had no effect on convulsions. The researchers concluded that the beneficial results of the ketogenic diet could not be reproduced by the simple introduction of ketones into the body.[34]

The second experiment at Elgin State Hospital involved snake venom. The researcher was determined to test the controversial assertion that crotalin (rattlesnake) injections decreased the severity and frequency of epileptic seizures, while enhancing general health. He did so in a systematic fashion. After selecting eight patients with frequent seizures, the researcher discontinued their medications, observed them for a week during which they received no treatment, and then injected them with a Moccasin-Mulford venom solution (he was unable to get rattlesnake venom). He increased the venom serum steadily. After nine weeks, the patients' seizures were so serious and frequent that the experiment was halted. Not only was venom therapy of no value, the researcher concluded, but it probably rendered epileptics more, not less, susceptible to fits. Although the subjects were all "deteriorated" epileptics, the researcher was certain that his results could be generalized to extramural epileptics as well.[35]

Conclusion

For the most part, although willing to use human subjects in risky experiments of uncertain value, the Northwestern researchers described their subjects in neutral, largely dispassionate language. A notable exception was Harry Paskind's discussion of those experimental subjects (roughly one-third of the whole) whose seizures did not respond to treatment. Ignoring the possibilities of inadequate drug dosages or treatment-resistant seizures, Paskind labeled these subjects "refractory epileptics" and resurrected the negative language of degeneration. "Refractory epileptics," he claimed, were almost all "irritable, egocentric, [and] quick-tempered." Many were feebleminded. They tended to have deviant physical characteristics, most notably the infamous "stigmata of degeneration."[36] The longer and more frequent an epileptic's seizures, the harder they were to control. What makes Paskind's negative assertions here even more surprising is that a number of them are contradicted elsewhere in the Northwestern report, including in an article he had coauthored. Their persistence well into what was supposed to be a period of medical enlightenment suggests the continuing power of older, more negative views of epileptics and epilepsy, especially when researchers had to explain therapeutic failures. This persistence of older views of the neurological patient is a theme that also appears in the chapters in this volume by Marjorie Lorch and Howard Kushner.

What more, if anything, did the Northwestern report reveal about the views of neurological patients as experimental subjects in the crucial decade of the 1930s? Frequently the Northwestern researchers had to weigh the potential benefits of experimental procedures against their potential harm to patients. Except in the case of surgical procedures, they always decided that the benefits outweighed the risks. They also felt free to repeat failed experiments, including those most painful for human subjects. For the most part, they seem to have asked potential subjects, especially the noninstitutionalized, for consent before involving them in research.

Perhaps the most striking aspect of The Northwestern Plan as it was executed is the differences in the way researchers treated institutionalized and extramural patients. In this respect, the Northwestern researchers resembled their colleagues elsewhere. For example, in one experiment run at the Craig Colony for Epileptics, an astonishing one thousand patients were involved in an experiment intended to test the hypothesis that epilepsy was an allergic reaction. The epileptics were given multiple skin tests involving protein extracts and then watched for positive reactions. The results were not only inconclusive but also useless, because the researchers failed to specify how many times they tested individual patients or the types of reactions they considered positive. Also conducted at Craig was a modified test of the high-fat ketogenic diet, along with the restriction of water. This experiment produced bitter complaints from patients and drove some to desperate stratagems, such as the drinking of drops of rain on the leaves of a vine and the sucking of a damp washcloth. The most successful subject who went nineteen days without a seizure had to be rehydrated when her temperature rose to 103.8 degrees, her pulse became rapid and weak, and the mucous membranes of the mouth and eyes dried.[37]

A number of questions about how neurological patients were treated when they became research subjects in the 1920s and 1930s remain unanswered. For example, what view of patients let researchers sit by and take notes while a patient deprived of oxygen tried to claw his way out of their anoxia chamber? Was the negative language of degeneration theory confined exclusively to Paskind's report on refractory epileptics or did it seep, almost invisibly, into other work? How many patients were subject to multiple experiments?

Despite these frustrating omissions and silences, the Northwestern report makes clear the importance of rereading the larger literature on the neurological experiments of the 1920s and 1930s, no matter how technical and dry. For example, after the graphic descriptions of the responses of Northwestern subjects to oxygen deprivation and dehydration, other more constrained accounts of the same procedures appear in a new, more negative light.

In addition, the Northwestern report suggests neurological researchers' relative lack of concern for institutionalized subjects. In contrast, because subjects recruited from clinics and hospitals could leave those experiments they found unpleasant (although not always fast enough), researchers had to get their consent. At Northwestern and elsewhere, this often involved substantial efforts to persuade them to continue. Perhaps the neurologist most skilled in the art of persuasion was William J. Lennox, whose long career at Harvard University spanned close to fifty years. At one point, for example, he managed to convince hospital patients to undergo repeated jugular punctures willingly on the grounds that their participation might increase neurologists' knowledge of intracranial circulation—or so he claimed.

At the end of his career, in the magisterial two-volume *Epilepsy and Related Disorders*, William Lennox professed great gratitude to the patients who had served as his "willing guinea pigs" in a wide range of experiments over many decades. With enthusiasm, he quoted William Osler: "To study the phenomenon of disease without books is to sail an uncharted sea, but to study books without patients is not to go to sea at all." He then extended the metaphor: "In past decades, students of epilepsy have been 'at sea' with no North Star books to guide them, but patients have always been in supply."[38] Lennox's description of patients as his research partners was an appealing conceit. Yet certainly in the 1930s and 1940s when Lennox was most heavily involved in experimental work, he did not speak of his human subjects in such warm and egalitarian terms. Their significance lay in their aggregate responses to experimental situations, not in a personal clinician-patient relationship.

Beginning in the 1920s and into the 1950s, William Lennox and his colleagues expressed much ambivalence about their epileptic research subjects. For example, Lennox wanted to eliminate the most disabled. Instead, he complained, "Society systematically and cruelly kills its best members by the means called 'war,' and unmercifully prolongs the lives of its hopeless liabilities."[39] Yet he simultaneously campaigned hard against negative stereotypes of epileptics and worked hard to promote the International League Against Epilepsy. He disparaged state colonies for epileptics as ineffective and wasteful even as he celebrated their value for researchers. (They held "collections of human material not to be matched elsewhere.")[40] These complex emotions colored the experimental work of most American neurologists, especially in the years before World War II. As a result, although they often asked private patients for permission before involving them in experiments, they seldom informed them fully of the hardships ahead. They ran and reran failed experiments in the hope of making neurological science more rigorous, ignoring the high costs to their human subjects. As the recent work of Lewis P. Rowland reveals, even neurological researchers as careful as H. Houston Merritt and Tracy J. Putnam could be dismissive of the toxic side effects of many anticonvulsants.[41] The voices of subjects never appeared in the many published accounts of the epilepsy experiments of the 1920s and 1930s. Perhaps most unsettling of all, the multiple tensions threading through so much research were seldom acknowledged, let alone resolved.

Notes

1. Susan E. Lederer, *Subjected to Science: Human Experimentation in America before the Second World War* (Baltimore: Johns Hopkins University Press, 1995), xii, 51–72, 89–100.

2. In print, neurologists seldom questioned even the most invasive experiments. During the discussion of a 1934 experiment that involved the repeated drawing of blood from subjects' veins and arteries, however, Tracy Putnam asked Abraham Myerson, the major investigator, if patients found the experiment "formidable." Myerson assured him that neurosurgeons need not worry about "little things like puncturing the jugular vein and carotid artery." They needed only to follow "the ordinary rules of asepsis and humanity." This discussion took place at the December 20, 1934, meet-

ing of the Boston Society of Psychiatry and Neurology, reported in Albert W. Steans, "Society Transactions: Boston Society of Psychiatry and Neurology," *Archives of Neurology and Psychiatry* 31 (September 1955), 686. A mere six months later, at the International Neurological Congress in London, William Lennox said of such work, "The theory [of generalized cerebral anaemia] is excellent; the experimental proof a failure." Hence, the theory "should be placed reverently in the museum of outmoded medical theories." William G. Lennox, "The Physiological Pathogenesis of Epilepsy," *Brain* 59 (1935): 113–14. That failed to happen, even in the work of Lennox himself.

3. Lederer, *Subjected to Science*, 126–38, xv. According to Lederer, some biomedical researchers first tried drugs and vaccines on themselves so as to dispel suspicion and public fears. This strategy was not common among neurologists, although the Johns Hopkins surgeon Walter Dandy claimed that the British neurologist Leonard Hill "with great fortitude [had] compressed one of his own carotid arteries and unilateral convulsions followed." Walter E. Dandy and Robert Elman, "Studies in Experimental Epilepsy," *Bulletin of the Johns Hopkins Hospital* 36, no. 1 (1925): 40.

4. Harry Marks, *The Progress of Experiment: Science and Therapeutic Reform in the United States, 1900–1990* (New York: Cambridge University Press, 1997), 1–129.

5. Ibid., 5, 21.

6. Ibid., 44–46.

7. As late as 1940, Alan Gregg still felt obliged to push hard for more scientific and interdisciplinary neuropsychiatric research. (Gregg himself was less interested in neurology than in psychiatry.) See Alan Gregg, "Present Day Trends in Neuropsychiatric Research: A Round Table Discussion," *American Journal of Psychiatry* 97 (1941): 780.

8. Like others, William Lennox and Erna Gibbs explained the need for human subjects in experiments in terms of the anatomical and physiological differences between laboratory animals, such as the cat, and human beings. See William Lennox and Erna Gibbs, "The Blood Flow in the Brain and the Leg of Man, and the Changes Induced by Alteration of Blood Cases," *Journal of Clinical Investigations* 11, no. 6 (1932): 1155–77. In 1934, H. Houston Merritt praised Abraham Myerson and his colleagues for having had the courage to carry on experiments involving humans "hitherto done only in animals" and, in the process, proving that even grueling experiments were "practical and harmless." See Oberndorf, "Society Proceedings," 686.

9. William G. Lennox, *Epilepsy and Related Disorders*, in collaboration with Margaret A. Lennox (Boston: Little, Brown, 1960), 1:x.

10. *Report on the Assistance of Indigent Patients Suffering with Epilepsy*, The Minnie Frances Kleman Memorial Fund (Ann Arbor, MI, 1936). Hereafter, *Report*.

11. For example, Lewis J. Pollock and Loyal Davis, "Studies in Decerebration. V. The Effect of Differentiation upon Decerebrate Rigidity," *American Journal of Physiology* 98 (1931): 47–49.

12. There is little published information on the Minnie Frances Kleman Memorial Fund, which seems to have supported only the Northwestern project. Yet in 1937, William J. Lennox described the fund as the largest in the country. Lennox, "The Campaign Against Epilepsy," *American Journal of Psychiatry* 94 (1937): 260.

13. *Report*, 26–35.

14. Ibid., 21.

15. Ibid., 65.

16. Ibid., 21.

17. Ibid., 32–33.

18. Ibid., 35.

19. Ibid., 69–135.

20. Ibid., 157.

21. Loyal Davis, "The Surgical Treatment of Epileptiform Seizures," *Report*, 187–212; and Loyal Davis, *The Principles of Neurological Surgery*, 2nd ed. (Philadelphia: Lea & Febiger, 1942), 428. Among the advocates of a more aggressive approach were E. F. Fincher and Charles Dowman, "Epileptiform Seizures of Jacksonian Type," *Journal of the American Medical Association* 97, no. 9 (1931): 1375–81. After surveying 130 cases from a ten-year period, Fincher and Dowman concluded that an "exploratory craniotomy is a justifiable procedures in all cases presenting epileptiform seizures in which the possibility of uncovering a removable lesion or destroying a demonstrable epileptic zone exists" (1380).

22. Wilder Penfield, "Surgical Treatment of Epileptiform Seizures," in Davis, *Principles of Neurological Surgery*, 428. See also Wilder Penfield and Lyle Gage, "Cerebral Localization of Epileptic Manifestations," *Archives of Neurology and Psychiatry* 30, no. 4 (1933): 709–27.

23. R. W. Waggoner, "Encephalography," *The American Journal of the Medical Sciences* 174, no. 5 (1927): 459–64.

24. W. Drayton, "Pneumocranium in the Treatment of Traumatic Headaches, Dizziness, and Change of Character," *Archives of Neurology and Psychiatry* (1934): 1302–99.

25. R. Cannon Eley, "Epilepsy: The Value of Encephalography in the Selection of Children for Ketogenic Diets," *Journal of Pediatrics* 3, no. 2 (1933): 359–68.

26. Reginald Steen and Mabel Matthews, "Encephalography," *Psychiatric Quarterly* 11, no. 1 (1937): 34–43.

27. Thomas Simpson and M. Herbert Barker, "Studies in Prolonged Anoxia," *Report*, 441–46.

28. Ibid., 452, 463.

29. Simpson and Barker cited fifteen other anoxia studies; ibid., 470–71.

30. Lennox, *Epilepsy and Related Disorders*, 2:741–44.

31. Theodore T. Stone and Harman Chor, "Water Metabolism and Epilepsy," *Report*, 178–79.

32. Ibid., 179–80.

33. Ibid., 180. Other researchers measured dehydration by weighing the gravity of the urine. As at Northwestern, the dehydration experiment failed to diminish seizures and proved unpopular with patients. "Even in hospitalized cases," the researchers noted, "it is sometimes difficult to combat thirst." J. L. Ketterman and H. J. Kumin, "Dehydration in Epilepsy," *Journal of the American Medical Association* 100, no. 13 (1933): 1006. For the translation of Hippocrates, see William G. Lennox and Stanley Cobb, "The Relation of Certain Physiochemical Processes to Epileptiform Seizures," *American Journal of Psychiatry* 85 (1929): 846.

34. Isidore Finkelman et al., "Ketosis in Epilepsy: Effects of Diacetone Alcohol on Institutionalized Epileptics, in *Report*, 154–55. The high-fat ketogenic diet worked to control seizures because it produced alkalosis in the body. It was notoriously difficult to sustain and generally was prescribed only to children. Several years after ketogenic

diets were first introduced, doctors began to report that their patients on the diet developed pellagra. See H. C. Sherman, "Some Recent Advances in the Chemistry of Nutrition," *Journal of the American Medical Association* 97, no. 20 (1931): 1429.

35. Isidore Finkelman, "Snake Venom (Moccasin) in Epilepsy, *Report*, 237–41. Although Finkelstein's experiments received little public attention, other trials of unconventional drugs attracted critical comments. For example, after a paper on the use of metrazol therapy at the 1939 meeting of the American Neurological Association, Stanley Cobb snapped, "The use of metrazol is the use of a perfectly dreadful drug." Cobb was followed by Erna Gibbs, who was much more accepting. Although she too had concerns about metrazol therapy, she held out hope for "the successful case." P. A. Davis and W. Suzlbach, "Changes in the Electroencephalogram during Metrazol Therapy," *Transactions of the American Neurological Association* (1939): 144–49. The experimental use of treatments designed for schizophrenics on epileptics was not uncommon; it suggests the continuing power of the idea that convulsive disorders were mental illnesses. See Grant E. Metcalfe, "Induced Hypoglycemic Shock in Crytogenic Epilepsy," *Psychiatry Quarterly* 2, no. 2 (1939): 348–56.

36. References to the so-called stigmata of degeneration first appeared prominently in the work on hereditary degeneration of the nineteenth-century French psychiatrist, Benedict Augustin Morel. For a succinct statement of Morel's writings on this topic, see Gregory Zilboorg, *A History of Medical Psychology* (New York: W. W. Norton, 1941), 42. Initially, in the late nineteenth century, medical professionals looked for these stigmata, which consisted of anatomical deviations from the norm, as well as some intellectual and moral deviations, largely in so-called mental defectives. Then, in the early twentieth century, neurologists in Great Britain, the United States, and France extended the search to individuals with epilepsy. A typical articulation of their findings can be found in the writings of William Aldren Turner, a major early twentieth-century British epileptologist. Turner observed that epileptics often had cranial abnormalities, facial asymmetry, and irregular and displaced teeth, which correlated with a poor prognosis. See William Aldren Turner, "The Influence of Stigmata of Degeneration upon the Prognosis of Epilepsy," *Medico-Churgical Transactions* 88 (1906): 127–45.

37. For an account of dehydration experiments at Craig Colony, see Glenn J. Doolittle, "Report of Results from Use of Ketogenic Diet and Ketogenic Diet with Water Restriction in a Series of Epileptics," pts. 1 and 2, *Psychiatric Quarterly* 5, no. 1 (1931): 135–50; no. 2 (1931): 225–52. To direct this work, Doolittle had enlisted the help of Irvine McQuarrie of the University of Rochester. At Craig Colony, McQuarrie oversaw twenty-five white female subjects who ranged in age from seven to twenty-eight. Besides occasional mentions of family problems, the patients' published profiles revealed little about them. For example:

> 7929. White, female, age 7 years. Native of U.S. Family history: Second in line of birth of 2 boys and 3 girls, all living. Personal history: measles and whooping cough, tonsillectomy at ages unknown. History of epilepsy: Onset at 3 years; no aura. (233)

McQuarrie's parallel work with pediatric patients at the University of Rochester suggests another research issue generally ignored by neurologists, although often a matter of public concern: the use of child subjects in physically stressful experiments. The difficult-to-sustain ketogenic diets most often were prescribed for very young children in hospitals and clinics across the country. There was a huge literature on the ketogenic diet during the 1920s and 1930s. For two examples, see H. F. Helmholz and H. M. Keith, "Ten Years' Experience with the Ketogenic Diet," *Archives of Neurology and Psychiatry* 29 (1933): 808–12; and F. B. Talbot, "The Ketogenic Diet," *Bulletin of the New York Academy of Medicine* 4 (1928): 401–10. The Mayo Clinic ran the largest number of these experiments.

38. Lennox, *Epilepsy and Related Disorders*, 2:756–57.

39. Lennox, "Campaign against Epilepsy," *American Journal of Psychiatry*, 94 (September 1937): 260. Several decades later, he repeated this sentiment word for word in a section called "Ethics Enters In," in *Epilepsy and Related Disorders*, 2:1046.

40. Lennox, "Campaign against Epilepsy," 260.

41. Lewis P. Rowland, *The Legacy of Tracy J. Putnam and H. Houston Merritt: Modern Neurology in the United States* (New York: Oxford University Press, 2009), 5–7.

Part Two

Public and Private Constructions of the "Neurological Patient"

Chapter Three

Speaking for Yourself

The Medico-Legal Aspects of Aphasia in Nineteenth-Century Britain

Marjorie Perlman Lorch

Introduction

Throughout the eighteenth and early nineteenth century there was consideration of the status of persons deemed insane. Two legal issues were relevant: acts of criminal behavior such as violent attack or murder leading to the possibility of prison or the death sentence, and more general aspects of social functioning and the question of confinement in asylums. With the emergence of the concept of a disorder of expression due to specific brain damage and the coining of the term "aphasia" in the second half of the nineteenth century, a new group of people whose civil rights required protection was identified: those whose ability to understand others' intentions and express their own had been compromised by illness. Although there is a large body of historical research into criminal law and insanity during this period,[1] very little work has been carried out with regard to mental deficiency and civil law. Peter Bartlett stressed the need for research in this area: "Study of the determination of civil competency has been marginal in the history of modern law and madness to the point of being almost ignored."[2] Bartlett expanded on this theme as follows: "Valuable work has been done on the history of criminal insanity, and work is beginning to appear regarding confinement in private madhouses and county asylums. The insights gained therein have not, by and large, been extended into the civil issues of competency determination nor have relations between law and medicine been theorized outside the context of criminal insanity."[3] This chapter examines a particular group of people whose civil identity was being redefined in Victorian England because of developments in both the medical and legal spheres.

At the beginning of the 1860s the clinical entity of aphasia was defined.[4] The focus of this syndrome was people who had suffered an illness that affected a particular part of their brain and were unable to express their thoughts through language, although their intelligence and muscular speech apparatus were intact. Previously this difficulty had been denoted as speechlessness, loss of speech, or defect of expression, and was regarded as a secondary symptom in those suffering typically from fever, epilepsy, or paralysis. The creation of this new syndrome spurred the reconsideration of the relationship between mind and expression, and the mental state of those people with difficulties in speaking. This reconceptualization of a clinical entity in the medical domain had consequences for the legal consideration of mental capacity in the civil courts. The legal status of aphasic persons in Victorian England must be viewed in the context of the particular developments in ideas regarding the term "mental defects" in British medicine and the term "unsound mind" in the British legal system, which were both undergoing refinement in the second half of the nineteenth century.

Defining Aphasia

In a series of case reports published over a period of four years, the French clinician Paul Broca attributed the long-standing speech production difficulties in a number of patients to lesions in the frontal lobes at autopsy. Broca's lectures and publications[5] stimulated others to pursue the idea that there was a specific part of the brain that was dedicated to language, and that this function would be compromised if the particular neuroanatomical location was damaged. Thus, language impairment was elevated to the status of a distinct clinical entity and a new term was coined, "aphasia." Before this time, people with difficulties in verbal expression were considered to have difficulties either with muscular control of the speech apparatus or a partial disorder of memory.[6] Only a few years after the appearance of the initial clinical descriptions of aphasic patients by Broca and colleagues in Paris, physicians in Great Britain began to consider the issue.[7] However, the work on language impairments in Great Britain followed a somewhat different trajectory than those on the Continent.[8]

Aphasia was being defined at a time when the British hospital system was undergoing dramatic change with the establishment of a large number of new hospitals dedicated to the treatment of particular illnesses or parts of the body. By 1860, there were sixty-six special hospitals listed in the *London Medical Directory*. The first British specialist hospital for the study of nervous diseases was The National Hospital for the Cure and Relief of Paralysis and Epilepsy, located in Queen Square, London, founded in 1859. This new hospital provided an opportunity for clinicians to observe and examine hundreds of patients a year with similar medical histories and patterns of impairment. A large portion of these patients had aphasic deficits.[9] It was in this context that the possibility that a defect in spoken expression could be independent from a loss of intellect was raised.[10]

The Victorian Legal System

Concurrent with these medical developments, there was evolving practice in Victorian jurisprudence; notions of mental capacity were being revised with respect to both criminal and civil law. There were both social and financial drivers to these developments. In criminal law, the Victorian period saw the emergence of the plea of not guilty due to moral insanity. At the same time, the expansion of middle-class wealth as a result of the industrial revolution triggered reform of the civil laws and court system for handling the growing significance of wills and inheritance. With the Probate Act of 1857, the jurisdiction over determination of wills was transferred from the ecclesiastical courts of the Church of England to state control. This also provided for the establishment of a new District Probate Registry replacing the traditional church records, and a Court of Probate that later became the probate division of the High Court.[11]

These state institutions were developed in response to the rising number of wills being made and of contested cases of inheritance. English law diverged from the convention followed by other European countries in allowing individuals full discretion to decide who would inherit their estate, what is called freedom of testamentary. In other countries a percentage of an individual's wealth would be inherited through a predetermined line of descent. Only in England was an individual allowed to completely disinherit family members and leave their wealth to whomever they wished. This circumstance naturally led to attempts to contest wills by those who felt they had been unjustly overlooked. At the same time, the judges made rulings that acknowledged that a distinction needed to be drawn between, for example, taking a dislike to a family member and choosing not to leave them money or leaving money to pets rather than people, which were within one's rights, and holding insane delusions that indicated a lack of testamentary capacity.

This widespread social change and the subsequent consequences for the legal system in Victorian England was illustrated in the literature and paintings of the day. Charles Dickens satirized the legal profession in his novels *The Pickwick Papers* (1837) and *Bleak House* (1853).[12] The whole of the plot of *Bleak House* is driven by a disputed will in which the question of who should receive a share of the legacy is argued through the courts over more than a generation. The ubiquity of this type of legal dispute is signaled in a passage of Dickens's earlier novel *David Copperfield* (1849):

I asked Mr. Spenlow what he considered the best sort of professional business. He replied, that a good case of a disputed will, where there was a neat little estate of thirty or forty thousand pounds, was, perhaps, the best of all. In such a case, he said, not only were there very pretty pickings, in the way of arguments at every stage of the proceedings, and mountains upon mountains of evidence on interrogatory and counter-interrogatory (to say nothing of an appeal lying, first to the Delegates, and then to the Lords), but, the costs being pretty sure to come out of the estate at last, both sides went at it in a lively and spirited manner, and expense was no consideration.[13]

Disputed wills figured in a number of other popular novels of the day. For example, in Trollope's *Orley Farm* (1862) there is a court case with a dispute over an inheritance by two sons with accusations that a handwritten codicil was forged. The emotionally charged event of the reading of a will to discover who would inherit was also represented in paintings. For example, "Reading the Will," painted by Frederick Daniel Hardy in 1870, was shown at a number of popular public exhibitions over this period, including the Royal Academy of Arts Exhibition in 1870, the Manchester Royal Jubilee Exhibition in 1877, and the Guildhall Exhibition in 1897. These various representations capture a widespread personal experience.

The Act of Will Making

In the early Roman Republic, wills were made orally before the *Comitia Curiata*, before the army assembled before battle or before five special witnesses. This form of oral will making, established by Julius Caesar, remained common practice in England up until the thirteenth century.[14] In the nineteenth century, practice was changed by statute, notably from oral to written will making. The Statute of Wills of 1838 required all English wills to be written and signed by witnesses.[15] In Victorian England, social change included increasing access to schooling and a huge rise in the portion of the population with literacy skills. The status of handwriting was extremely high; it was viewed as a marker of social status and identity and directly linked to employment prospects and wealth creation. The anthropologist Edward Burnett Tylor's comments reflect a general social attitude in this regard: "We English are perhaps poorer in the gesture-language than any other people in the world. We use a form of words to denote what a gesture . . . would express. Perhaps it is because we read and write so much, and have come to think and talk as we should write, and so let fall those aids to speech which cannot be carried into the written language."[16] Indeed, the ability to write had such high social currency that it was taken as evidence of mental capacity. Wharton and Stillé state: "The fact of the paper being entirely in a party's handwriting gives a strong presumption of sanity, which is not effaced by proof of generally impaired intellect, nor by the fact, that when the paper is a will, in it omissions of property exist."[17]

The importance of the manner in which a will was communicated is also reflected in the exceptions made for those who were illiterate, deaf, dumb, and blind. In the case of illiterate or blind persons, the matter was fairly straightforward; they could dictate their will to a lawyer who would transcribe it in front of witnesses. In contrast, the civil rights of people who were deaf were renegotiated throughout this period. The prevailing view up to this time had been that deaf persons did not have mental capacity (i.e., they were considered as idiots) because they could not speak intelligibly. Subsequent legal precedents were set that acknowledge the possibility that deaf and dumb persons could have testamentary capacity. In their treatise on estates and probate, Edward Williams and colleagues set out the issues regarding such a determination:

> One who is deaf and dumb from his nativity is, in presumption of law, an idiot, and therefore incapable of making a will; but such a presumption may be rebutted, and if it sufficiently appears that he understands what a testament means, and has a desire to make one, then he may by signs and tokens declare his testament. One who is not deaf and dumb by nature, but being once able to hear and speak, if by some accident he loses both his hearing and the use of his tongue, then in case he shall be able to write, he may with his own hand write his last will and testament. But if he be not able to write, then he is in the same case as those which be both deaf and dumb by nature, i.e., if he have understanding he may make his testament by signs, otherwise not at all. Such as can speak and cannot hear, they may make their testaments as if they could both speak and hear, whether that defect came by nature or otherwise. Such as be speechless only, and not void of hearing, if they can write, may very well make their testaments themselves by writing: if they cannot write, they may also make their own testaments by signs, so that the same signs be sufficiently known to such as then be present.[18]

It is interesting that for these people with sensory impairments what was crucial was the establishment of evidence of intelligence and education. The use of signs and the need for interpreters was seen to be less of an obstacle to gaining their rights.[19]

Changing Views on Mental Capacity: Defining Idiots, Imbeciles, and the Elderly

The notion of insanity and being of unsound mind was based on the assumption of the unitary nature and indivisibility of the mind. In the nineteenth century, the idea of partial insanity, monomania, or partial mental defect developed through the accumulation of case descriptions of acquired disorders in adults and the differentiation of these from natural aging and mental deficits in the elderly.[20]

The notion of who had testamentary capacity in legal terms underwent refinement throughout the century as medical practitioners began to draw distinctions between (1) those who had been born with mental defects, (2) those who had acquired them later in life, (3) those who were compromised through advanced aging, and (4) those who were termed insane. This growing appreciation of the significance a patient's age with respect to their diagnosis and prognosis for neurological disorders was a trend at this time.[21]

There were several categories of people who were deemed not to have testamentary capacity. One was infants; at this point the legal age was twenty-one, having been set at fifteen at the beginning of the century. A second group who were considered not to have testamentary capacity was so-called idiots. Idiots were traditionally considered to be those deprived of intellect from birth. In Victorian England, it became acknowledged that the development of intellect could suffer as the result of childhood illness or accident, and did not have to be present from birth. In this context, the limitation of the development of intellect was tested by such things as a failure to learn the names of family members, and an inability to count to twenty or name the days of the week.

With respect to those deemed to be insane, up until the Victorian period insanity was considered solely as an impairment of the intellect. The legal evidence required for the determination of insanity was the presence of delusions.[22] However, the inability to know the difference between right and wrong was introduced as another criterion for insanity in the law courts at this time. In 1835, James Cowles Prichard wrote *A Treatise on Insanity and Other Disorders Affecting the Mind.* Prichard proposed a novel, distinct mental disease: moral insanity, which involved an impairment of the emotions and an inability to know the difference between right and wrong. He defined it as "a morbid perversion of the natural feelings . . . without any remarkable disorder or defect of the intellect or knowing and reasoning faculties . . . the individual is found to be incapable, not of talking or reasoning upon any subject . . . but of conducting himself with decency."[23]

This notion of moral insanity became a significant source of legal argumentation in the case of Daniel M'Naghten in 1843,[24] which is still a significant precedent in today's case law. M'Naghten had assassinated Edward Drummond, whom he had mistaken for Prime Minister Robert Peel. The court found him to be suffering from moral insanity, and committed him to an asylum rather than executing him for murder. The test of insanity for the purpose of defense in criminal law was established by Chief Justice Tindal in this case, which still stands today: that the person must be proved to have a defect of reason, from a disease of the mind, as to not know the nature and quality of their behavior or not know it was wrong. This development had great significance in criminal law but held implications for civil law to a lesser extent.

As Bartlett pointed out, for English law insanity was not viewed as intrinsic to the individual, but was determined by the abilities of the individual in the context of the specific situation.[25] With respect to the confinement of the insane to asylums and the loss of their legal responsibilities, the Commission of Lunacy was responsible for such determinations.[26] Because of perceived abuses to the system, the determination of unsound mind was being refined by statue for the Commission of Lunacy, which decided the fate of those individuals to be confined to an asylum.[27]

An interesting case that demonstrated the difficulties that such a system led to was discussed in the medical community in the mid-nineteenth century. Reflecting on this some decades later, Alfred Taylor and John Reese point out: "Only in cases where the person is wealthy can a commission of lunacy be used to inquire about capacity to manage one's affairs (*non compos mentis*) or to be placed under interdiction (have finances and estate managed by others)."[28] However, the determination of unsound mind with respect to testamentary capacity was not regulated by statue, then or now; rather, it was dealt with by legal precedent. In ruling on the case of *Waring v. Waring*[29] in 1848, Lord Brougham decreed that mental disease could not be safely defined by legal tribunal; therefore it was necessary to hold *any degree* of insanity as unfitting to testamentary capacity. At the time, this judgment reflected the assumptions that insanity is not a physical disorder, that idiocy and insanity are the same, that the presence of insanity can be determined by the judge, and that the knowledge of right and wrong is the test both of soundness of mind and of responsibility. Taylor and Hartshorne cite a case in which a Mrs. Cummings's estate was exhausted by the court costs for numerous appeals over her will because of disagreement by medical experts for and against a finding of insanity, so that in the end there was nothing left to inherit.[30] As will be discussed below, over the next three decades each of these assumptions would be revised and illuminated by growing clinical evidence and changing conceptualizations of language and thought. This specific development occurred within the larger context of increasing somatization of psychiatric disorders in Britain over this period.[31]

The views expressed by Lord Brougham in 1848 regarding the unity of sanity were substantially overturned in the ruling by Chief Justice Cockburn in the case of *Banks v. Goodfellow* in 1870. That mental disease could be selective was acknowledged for the first time: "The pathology of mental disease and the experience of insanity in its various forms teach us that, while on the one hand all the faculties, moral and intellectual, may be involved in one common ruin (as in the case of the raving maniac), in other instances one or more only of these faculties or functions may be disordered while the rest are left unimpaired and undisturbed."[32] The determination of mental capacity for those allowed to make a will became more explicit following the precedent of the case of *Banks v. Goodfellow*, which still serves today:

> It is essential to the exercise of such a power that a testator shall understand the nature of the act and its effects; shall understand the extent of the property of which he is disposing; shall be able to comprehend and appreciate the claims to which he ought to give effect and, with a view to the latter object, that no disorder of mind shall poison his affections, pervert his sense of right, or prevent the exercise of his natural faculties—that no insane delusion shall influence his will in disposing of his property and bring about a disposal of it which, if the mind had been sound, would not have been made.[33]

Interestingly, through this new distinction, it became possible that an individual who was unable to manage his or her own affairs and thus be committed to an asylum could still be deemed competent to make a will.

In their consideration of the requirements for determining if an individual was of disposing mind, Taylor and Reese suggest that a good test in those who are aged and infirm is to get them to repeat from memory the contents of their will.[34] If a person cannot do this, it should be taken as evidence that they do not have a sane and disposing mind. It was further specified that the ability to answer yes-no questions regarding the contents of the will should not be taken as evidence of understanding. Up to this point, legal tests of a sound and disposing mind implied that intact linguistic function was synonymous with sanity.

Aphasia, Soundness of Mind, and Testamentary Capacity

From the moment that aphasia became a recognized medical category, the question began to form whether a person suffering from aphasia had an impairment limited to language or was more broadly affected in general intelligence, reasoning, memory, and so on. The legal significance of this distinction between language and intelligence was the bearing it had on the determination of mental soundness and testamentary capacity. Shortly after the first papers reporting cases of the new syndrome by British clinicians began to appear in the mid 1860s, discussion of the medical and legal issues concerning these patients were published in both the medical and lay press. The first notable report appeared in the *British Medical Journal*; it was written by a clinician about a case he had seen four decades before and that he now viewed in this new light. Bramwell retells a case of attempted murder in which the victim, who his patient, was rendered aphasic and served as a prosecution witness at the criminal trial.[35] As Paul Foley shows in his chapter in this volume on encephalitis lethargica, physicians often relied upon patient narratives. Yet the report of this case is unusual in that it presents the patient's own recorded words with commentary provided by the physician. Immediately after the attack the patient reports:

> To my surprise and horror, I found I could only utter unintelligible sounds. . . . Notwithstanding all my efforts to speak, my recovery was so slow that I could converse with none but a man who had been in my employ previously and was my constant attendant after the accident, to whom I communicated my ideas and desires, partly by gestures and partly by my attempts at speech. So much was this the case that, at the trial of Wilson [the accused], which occurred nearly 3 months after my injury, he had to be sworn as my interpreter. My examination in court, on account of this, was so grotesque, and at the same time interesting to the members of the bar, that it was continued till I was quite exhausted; and it affected the audience as laughable or deplorable, according to their different bent of mind.[36]

Bramwell's analysis outlined succinctly the debate as to whether aphasia was a strictly language disorder or symptomatic of a more general disorder of intellect. Bramwell commented: "Although cases of aphasia are often associated with impaired mental powers, simply because a pure case of this disorder is rarer than a complicated one, we believe that, in simple aphasia the reasoning powers are quite intact, and that in cases where it is otherwise, the brain has sustained a complex lesion."[37] This case is notable in that a medical practitioner is presenting a retrospective reevaluation of a case in light of contemporary developments. The patient is now viewed as suffering from the new syndrome of aphasia. Moreover, the medical expert made his analysis of the witness's mental capacity through consideration of the witness's narrative—the complex relationship between patient narratives and medical discourse is a theme reiterated throughout this volume.

The following year, another court case concerning an aphasic person with legal consequences was reported in the daily British newspaper the *Times:* "For some months before his death [Maurice Peter Moore] had been suffering from what is called 'aphasia,' a disease which renders the patient unable to express in words the ideas which pass through his mind, and the question was whether in addition to this disease his mental capacity was affected."[38] The daughter of the deceased contested the will on the ground of incapacity, alleging the deceased was of unsound mind at the time of the execution of the will. The contested question was raised on the basis of conflicting spoken and written expression. While several witnesses testified to his ability to converse on various topics in a rational manner as evidence in support of his testamentary capacity, written specimens were shown as evidence of mental incapacity: "The witnesses described him as being often unable to give utterance to the proper words to express the ideas passing through his mind until he heard them spoken or saw them written. He had a number of cards printed with the names of articles in common use and he carried about with him books containing lists of proper names to which he referred when at a loss for a word. A number of memorandum books and scraps of paper were produced, on some of which he had written unintelligible and unconnected words."[39] Several testified that they had received letters from the deceased "expressing a decided opinion of his [own] unsoundness of mind and of his [own] incapacity to make a valid will."[40] The family solicitor was persuaded that the deceased man did have testamentary capacity when he had interviewed him and received verbal instructions that were then written up in a will and signed. The interesting thing in this case was the discrepancy between the spoken production, which was viewed as defective but rational, in contrast to the written production, which was viewed as defective but irrational. On summing up to the special jury the judge, Sir J. P. Wilde, stated that "the ambiguous conduct of Mr. Peake, coupled with his condition as a testator, might fairly raised doubts as to his mental capacity in the minds of those who only saw him occasionally and for a short time, and who had not the opportunity of forming an opinion as [family friends] Mr. Nisbet-Hamilton and Archdeacon Trollope and others."[41] The court pronounced for the will.[42]

In a significant contribution to the English medical literature on aphasia, Henry Charlton Bastian pointed out: "Then, with regard to the degree of general *mental impairment* existing in aphasia, there cannot be a doubt that here also the widest latitude of variation is met with."[43] In Bastian's classification the relation between speech and intellect is confounded. He proposed that aphasic symptoms should be classified by degrees of severity, defining "very severe" patients as those in whom the amount of mental impairment is generally so great that inability to speak is only one factor, while "typical cases" were those persons who could think but not speak or write. However, he himself pointed out the need for a theoretically motivated distinction between language and thought in a subsequent passage: "The theories that have been put forward in explanation of the 'aphasic' state are numerous, but owing to the various allied conditions not having been clearly distinguished from one another by some writers, and owing, as I think, to some others not having properly apprehended the kind and degree of relation existing between Language and Thinking, no small amount of confusion and contradiction is to be met with amongst these various explanations."[44]

The next case that has bearing on the factors perceived by the judiciary as setting a precedent on the determination of mental capacity is *Boughton and Another v. Knight and Others*, 1873, which was reported in the *Times*. The judge, Sir James Hannen, in summing up the case stressed that it "involved the question of what was the amount and quality of intellect necessary to constitute testamentary capacity? In his [Hannen's] opinion that question was eminently a practical one, to be decided by the good sense of men of the world rather than by legal definitions. It was a question of degree, to be determined by the jury."[45] This followed the ruling in *Banks v. Goodfellow* three years earlier. However, Judge Hannen went further. He considered the degree of mental capacity required for will making to be higher than for other functions. Hannen ruled: "A sound mind in contemplation of law does not necessarily mean a perfectly balanced mind, and large allowance must be made for the differences of individual character, habits, and mode of living. It must not be assumed that because a man acts in unaccustomed ways he is, therefore, of unsound mind. The burden is on those propounding a will to satisfy the court that when the will was made the testator was of sound and disposing mind. . . . Mental capacity is a question of degree, but the highest degree of capacity is required to make a testamentary disposition, inasmuch as it involves a larger and wider survey of the facts than is needed to enter into the ordinary contracts of life."[46]

Many cases of aphasia published in the literature of this time included descriptions of the patient's mental capabilities. However, as Stephen Casper discusses in his study of the neurological examination of the patient in this volume, no standard system of clinical assessment existed, and there were inherent difficulties in accurately determining the extent of the language disturbance and mental impairment in a given patient. While initial publications on aphasia focused on the difficulties aphasic patients had with expression of their intentions, others raise the issue of how to determine that patients understood what was being said to them as an issue distinct from general intellectual difficulties such as remembering. William Tennant Gairdner is one of the earliest clinicians to raise this consideration. In discussing one such aphasic patient, Gairdner commented on the difficulties for clinicians in this regard: "It cannot be distinctly affirmed that she has clearly understood anything spoken to her, except in so far as the general sense may have been apparent to her through surrounding circumstances and gestures."[47] That mental competence was typically judged through the medium of language posed an obvious problem for those attempting to gain an accurate assessment of aphasic patients' mental capacity.

In his book *Responsibility in Mental Disease*, the clinician Henry Maudsley addressed this question directly: "It is obvious that difficult questions must sometimes arise with regard to the amount of understanding which a person who is in this aphasic state actually possesses: having lost the usual means by which intelligence is manifested, there will necessarily be a difficulty in gauging the measure if it."[48] At various points in his discussion of aphasic patients' ability to express themselves, he pointed out that the patient may be unable to recall any word or may "substitute wrong words for those which he wishes to use." Or, the patient "may understand words written as well as words spoken, but he cannot express himself either in the one way or in the other." Maudsley was clear that "the practical question [is] whether an aphasic person is competent to make a will. It is quite possible that he might not be capable of sustained thought, might have suffered some impairment of thought, feeling, and will, and yet might know the nature and amount of his property, and be competent to express his wishes with regard to the disposal of it."[49] This passage highlights the dual questions with regard to ascertaining aphasic patients' testamentary capacity: on the one hand there is the need to demonstrate their ability to comprehend discussions about the details of their estate and the relevant people involved, and on the other is their ability to successfully express their intentions and desires. With a deeper understanding of the nature of aphasia and the variety of dissociated manifestations for both expression and comprehension, clinicians began to develop more refined subcategories and classifications.

At the same time, clinicians were becoming concerned with dual responsibilities in this regard. First, to counsel patients and their families regarding will making in cases where the ability to express one's wishes was compromised, and second, to be called as court witnesses in civil disputes that arose in consequence. This growing matter of professional concern is highlighted in an editorial that appeared in the *British Medical Journal* in 1877. As with the assessment of sanity in criminal cases, medical experts were increasingly being called upon to testify in civil court as to aphasic patients' mental competence. The editorial discussed the difficulties faced by medical practitioners called to give their expert opinion in such cases:

> Questions of the law are often likely to arise, as they have indeed already arisen, in connection with aphasia; and they are of a nature to give much trouble to practitioners. The greater number of aphasic persons has undergone a certain intellectual depression, dating from the attack, but nevertheless they preserve, in many cases, enough intelligence to express themselves by gestures when they cannot do so in writing, either because of paralysis of the right arm or because they have lost the power of expression. Such persons, however, still have enough intelligence and will to interest themselves in the carrying on of their affairs and to take an active and useful part in them when they become able to make themselves sufficiently understood to get their injunctions obeyed. Often, however, in these cases, interested persons demand the sequestration of the estates of such "aphasics" but this is only legally justifiable when the individual is in an habitual state of imbecility, dementia or mania, either with or without lucid intervals. These conditions often do not exist in the aphasic.[50]

In direct response to this editorial, a regional clinician attending at a district asylum submitted a case report for publication in the *British Medical Journal*. This article exemplifies the burden of legal responsibilities felt by clinicians at this time with regard to their aphasic patients. O'Neill's case was of a fifty-five-year-old man with right hemiplegia and aphasia who was a patient in the Lincoln Lunatic Hospital. He described the patient as follows:

"He could say 'yes' or 'no' distinctly but these were the only intelligible words he could utter . . . he seemed to be quite rational and to understand everything that was said to him and of him. He attempted to answer questions . . . but intelligent speech failed him and he gave utterance to an unintelligible jargon." What is relevant about this report is the clinician's telling remark at the very end that "had he been called upon to make a will at the time I saw him, I believe he would not have been competent to do so; for although his intelligence might have been adequate to the task, he had not power to explain himself so that his wishes might be understood."[51]

In his wide-ranging paper "On Affections of Speech," which appeared in several parts in *Brain* throughout 1878–79, John Hughlings Jackson also raised the question, "can an aphasic make a will?" In response, he remarked that it cannot be answered any more than can the question, "will a piece of string reach across this room?"[52] Jackson insisted that because there is a large degree of variation in the manifestation of aphasia, this question can only be decided on an individual case basis. In an editorial review of Jackson's paper in the *British Medical Journal*, this point was picked up:

> The practical aspect of this disease [aphasia] has never been so clearly enunciated by any previous writer. We confess that we have hopes that, before Dr. Hughlings Jackson has finished with the subject, he will leave us a few suggestions as to the medico-legal importance of the most prominent symptoms detailed above. A few simple tests of the patient's capabilities of articulation, pantomime, recognition, writing powers, ability or not to sign his name, emotional language as expressed by ejaculation, and general signs of intellectual capacity, would be most welcome from the pen of so experienced a practitioner . . . and would probably, in such able hands, be fashioned into weapons sufficiently keen and powerful to enable us to determine exactly the medico-legal position of any given case of aphasia.[53]

Although Jackson did not take up the challenge, some of his medical colleagues, notably Samuel Wilks, William Gowers, and Henry Charlton Bastian, did make certain attempts decades later.

Another offhand comment that reflects a similar concern with distinguishing speech defect from mental impairment comes from John Syer Bristowe in his Lumleian Lecture the same year at the Royal College of Physicians London on the pathologies of voice and speech. In his discussion of the case of an aphasic fifty-year-old woman, Bristowe included the pointed remark that "her general intelligence was much less seriously impaired than her knowledge of language might have led one to suppose."[54]

By the end of the nineteenth century, medical practitioners' concerns about their responsibilities to their aphasic patients and their role as medical witnesses in cases of contested wills combined with a theoretical interest in the relation of language to intellect. As Bartlett pointed out: "This complexity of legal and medical relations exists not merely on a theoretical, but also on a practical level. Certainly, there are cases of legal and medical antagonism; but the nineteenth century shows equally increasing reliance of the law on doctors and of doctors on the law."[55]

The first notable medico-legal commentator on aphasia was Frederic Bateman, who added a new chapter dedicated to the topic in the revised and enlarged edition of his groundbreaking book *On Aphasia* (1870). Bateman asserted: "I am not aware that this important and interesting subject [of testamentary capacity in aphasia] has been treated by any British writer; at all events, no systematic essay on the legal aspect of aphasia has come under my notice."[56] Reviewing the issue of jurisprudence with regard to aphasia, Bateman stated that there is "no code or law as to the legal capacity of aphasics in this or any other country" such that "each particular case would have to be judged on its own merits."[57]

With respect to testamentary capacity in aphasic patients, Bateman noted that while there may be issues regarding criminal and civil responsibility, the most frequent instances involved the question of the management and disposal of property and the validity of a will. Bateman delineated the question clearly by asking "what modifications, if any, the aphasic condition may necessitate in the civil rights of the individual affected with this infirmity. Questions of law have often arisen in our courts of justice in connection with persons deprived of the faculty of speech whether such persons are to be considered to possess testamentary capacity; and whether, also, in other respects, they are legally responsible units in the social scale."[58]

Conclusion

By the time aphasia became recognized as a syndrome in the 1860s, clinicians in Britain already had expertise in assessing mental competence for purposes of the law with respect to criminal insanity. As the consideration of whether patients with aphasia were suffering from a language disorder as distinct from a thought disorder was being debated in 1860–90, courts were engaged in the refinement of notions regarding testamentary capacity and soundness of mind. This chapter has reviewed the evidence from the period of syndrome definition for aphasia in the 1860s through several decades of elaboration, which reflect the way the medical and legal establishment viewed the civil status of those people affected with an acquired disorder of language. It has also demonstrated the ways in which the status of this group of patients changed as ideas about the relationship between language and thought and mind and brain developed in parallel with the social need for a refinement of criteria for legal determination of mental capacity.

The medico-legal aspects of aphasia have received very little attention from historians in contrast to medico-legal issues regarding insanity. Even in the contemporary literature there has been almost no consideration of the civil issues of mental soundness and testamentary capacity of aphasic persons. Ferguson and colleagues, reviewing a recent legal case involving a challenge to the will of a woman with severe aphasia, assert that "no previous empirical research has been reported that investigates issues directly related to testamentary capacity and aphasia . . . [and] there is no discussion regarding assessment of the communication abilities relevant to testamentary capacity."[59] Although there was active examination of these issues toward the latter part of the nineteenth century, surprisingly little has been written since then to further develop these ideas.[60] There is a further future consideration to be pursued: why did this question of aphasia and the determination of testamentary capacity disappear from the research landscape in the ensuing years? And why is there so little concern about it now?

Notes

I would like to thank Dr. Paula Hellal for her contribution to the early stages of development for this project.

1. For example, see Joel Peter Eigen, "Historical Developments in Psychiatric Forensic Evidence: The British Experience," *International Journal of Law and Psychiatry* 6 (1983): 423–29.

2. Peter Bartlett, "Legal Madness in the Nineteenth Century," *Social History of Medicine* 14 (2001): 117.

3. Ibid., 130.

4. Armand Trousseau, "De l'aphasie, maladie décrite récemment sous le nom impropre d'aphémie," *Gazette des hôpitaux civils et militaires* 37 (1864).

5. Paul Broca, *Sur siége de la faculté du langage articulé avec deux observations d'aphémie (perte de la parole)* (Paris: Victor Masson et Fils, 1861); Paul Broca, *Nouvelle observation d'aphéme: Produite par une lésion de la troisième circonvolution frontale* (Paris: Victor Masson et Fils, 1861); Paul Broca, *Remarques sur le siége, le diagnostic, et la nature de l'aphémie: Extrait des Bulletins de la Société Anatomique, etc.* (Paris, 1863); and Paul Broca, *Du Siége de la faculté du langage articulé dans l'hémisphère gauche du cerveau: Extrait des Bulletins de la Société d'Anthropologie, etc.* (Paris, 1865).

6. For overviews of this period, see, for example, Robert M. Young, *Mind, Brain, and Adaptation in the Nineteenth Century* (Oxford: Oxford University Press, 1970); Anne Harrington, *Medicine, Mind, and the Double Brain: A Study in Nineteenth-Century Thought* (Princeton: Princeton University Press, 1987); L. Stephen Jacyna, "Somatic Theories of Mind and the Interests of Medicine in Britain, 1850–1879," *Medical History* 26 (1982): 233–58, Marjorie Perlman Lorch, "The Merest Logomachy: The 1868 Norwich Discussion of Aphasia by Hughlings Jackson and Broca," *Brain* 131, no. 6 (2008): 1658–70.

7. Marjorie Perlman Lorch, "The Unknown Source of John Hughlings Jackson's Early Interest in Aphasia and Epilepsy," *Cognitive and Behavioral Neurology* 17, no. 3 (2004): 124–32.

8. Lorch, "Merest Logomachy."

9. The National Hospital in Queen Square was initially established for the treatment of individuals with paralysis. However, the founding physician, Jabez Spence Ramskill, had a particular interest in epilepsy and caused this group of individuals to be included in the hospital's mission. Although he primarily dealt with the epileptic patients, a survey of Ramskill's casebooks for the years 1863–65 included thirty-five aphasic individuals. Once John Hughlings Jackson and others joined the growing staff, the percentage of aphasic patients continued to increase. Lorch, "Unknown Source," 126.

10. For a review of this issue, see Frederic Bateman, *On Aphasia, or Loss of Speech, and the Localisation of the Faculty of Articulate Language* (London: J. Churchill & Sons, 1870).

11. Probate Records: Legal Records Information Leaflet 23, Online Catalogue Research Guide, 2003, The National Archives, Kew, Surrey.

12. William Searle Holdsworth, *Charles Dickens as a Legal Historian* (New Haven: Yale University Press, 1928).

13. Charles Dickens, *The Personal History of David Copperfield* (London: Bradbury and Evans, 1850), 273.

14. Bernard J. Hibbitts, "Coming to Our Senses: Communication and Legal Expression in Performance Cultures," *Emory Law Journal* 4 (1992): 874–959.

15. The statute still allowed for nuncupative (i.e., orally given) wills to be made in certain exceptional circumstances such as soldiers engaged on expedition or the field of battle and sailors at sea.

16. Edward Burnett Tylor, *Early Researches into the History of Mankind and the Development of Civilization* (Boston: Estes & Lauriat, 1878).

17. Francis Wharton et al., *A Treatise on Medical Jurisprudence [Electronic Resource]*, 2nd rev. ed. (Philadelphia: Kay & Bros., 1860), 7.

18. Sir Edward Vaughan Williams, *A Treatise on the Law of Executors and Administrators*, 7th ed., by Sir Edward Vaughan Williams and Walter V. Vaughan Williams; 6th American ed., in which the subject of wills is particularly discussed and enlarged upon, by J. C. Perkins (Philadelphia: Kay & Bro., 1877), 21–22.

19. Christopher Stone and Bencie Woll, "Dumb O Jenny and Others: Deaf People, Interpreters, and the London Courts in the Eighteenth and Nineteenth Centuries," *Sign Language Studies* 8, no. 3 (2008): 226–40.

20. An example of this is represented in the treatment given by Maudsley with separate chapters dedicated to general insanity, partial affective insanity, partial intellectual insanity, and senile dementia. Henry Maudsley, *Responsibility in Mental Disease*, 2nd ed. (London: Kenry S. King, 1874).

21. Paula Hellal and Marjorie Perlman Lorch, "The Emergence of the Age Variable in Nineteenth-Century Neurology: Considerations of Recovery Patterns in Acquired Childhood Aphasia," in *Handbook of Clinical Neurology*, ed. S. Finger, F. Boller, and K. L. Tyler (Edinburgh: Elsevier, 2010), 845–52.

22. Peter Bartlett, "Sense and Nonsense: Sensation, Delusion, and the Limitation of Sanity in Nineteenth-Century Law," in *Law and the Senses*, ed. Lionel Bendy and Leo Flynn (London: Pluto Press, 1996), 21–41.

23. James Cowles Prichard, *A Treatise on Insanity and Other Disorders Affecting the Mind* (London: Sherwood, Gilbert, and Piper, 1835), 4.

24. 10 Clark and Finnelly 200 (1843).

25. Bartlett, "Legal Madness in the Nineteenth Century," *Social History of Medicine* 14: 107–31.

26. For discussion, see Peter McCandless, "Dangerous to Themselves and Others: The Victorian Debate over the Prevention of Wrongful Confinement," *Journal of British Studies* 23, no. 1 (1983): 84–104.

27. For example, the Lunacy Regulations Act of 1862.

28. Alfred Swaine Taylor and John James Reese, *A Manual of Medical Jurisprudence* (Philadelphia: H. C. Lea's Son, 1880).

29. 6 Moore's Privy Council Cases 341, 356.

30. Alfred Swaine Taylor and Edward Hartshorne, *Medical Jurisprudence* (Philadelphia: Blanchard & Lea, 1856), 640.

31. Jacyna, "Somatic Theories of Mind."

32. 5 Queen's Bench, 549.

33. Taylor and Reese, *Manual of Medical Jurisprudence*, 565.

34. Ibid.

35. J. P. Bramwell, "Case of Traumatic Aphasia: Recorded by the Patient with Remarks by J. P. Bramwell, M.D.," *British Medical Journal* 2, nos. 180–81 (1867): 180.

36. Ibid., 180–81.

37. Ibid., 181.

38. "Court of Probate and Divorce, Feb. 26," *Times*, February 27, 1868. The case was Peacock and Another v. Lowe and Others.

39. "Court of Probate and Divorce, Feb 27," *Times*, February 28, 1868.

40. Ibid.

41. "Court of Probate, Feb. 29," *Times*, March 2, 1868.

42. This case is also discussed in Maudsley, *Responsibility in Mental Disease*, 267.

43. Henry Charlton Bastian, "On the Various Forms of Loss of Speech in Cerebral Disease," *British and Foreign Medico-chirurgical Review* 43 (1869): 218.

44. Ibid., 470.

45. "Court of Probate, March 31," *Times*, April 1, 1873.

46. Boughton v. Knight and Others, LR 3 P & D 64 (1873).

47. William T. Gairdner, "Report of a Case of Aphasia," *British Medical Journal* 1 (1875): 568.

48. Maudsley, *Responsibility in Mental Disease*, 265.

49. Ibid., 266.

50. Anonymous, "The Jurisprudence of Aphasia," *British Medical Journal* 2 (1877): 386.

51. William O'Neill, "A Case of Aphasia," *British Medical Journal* 2 (1877): 476.

52. John Hughlings Jackson, "On Affections of Speech from Disease of the Brain," *Brain* 1, no. 3 (1878): 314.

53. Anonymous, "The Pathology of Speech," *British Medical Journal* 2 (1879): 379.

54. John Syer Bristowe, "The Lumleian Lectures on the Pathological Relations of the Voice and Speech," *British Medical Journal* 1 (1879): 733.

55. Bartlett, "Legal Madness in the Nineteenth Century," 129.

56. Bateman, *On Apasia*, 301–2.

57. Ibid., 301.

58. Ibid.

59. A. Ferguson et al., "Testamentary Capacity and Aphasia: A Descriptive Case Report with Implications for Clinical Practice," *Aphasiology* 17, no. 10 (2003): 967.

60. Extensive searching through the research literature on aphasia from the past fifty years has identified only one other treatment of this topic. Pamela Enderby, "The Testamentary Capacity of Dysphasic Patients," *Medico-legal Journal* 62 (1994): 70–80.

Chapter Four

The Spouse, the Neurological Patient, and Doctors

Katrina Gatley

Introduction

The period spanning the late nineteenth and early twentieth centuries might be described as the age of the "specialist patient," if only in response to the emergence of institutions and specialist doctors that required such bodies. In the case of nervous disorders, the Great War aided and abetted this development.[1] The neurological patient of this paper—the Anglophile Frenchman Jacques Raverat (1885–1925)—and his illness narrative are also intertwined with the Great War. It was his failed attempt to enlist in the armed forces that precipitated his diagnosis by a specialist in nervous diseases of a central nervous system disease known as disseminated sclerosis.[2] Patients such as Jacques, and those that returned from the war with head injuries and shell shock, were, like many with chronic or debilitating conditions, cared for in their homes, not hospitals. They were attended by family members and not by qualified specialist doctors and nurses. Caregivers were frequently spouses such as Gwen Raverat (1885–1957), whose chosen career was wood engraving, not caregiving. Malcolm Salaman, a well-regarded art scholar and critic, considered her "the most gifted and original artist using the medium creatively."[3]

These caregivers and modes of informal care often are absent from the literature of the history of medicine because, in the face of the welfare state, their provision was thought to have been dwarfed and subsumed by the political state. Their role was overlooked or, at most, considered through the prism of their absorption into formal systems of care.[4] In the Western world, the late nineteenth to early twentieth century might be described as a period that saw the dissolution of informal care; its final blow was the introduction of the United Kingdom National Health Service. Feminist historians in the 1980s have, however, argued that "despite its place in all of our lives, caregiving receives little social recognition, [as] the dominant culture . . . trivialises most unpaid work done by women in the home."[5]

Jane Lewis claimed, "There is little evidence that informal care by families decreased after the Second World War in Britain." Her view is that informal family caregivers, as agents of health or providers of health care, have been ever present throughout the twentieth century.[6] In *Hearts of Wisdom*, Emily Abel uncovered the history of home care for an earlier period, 1850–1940. She demonstrated that when a traditional American female role—caring for sick and debilitated family members—intersected with an emerging and expanding medical and health profession, these untrained yet "empathically knowledgeable" caregivers did not vanish despite the derision of their caregiving by an increasingly authoritative medical profession. She argued that their role altered, albeit unevenly across ethnic and class lines, and that while spending less time as "hands-on carers," female caregivers continued to and insisted on acting as their ill family member's health and illness advocate.[7] This transition of role may explain why for the latter half of the twentieth century medical and social histories of multiple sclerosis (MS) have featured family and spouses of the ill as lay activists and outward-looking political bodies, not care providers in domestic settings.[8] Moreover, histories of informal care related to MS in the first part of the century total pages rather than papers or chapters.

This chapter is concerned with the first quarter of the twentieth century. Its focus is the caregiver and care receiver rather than the neurologists with whom they interacted. Primary sources from caregiver-spouses (i.e., those who gave and managed the care of their spouses with MS at home) are uncommon, especially in the first half of the century. Nonetheless the Gwendolen Raverat (née Darwin) archive at Cambridge University Library is a rich resource that encompasses the majority of her life and all of her married life.[9] Gwen was a granddaughter of Charles Darwin, the daughter of George Darwin and the well-connected American Maud De Puy. Additionally, this archive includes her husband's letters, allowing an exploration of receiving care as well as caregiving. It also includes letters sent to the Raverats by their doctor friends Oliver Gotch (1889–1973?) and Geoffrey Keynes (1887–1982).

Oliver Gotch was the eldest child of Francis Gotch, professor of physiology at Oxford, and Rosamund Horsley, the sister of Sir Victor Horsley, with whom Francis worked. Oliver Gotch and Jacques Raverat met as pupils at Bedales, an English public school that overlooked the Sussex Downs.

Jacques' haute bourgeois parents, Georges and Helena, who owned a second-generation family construction firm (which had built Le Havre port), sent their thirteen-year-old-son across the channel to school in England for two reasons. First, the local Le Havre lycée did not seem to suit Jacques. At the age of twelve his health had collapsed and he spent a year away from school. Second, Georges had learned about Bedales from an acquaintance, Edmond de Molins, who had sent his son there.[10] De Molins considered that the English had been more successful than the French at empire building and trade because of their educational system.[11] Georges wanted to instill such an ethos in his son.[12] This appealed to Georges, as he had extended the family business into overseas rice trade and significantly contributed to the commercial growth of Le Havre (which was officially recognized when he became a *grand maître du port du Havre*).

Geoffrey Keynes met Jacques in 1906, while both were studying at Cambridge University. Geoffrey was reading natural science at Pembroke College and Jacques attended Emmanuel College as an advanced mathematics student. Geoffrey met Gwen much earlier. Throughout their younger years they attended the annual dance for children of Cambridge academics, arranged by Gwen's aunt, Bessie Darwin. Geoffrey was the son of John Neville Keynes, who lectured in economics at the university.

Gwen Raverat was not unique in sharing her home with a debilitated relative. With the return of soldiers from the Great War, many women found that their partners were in sickness rather than in health.[13] Moreover, at this time the actual caring of family members was considered to fall within women's domestic remit of work and duty.[14] Even with the increasing number of hospitals and people trained in the care of the ill, access to those institutions and their personnel came at a cost, financial, social, and emotional. Gwen was unusual in that she was a relatively wealthy woman who was independent and could afford to hire help in the home—and so she did not have to consider the perils of hospitalization for Jacques. Thus Jacques was never a patient of any institution in that sense.

Till Death Do Us Part

When Gwen married Jacques at the South Kensington registry office in June 1911 she was aware of his "adventures," her pseudonym for periods past during which Jacques typically escaped to the English countryside to recover his health. The cause of his problems was not clear. He seemed to have suffered from three or four episodes of nervous collapse. His friend Keynes, then a trainee surgeon, observed one such episode en route to the Swiss Alps in 1907, which he described as "maniacal."[15] Nevertheless, whatever it was, by the time of the wedding, Jacques had been well for a year or two. Furthermore, before the impending marriage, Jacques' father, Georges, had insisted that Jacques revisit the only medical specialist that we know he had consulted, Dr. John Milne Bramwell, to seek assurances that his son's tendency to nervous weakness was behind him. Jacques' adventures were if anything thought to be functional, and Bramwell, a well-reputed physician with a speciality in hypnosis, had taken Jacques through a course of suggestion therapy. Gwen felt she was to marry a wonderful man, "with guts and [who was] awfully clever," and was not concerned about his health.[16] Her father, in asking a Parisian friend if he could ascertain a little of the family by way of introduction, wrote, "Young Raverat is a man of unusual ability and after taking his *bac[calauréat]* in maths and physics is now devoting himself to art. I don't think he cares at all for 'mondaines' affairs, . . . we both like him very much."[17] Health was not mentioned nor inquired about. Others considered him a rare intellectual match for Rupert Brooke,[18] and that Jacques and Gwen "answer[ed] each other from top to bottom of the piano."[19] They shared a passion for English literature, art, theater, and testing conversation.

Yet six months into her marriage, Gwen wrote to her mother, "It is so difficult to understand his health and his nerves: they puzzle me more and more, I feel awfully stupid in taking care of him."[20] This letter suggests that Jacques' adventures were not entirely a thing of his past and that Gwen, now his wife, accepted without question that it fell to her to look after him, which only served to highlight her self-doubt. Gwen was not just reflecting the uncertainties of a newlywed; she had her reasons to worry. They had abandoned the plan to live in Paris. Even three months of living in London proved too much for his health. The winter saw them take a break in Dorset, a repetition of the strategy that Jacques had used in the past to regain his health. In January 1912 Jacques drew up a spoof document giving Gwen powers of attorney with respect to his health.

> I the undersigned Jacques Pierre Paul Raverat being of very sane in mind [*sic*] hereby declare that being totally incompetent to take care of my own health I resign all power over it to my wise and beloved wife Gwendolen Mary Raverat and that I will hereafter always eat, sleep, drink, smoke, walk, work and contemplate only as she desires.[21]

Even as a spoof document it illuminated a reality: Gwen was already his informal caregiver. Her wedding vow, in sickness and in health, had come into operation. Gwen's letter to her mother suggests that Gwen felt out of her depth, and Jacques may have wished his document to amuse and signify his trust in her or bind her into caring. They were, after all, in it together, and six months into their marriage Gwen's role as primary caregiver was established.

Over the next couple of years Gwen did take to her power of attorney. According to Gwen, it was she who decided, during the autumn of 1912, that Jacques should not do heavy labor because she linked his exertions with worsening leg spasms. In the spring of 1914 she wrote crossly to her mother, "I really believe the less he does walk the better. . . . I only write this because I don't believe you have ever understood how ill he is."[22]

Gwen's frustration with her mother stemmed from Darwin family life. Gwen and her mother were not naïve about illness. Gwen thought her family nurtured a cult of illness. She found the "attitude of the whole Darwin family to sickness . . . most unwholesome. At Down, [her grandparents' home], ill health was considered normal."[23] She and her mother concurred in this opinion. Gwen was as dismissive as her mother of pampering when she thought it beyond the requirements of the sickness and especially if she felt it was not a proper sickness. Familiarity with illness left Gwen and her mother rather impervious to anything that was not current or proper.[24] Gwen suspected her mother was casting Jacques in the same light as not really or properly ill—and without an attached disease label of any ilk, her mother, Maud, might have claimed a certain justification. Gwen said this was unfair—on Jacques and her.

The Implications of a Diagnosis

When it came, Jacques' diagnosis was useful to Gwen, especially because it came from the neurological branch of medicine, which concerned itself with functional and organic nervous disorders. In giving Jacques his diagnosis, the neurologist J. S. Risien Russell set out Jacques's situation as a neurological patient. Jacques recounted the event to his father:

> Regarding the doctors, I have not only seen the hypnotist that I've told you about but also an (orthodox) neurologist, the best known in London, the renown [sic] Risien Russell. For 3 guineas (!) (what Jews doctors are). He made my diagnosis with a remarkable certainty. He said that without any doubt I have disseminated sclerosis, that is to say not a continuous but a dispersed thickening of the spinal tissue. The thickening is caused by a poisoning of the nervous tissue and is definitely not caused by syphilis, that's all he could say about it. At the moment there are no signs that this organic disease is worsening. The treatment he suggested is as follows: 1) Suggestion for several weeks to try to help combat the functional problems that are associated with the organic disease. 2) Then (after another 3 guineas consultation with him) a physical treatment, a series of injections to try to tone the nervous tissue. He said that my condition [symptoms] might much improve but that the underlying disease will always be there. . . . I am a little disappointed because I had really hoped that there would not be an organic cause for my problems; but then . . .
>
> Love to Mathilde
> Jacques[25]

This diagnosis gave Gwen evidence to use against the likes of her mother. Gwen evoked medical authority in her indignant letters to her mother. She insisted "the doctors all say that every time he has a bout of illness—every time he gets exhausted mentally and physically—he loses a certain amount which he does <u>not</u> regain—ever."[26] It also put paid to any suspicion that

Jacques had evaded enlistment. During the war years, Gwen and Jacques were caught up in the wave of patriotic sentiment, and both were sensitive to the accusation of not contributing. Gwen did not really expect Jacques to pass a military medical, but with this diagnosis in hand, he and Gwen were exonerated.[27] Jacques and Gwen did not, like their Bloomsbury group of friends, fret over the wrongness of the war, and did not want Jacques to be thought of as avoiding service by obtaining a functional diagnosis, a tactic that they considered Leonard Woolf had deployed.[28]

The division of Jacques' illness into two parts, organic and functional, was significant. First, it squashed the idea that Jacques primarily had a functional disorder—an idea that had been discussed, even if Keynes was not convinced. Keynes felt a purely functional explanation of Jacques' illness did not sufficiently encompass his symptoms. "I must have expressed this puzzlement to you I think; anyway I know I have to one or two other people," wrote Keynes on hearing of Risen Russell's more compelling diagnosis.[29] Clearly there had been talk of Jacques possibly having a nervous disorder, but there appears not to have been, up until this point, any formal diagnosis of functional disorder, more a suspicion.

From this time on Gwen no longer used the term "adventures" to describe Jacques' condition. The diagnosis led Gwen to modify her understanding of Jacques' illness, particularly its division into two categories. In casting Jacques' functional problems as associated with his organic disease, Risien Russell rendered the organic disease the primary cause of his functional problems. Gwen assimilated this separation and the implied hierarchy and used it to defend Jacques' behavior over the coming years, albeit in subtly different ways. As already noted, Gwen had, prior to their marriage, used the term "adventures," not "holiday" or "*remise en forme*" or anything that suggested a slowing down, hiding away, or health-promoting regime. Her term, "adventure," suggested an exciting, interesting, possibly hazardous incident that required one to live by one's wits. Perhaps Gwen did think his trips into the English countryside were dangerous and challenging, but Jacques' letters from these trips away were filled with his accounts of hours spent walking, alone, and appreciating the unspoiled beauty and tranquility of his rural surroundings. After the diagnosis, Gwen recast these trips; now they were necessary breaks from people and especially cities to rural idylls. They stayed frequently in the homes of friends and family while their owners were away.[30] These were places and times of sanctuary, not adventure. Gwen changed her representation of Jacques' use of and need for the countryside in line with her adapted view of her husband and his medical diagnosis and prognosis. Rest replaced adventure.

Gwen also began to acknowledge the separate yet dual aspect of his illness. She began to describe his health more explicitly. "He's a good bit better than he was, mentally & nervously & in his arms, but his legs are still very wobbly"[31] displaced earlier less specific and amorphous references, such as to "his nerves."[32] Gwen was not alone in reframing her view of her husband's illness. Keynes wholeheartedly applauded Risien Russell's diagnosis and treatment plan.[33] Keynes's endorsement could only have added to the Raverats' good impression of Risien Russell and his medical ideas.

In 1899 Risien Russell had set out his thoughts concerning the disease in the chapter "Disseminate Sclerosis" in *A System of Medicine*. He thought the cause of MS was "shrouded in great obscurity" and did not favor any one of the prevailing etiological theories.[34] Risien Russell's explanation to Jacques that his disease was "caused by a poisoning of the nervous tissue and is definitely not caused by syphilis" suggests that, by late 1914, Risien Russell still held that the cause of MS was "some toxic agent."[35] As for prognosis, he had noted "how hazardous it was to express too confident a prognosis," such were the exceptions to a "general rule" that "life is not usually prolonged beyond two or three years after the clinical picture is sufficiently characteristic to leave no doubt as to diagnosis."[36] In 1899, Risien Russell held that treatment "prospects were gloomy in the extreme" and that subcutaneous injection of silver or arsenic might be worth a trial, although he was doubtful if this mode had any advantages over oral administration.[37] In the intervening years Risien Russell had changed his therapeutic stance a little. He offered Jacques a series of injections rather than any oral formulations and advocated suggestion therapy, which was not mentioned in his 1899 treatise, although he did note that "all depressing influences must be removed as far as possible."[38]

Gwen followed the implications of Risien Russell's diagnosis with respect to modes of therapy. Gotch's letter of reply to Gwen, cited in part below, suggests she had written to him using the division of Jacques' symptoms into functional and physical. First he commented on her thoughts about massage, and then he explained why suggestion therapy would also be useful. His helpful letter explained:

> I entirely approve of your suggestion about having his arms gently massaged, and I should certainly start it as soon as possible. There is very good grounds for supposing that a lot of the stiffness of neuritis in his arms is the result of a defective circulation owing to his being unable to take any active exercises. As long as the massage is undertaken with that end in view nothing but good can come of it. It mustn't however tire him. I don't think there is any need to write to Dr Head. Let me know what you settle to do. There is no harm in waiting till [you have] weaned Eliz[abeth] in order to take J[acques]. up to London for suggestion treatment—but I should certainly take him up. . . . I believe that that does him more good almost than anything else. People with nervous disease of any sort who are incapable of leading the life of other people are extraordinarily liable to become irritated and worried—by the common little day to day things of life; . . . and the suggestion treatment course was successful last time wasn't it?[39]

Gotch's reply also illustrated his physical explanation of why massage would be useful, followed by a behavioral explanation of why suggestion therapy would do Jacques more good almost than anything else. Gotch's detailed reply underpinned the double sidedness of Jacques' treatment plan should Gwen have needed it. Gotch also promoted the idea that nervous disease of any sort would by default have a functional aspect, therefore justifying the use of suggestion therapy. In doing so, Gotch endorsed a general principle that divided nervous disorders in two while acknowledging their inherent association. Keynes had also noted that "it is an excellent thing that these folk should at last be trying to dissociate and attack separately the functional and organic elements."[40] Gotch and Keynes underpinned Risien Russell's authority in particular, and neurologists ("these folks") in general, with their ideas of "attacking separately the functional and organic elements of disseminated sclerosis." Gwen's doctor friends supported her modified reading of Jacques' illness.

Gwen negotiated Jacques' illness in light of this modified reading. Thus her aim was to ensure "home care and periodic enforced periods of rest" by which she meant physical and mental rest, for by this means she considered that both mental and physical exhaustion were avoided.[41] Each type of excess was understood to harm the other; they were different and yet inextricably linked, and this mantra ruled their lives. The Raverats thought of Jacques as having a finite supply of energy and that he must not outstrip it; he had to limit and ration its use to safeguard his basic level of function.[42] Consequently, Gwen thought of the immediate and midterm management of his health. "He shall have to be careful with his arms," wrote Gwen in the middle of one relapse, before reporting on the current situation, "however rest is making him better & will go on doing so I think."[43] Wherever and whenever Gwen and Jacques thought it was needed, they rallied medical authority to support their attitude. In April 1915, Jacques told André Gide, "I have had a long conversation with one of my doctor friends. He tells me that it is necessary to take precautions and to avoid painstakingly all types of fatigue."[44] It was the use of the word "all" that is significant here. Gide and Jacques had enjoyed each other's mental gymnastics in the past.[45] In this context Gide was being forewarned that physical rest alone was insufficient to avoid aggravating "significantly [Jacques'] illness in a fashion that would be definite and permanent." Similarly, soon after arriving in Vence, in southern France, in 1920, Gwen managed the expectations of others by announcing that she did not think they would often return to England, as "Jacques could not do the journey."[46] At times she delayed others from visiting.[47] But as friends and family came to know Jacques' progressive illness, Gwen's recourse to medical authority became less necessary and less frequent.

More marked, however, than Gwen's dual vision of Jacques' symptoms in formulating her understanding of how best to manage his illness was her use of the functional aspects of Jacques' illness to both explain and seek acceptance, forgiveness even, of Jacques' behavior. Before Jacques' diagnosis friends thought very fondly of him but also acknowledged his periods of misanthropy.[48] He had a prickly personality. Virginia Woolf referred to him as the "Volatile Frog," Jacques' dramatic (and unfavorable) response to Duncan Grant's "Adam and Eve" exhibited at the Alpine Club in early 1914 being a good example.[49] His in-laws, particularly Maud, also found him difficult to accommodate.[50] Even Keynes, while having acknowledged the dual aspects—organic and functional—of his illness, still thought of Jacques' tendency to rages and bleakness as essentially part of the man, and especially the young man. In 1916, nearly two years after Jacques was diagnosed, Keynes wrote: "I hope your tempers are getting better; you will probably mellow with age, and you will find your tempers getting better rather than worse. The fact that you can read Trollope is a sign of it."[51] Furthermore, the war made people in general pretty gloomy. Jacques was not alone.[52]

Jacques' diagnosis lent itself to a different conception of his prickly and not infrequently morose personality. It became a product of his organic disease. Thus when the Marshall family was planning to visit the Raverats in Vence, Gwen apologetically but assertively wrote:

> I am afraid you had better not count on us for your holiday, because J[acques] is much too ill for us to make any plans at all. He hasn't got any better since the beginning of this illness, he only adapted himself to the conditions & now (I think) he's worse. But with all the ups and downs it is very hard to judge which way he is going; only anyhow he's not fit for company. . . . Of course he <u>might</u> be better by Xmas—or worse & it makes everything so unsettled and upside down in the house that its no use my asking you to come to see me much as I should like to see you and The Lady.[53]

Gwen began to see his misanthropy as accompanying a relapse of his physical symptoms,[54] and when it did not, this in itself became noteworthy and a source of puzzlement. "J[acques] has been much happier lately though there doesn't seem any physical reason for it," she noted to Nora.[55] As Jacques became less able, Gwen continued to interpret his state of mind within this framework. In 1924 she implored her cousin Nora Barlow:

> I don't suppose I can make you quite understand about Jacques: but though you perhaps don't see it because he seems so alive on the outside, his spirit is half-dead, as well as his body half numb & all tortured; & built round with a wall between him & all real people.[56]

A month later, while away on a holiday with her daughter in Peira Cava, Gwen reiterated to Nora: "I don't think you <u>any of you</u> have the least idea of the effect of the sort of death-in-life of his illness upon him. He can never be just nor reasonable, nor sane, neither to me nor to anyone else. He can't help it."[57]

Furthermore, in this letter and other letters, Gwen expatiated on additional and consequential themes, not least that his illness had a marked impact upon Gwen herself.[58] Her Peira Cava letter to Nora of five pages continued:

> You [Nora] say something about the bitter unhappiness which has sometimes come between us (meaning J[acques] & me, you & R[uth]. & F[rances]. & K[a].) I want to explain that I believe it is all or very nearly all a sort of reflection of J[acques]' illness. I've been away from him for a fortnight & I begin to see things a little more clearly. I get all warped, inevitably I suppose, when I'm with him. . . . I suppose the appearance of logic & truth makes one doubt but Nora, he's all warped crooked with bitterness & suffering. And when I am with him night & day, night & day I get crooked too. So you must try & forgive us both. He has such an influence—very subtle on me. Sometimes he talks and talks to me & says things, each half true, or with one grain of truth in them, & I listen & believed; and afterwards when I get away, I think that's not the truth; & in fact often, its perfectly absurd, & any outside sane person would say so at once. . . . This sounds as if I wanted to put the blame on him: I don't, I ought to have keep [sic] steady myself. He can't help it. The real difficultly of my life is keeping sane myself & also sharing with him. . . . It's very difficult to keep sane as you get on in life I think. Its no good writing more about this only you & R[uth]. must realise this. His intelligence is untouched, of course.[59]

By this stage Jacques' illness had become the reason for their emotions. It explained his temperament—volatile, irritable, miserable. It explained, she said, her bitterness, as his bitterness had rubbed off on her.[60] In some sense, his illness had pervaded her. All of which her friends, family, and strangers could accept as understandable; and without detracting from their anguish, this attribution of emotions and faults to his organic illness allowed them to ascribe traits that had hitherto been thought of as essentially those of the Cambridge graduate "Jakes," and to blame his disease for them.

Gwen's observation that despite all the bitterness and crookedness, his logic was solid—"his intelligence untouched"—was supported by an expectation, among their medical friends, that the nature of his illness would not attack his intellect. This added credibility to her claim that Jacques was still such an influence over her, an influence that others could also see in her paintings and wood engravings persistently from their early married days.[61]

Living with Jacques—his temperament, his decreasing abilities, yet his insistent and apparent subtle influence, or perhaps manipulation—was not easy. When she described him more as a neurological patient, she said she could accept his unreasonable behavior and pleaded that others should too. When she could not describe him as a neurological patient she contemplated divorce.[62] And that is the point: Gwen, for all her assimilation of medical knowledge and employment of its authority, also saw Jacques as her husband, a man, a forceful intellect, and painter. Neither she nor he made claims that somehow the tragedy or adversity of his illness, in its organic or functional guise, had given rise to his best art.[63] It only cut short his time. It imprisoned him. She wrote to her sister, Margaret Keynes, "I wonder if you can guess how much more wearisome all these little disabilities make things. You wouldn't think, till you've tried, what difference in freedom there is, between being able to walk three steps alone, and not being able to; everything you lose is such a loss of liberty";[64] and a month later, "and it's impossible [for Jacques] to rest more and remain alive."[65]

Shortly after Jacques' death, Gwen too noted how events that might have been considered significant from a neurologist's point of view went by completely unremarked, such was the insignificance of the specialism in practice in their lives. In her letter to Virginia Woolf she wrote:

> The worst was over long ago I think—or perhaps about two years ago was the worst of all. The day I gave all his boots away & knew he would never walk again—ages ago—there ought to have been a hearse & undertakers to take them away, but no one knew of course.[66]

For all of Gwen's assimilation of the medical understanding of a neurological patient, neurologists offered little in the way of treatment and left her, she said, standing alone, with "the worse thing in the world to watch suffering in helpless understanding,"[67] and to conclude that "physical pain [was] awful & degrading, and so hopeless and useless."[68] But these were human losses and emotions not unique to neurological patients, and her husband was not simply and wholly reducible to a neurological entity. To what extent and how Jakes fitted that construction, and how it aided Gwen, was in his final few months of little import. Jacques was dying.

Gwen's visual depictions of Jacques at this time reflected her pain. The ink and pencil sketch (fig. 4.1) was not initialed or signed and is on feint-lined, lightweight writing paper. It is not in an artist's sketchbook. Jacques' head is the entirety of the piece. One can surmise he is lying on his side, although his body is absent and the bedding detail minimal. The directness of the gaze is forceful in this study. The almost complete lack of visible muscular effort perhaps encourages the viewer to be drawn into his gaze. Apart from open eyelids and perhaps a slightly raised eyebrow there is no muscle activity. Jacques appears weary.

Her focus upon his head may also be intended to suggest that although drawn and tired, his mind continued to exist.[69] The lack of physicality in this illustration might suggest the effects of his disease, but equally there is no hint of the body "all tortured" that she had described six months earlier.

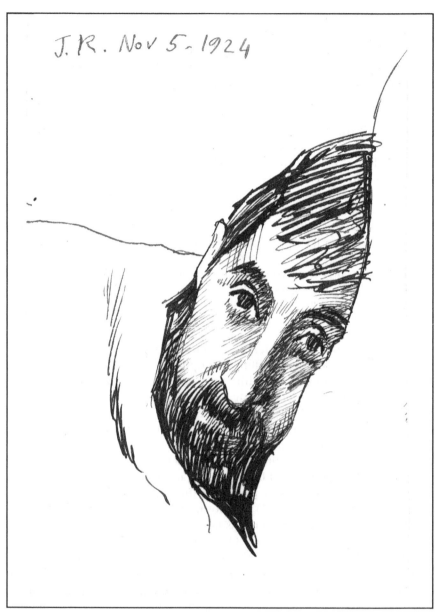

Figure 4.1. "Jacques Raverat (1924-11-05)," by Gwen Raverat, drawing (pen and ink on paper), museum accession number: PD.202-1994. © Estate of Gwen Raverat. All rights reserved, DACS 2010. Reproduced with permission of the Syndics of the Fitzwilliam Museum, Cambridge.

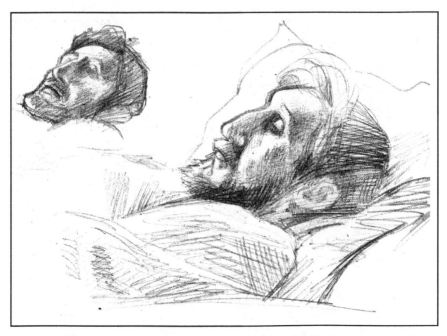

Figure 4.2. Untitled sketch by Gwen Raverat, graphite on off-white paper, Sketch-book 1924, museum accession number: PD.66-1994. © Estate of Gwen Raverat. All rights reserved, DACS 2010. Reproduced with permission of the Syndics of the Fitz-william Museum, Cambridge.

This sketch speaks of stillness rather than muscle tremor or spasm. Gwen sketched this around the time of her hurried return from England to Vence, prompted by the news that Jacques was very unwell with cystitis.[70] She "thought he was going to die," and this may explain why, unusually, she dated the sketch.[71] It was not a sketch of a neurological patient, but rather one of a dying person.

These were sketches in essence that she returned to and reiterated on March 7, 1925.[72] These pencil sketches (fig. 4.2) are less haunting and sparse in their line detail, which suggests that Gwen may have been tired. Others have noted that, unusually, she used "a thick, soft pencil," and that "her summary style betrayed emotional exhaustion."[73] Gwen did these sketches after her final four days of sitting with Jacques day and night, and they do not communicate anything particular to the neurological patient or speak specifically of his disease.

In contrast, Gwen's wood engraving and sketches, which were worked into prints and oil on canvas portraits completed in 1924, were neither of the dying person nor the neurological patient. They were depictions of a man who was not overtly ill. Furthermore these were the images of Jacques

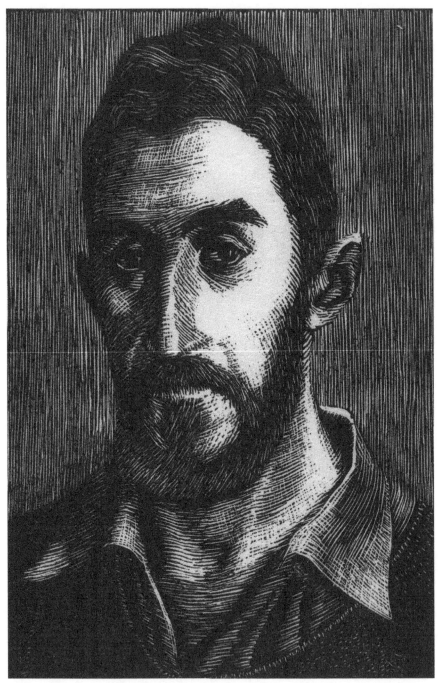

Figure 4.3. "Portrait of Jacques Raverat I (1925)," by Gwen Raverat, print, museum accession number P.585-1974. Reproduced with permission of the Syndics of the Fitzwilliam Museum, Cambridge.

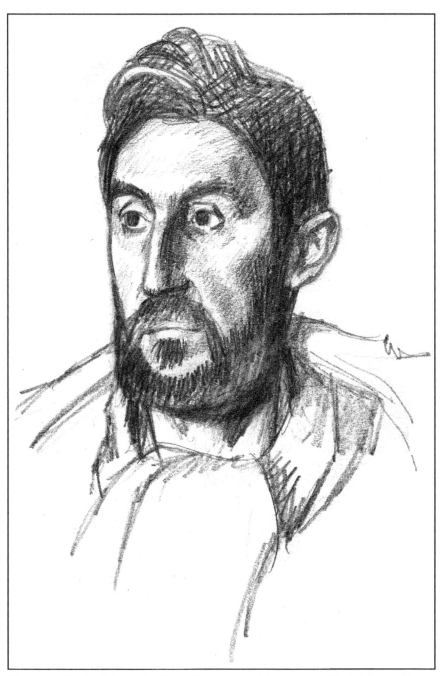

Figure 4.4. Untitled sketch by Gwen Raverat, graphite, pen and black ink on off-white paper, Sketchbook, 1924/25, museum accession number: PD.67-1994. © Estate of Gwen Raverat. All rights reserved, DACS 2010. Reproduced with permission of the Syndics of the Fitzwilliam Museum, Cambridge.

that she selected to distribute by print series and photograph.[74] In the examples shown here (figures 4.3 and 4.4), a print from the wood engraving "Portrait of JR" and an untitled pencil sketch, there is no guide to whether the subject is standing or sitting, but he is upright. He is not particularly ill looking, weakened, or haunted. These portraits do not illustrate pain—his or hers—or his discomfort, his volatile nature, and his decline. The direct gaze in figure 4.3, as opposed to that in the ink and pencil sketch, is inquiring rather than pleading. Perhaps the lack of artifacts—there is not even a suggestion that he was a painter himself—is suggestive of a lack of, or loss of, purposeful endeavor that both Gwen and Jacques recorded.[75] The scarf, shown in figure 4.4, is also potentially symbolic of his need for warmth and protection, yet it also creates a sense of movement in the piece. On balance, there is little in these portraits that speaks of Jacques' illness or disease, functional or organic.

In Gwen's varying images of Jakes during his final year, she chose to highlight the person rather than the disability or disease; the construct of "neurological patient" was not illustrated. Moreover, it was only when she believed he was dying that she showed the ill man in her art.

This perception of her husband's identity was also reflected in her correspondence with Virigina Woolf during Jacques' final years, and significantly for Gwen it was affirmed by Virginia. At the end of 1922 Virginia wrote to Jacques, thanking him for his valued and insightful comments concerning *Jacob's Room*, which Jacques had dictated to Gwen, and she reported to Gwen and Jacques that she had "heard praises of [Jacques'] pictures from Roger Fry the other night. He thinks [Jacques is] now doing the interesting things."[76] It is not known if Roger Fry or Virginia Woolf knew that Jacques created these works with his left hand; the significance for Gwen, however, was that others shared her view that Jacques was (still) creative and intellectually alive. Furthermore, late in 1924 Virginia asked Jacques to review a draft of *Mrs. Dalloway*. His correspondence to her during the intervening two years, via Gwen's hand, had presumably not altered Virginia's view of him as a valued literary critic. This chimed with Gwen's view that he was not destroyed or consumed by his disease. Moreover, Gwen only shared the misery of Jacques' final months with Virginia after he had died.[77]

Conclusion

In Jacques' final days Gwen continued to be his primary caregiver, helped by the team she had assembled over the recent years. Babette Giroux, the woman she had employed as nanny to her children, Jean Marchand, her artist friend, and toward the end an experienced Italian nurse. There had been almost no collision of caregiver-spouse with medical or nursing authority over the course of Jacques' illness. Nurses were not part of the array of support that Gwen sought, until the final six weeks. She managed. Their resorting to neurologists was also infrequent.[78] Once they had the diagnosis and had tried Risien Russell's duo of suggestion therapy and injections to little affect, they sought advice from other neurologists. Both Edgar Adrian and Henry Head consistently advised rest. Nothing else. Despite the Raverats coming to the view that even rest was of limited benefit, and that indeed to rest more and remain alive was becoming an oxymoron, they did not dismiss the advice or turn to other neurologists or specialists. Gwen did not rail against expert opinion. She accepted that "things must just go on as they may."[79] But this was not just a mutual default, a passive standoff between geographically separated patient, caregiver, and specialist. Gwen's acknowledgment of the status quo, deeply disappointing and distressing, was not simply resignation or deferential.

Gwen and Jacques had chosen one of the most reputable neurologists of their day. The couple respected and supported professionalism, with its inherent arcane knowledge, behavioral codes, and general cultural awareness, across all types of activity: Roger Fry as art critic, André Gide and Virginia Woolf as writers, Paul Desjardins as academic, and George Darwin as scientist (latterly geophysicist).

There were clashes only when the medical men they encountered did not match up to the Raverat ideal of professional men. Haydn Brown, the suggestion therapist, seen just after his diagnosis in early 1915, was one such character. Brown's lack of broad knowledge underwhelmed Jacques and he was put off by his boastfulness and vulgarity.[80] He was not sufficiently professional.[81] The local doctor in Vence was similarly not thought by the Raverats to be up to standard. Gwen wrote of an encounter with him, "he wouldn't come till I made him, and then wouldn't look or help and got away as quick as he could. He was frightened and upset I think, but I do think he might have been more use."[82] In another letter she relegated the local doctor to "the man here" denying him his professional title and referred to his words as "vague doctor-jargon."[83] She found his prognostic optimism, as late as January 1925, ridiculous. Gwen was not deferential toward medical men per se.

The medical men they trusted and believed in were the likes of Risien Russell, Edgar Adrian, and Henry Head. As already noted, these were neurologists of very positive repute, and with Adrian and Head they also shared an appreciation of the arts and literature.[84] Given these shared interests, as well as a respect for their chosen professional specialists, it was unlikely that there was going to be a collision of views when it came to Jacques' therapies and care. Moreover, Gwen had two very good friends in Gotch and Keynes, as physician and surgeon (not neurologists) who interpreted, engaged, and supported Gwen in her understanding and care of Jacques in his illness. Furthermore, Keynes was not only a friend of longstanding; they had known each other since childhood and he had married Gwen's younger sister Margaret in 1917.

Thus, despite Gwen's initial uncertainty of her abilities to understand and care for Jacques, Gwen became, to use Abel's term, "empathically knowledgeable," and moreover confident in her care of Jacques. Additionally, in light of her construction of the concept of the "neurological patient," she confidently asserted how others should see him. She took the authority of arcane medical knowledge for her own. From this basis she dismissed doctors she considered not up to the task. She felt little need for ancillary day-to-day medical or nursing assistance. In light of their shared understanding of the duality of Jacques' nervous disease—its organic and functional aspects—she sought out information about therapies and care from her doctor friends. Neither did she hold out hopes for some new treatment that she ought chase after. She accepted "the state of the science" as Jacques called it.[85] This may have in part reflected her scientifically endowed background, not, however, because she simply accepted the authority of science and family. Gwen was an artist, despite her parents' misgivings. She contemplated Catholicism and came to her own view. Gwen's scientifically minded father and forthright American mother endowed her with an attitude, which was to question and inquire. Thus in contrast to Abel's findings in *Hearts of Wisdom*, in which the collision between trained and untrained caregivers frequently led to derision of the untrained by the trained and conflict between the two groups, here it was the medically untrained Gwen who dealt out the derision. But that she did so may also explain, using Abel's argumentation, why Gwen remained Jacques' primary caregiver. Gwen overcame any lack of formal medical training by her diligent deployment of her social status and assimilation of specialist medical knowledge.

Moreover, although she could have afforded to choose differently, Gwen chose to be his hands-on caregiver. Like the women in Abel's studies of the late nineteenth to early twentieth century, Gwen was expected to (and Jacques wanted her to) be his primary caregiver, with him day-in, day-out. For whatever reasons she undertook this duty, despite her physical and emotional exhaustion and the fact that it took her away from her children and wood engraving.

Furthermore, like the women in the later period of Abel's study, Gwen was also Jacques' advocate. She explored therapy options with her doctor friends based on her understanding of his medical condition, and she constructed an interpretation of Jacques' at times testing behavior, which she promulgated to their friends and family. This advocacy also served their marriage. As his illness progressed she became the interlocutor in the doctor-patient relationships, indeed nearly all his relationships. All his letters came via her pen, but she did not become his voice—she represented it, conveyed it—she did not silence him, and in that she truly was his advocate. Throughout, she juggled her accounts of Jacques as neurological patient and of him as her husband. But she used the representation of the neurological patient less frequently as his illness progressed. The construct had served her purpose. Her final act for him was one that spoke of her advocacy, her care and compassion, her autonomy, and of him as her husband. She suffocated him.[86]

Gwen was not a passive bystander, simply enacting instructions from the professionally qualified. The degree of her influence was contingent upon her social standing and was variable with the status of Jacques' health. That Gwen had doctor friends and the skills to engage with medical specialists, and particularly those with shared cultural interests, was key to her role as caregiver and advocate and the influence she carried in those roles. Whether, more generally, this influence would be significantly different if it were the women who were unwell or the men who were the informal caregivers cannot be judged. The issue of gender in influencing, deciding, and delivering the home care and medical care needs of ill spouses in this period, should the archives exist, is worthy of exploration. This question is all the more of interest given that in the United Kingdom, it was Richard Cave—whose wife, Mary, suffered from MS—who established the MS Society in Great Britain and Northern Ireland in 1953, a charity devoted to the amelioration of welfare for those with MS and the sponsorship of research.

Malcolm Nicolson and George W. Lowis have studied the MS Society as a locus for the interaction between neurologists and the laity.[87] Gwen's interaction and experience of MS predates the social tensions that Nicolson and Lowis argue gave rise to the controversies that dogged the early decades of the MS Society. Conflicts that arose as lay members collectively challenged the authority and hierarchical dominance that the medical profession had been ascribed at the Society.

Gwen's experience also predated what Nicolson and Lowis identified as "structural causes of tension between lay person and profession found in modern medicine and health care."[88] Like those with MS in the 1950s, orthodox medicine dominated Gwen's experience of medicine. However, Gwen and her family were not, according to their correspondence, given to hope in claims for cures that were just around the research corner by Risien Russell, Adrian, and Head, as noted by Nicolson and Lowis of later neurologists. Thus Gwen is set apart on two counts from many of the early lay members of the MS Society and their discontentment with the profession. First, she occupied the same social, economic, and intellectual space as the medical profession of her day. Second, the profession, at least those consulted by Gwen and Jacques, did not engender the undeliverable and contradictory expectations that Nicolson and Lowis relate, and that rose to a lay questioning of the authority of medical men and medicine itself.

Yet, as has been noted, Gwen's respect for the authority of medical men was undermined when they failed to meet her expectations of professional behavior. It would appear that failure by the medical profession to meet patient or spouse expectations, albeit different expectations in different epochs, nonetheless resulted in a questioning of medical authority. But Gwen was not, as argued by Nicolson and Lowis for the later period, part of a collective that questioned the dominance of orthodox medicine, or the changing place of the chronically ill and their carers in British society. Gwen's collision was with doctors who failed to come up to her standards, not with neurology or medicine itself.

It could be argued that Gwen was more akin to the policy-making and executive hierarchies at the MS Society in its early years than to the ordinary lay membership. Richard Cave upheld and promoted an organization that "derived much of its character from taken-for-granted patterns of authority and deference"; its sponsors were drawn from the titled and its executive from the higher ranks of British society.[89] Cave attracted these types of people to the Society, aided by his employment in the House of Lords. It is not known, however, if in her later years Gwen took an interest in or contributed to the nascent MS Society. Her name does not appear in the Society's archives held at the Wellcome Library for the History of Medicine, London, or early editions of *MS News*, a regular publication for members of the charity.

It may also be suggested that Gwen had much in common with Cave. Both were of the British establishment. She was bound by a sense of duty to be her husband's primary caregiver, and he was duty bound to acquiesce to medical advisors within the context of the MS Society. But Gwen did not share Cave's devout Roman Catholicism, nor did she share the deference that Nicolson has ascribed to Cave. Significantly, Gwen's experience of caring for her husband preceded World War II, which precipitated major changes in British society and gave rise to a new hope, belief even, that science would deliver new treatments and a cure for MS and many other diseases. In different social climates, however, both individuals, as spouses of MS sufferers, used the social status and connections they possessed and their intellectual skills to engage with the medical knowledge of their era and act as committed advocates for their partners.

Notes

This study is heavily dependent on the Gwen Raverat papers in the Cambridge University Library. I wish to thank Godfrey Waller in the Department of Manuscripts and University Archives at the library for his learned assistance as I explored the collections. I am grateful also to Marit Gruijs and Emma Darbyshire at the Fitzwilliam Museum for their guidance in the reproduction of the images used within this text. Stephen Jacyna and Stephen Gatley read earlier versions of the paper and offered many useful criticisms, as did the attendees at "The Neurological Patient" workshop held at the Wellcome Trust Centre for the History of Medicine at University College London.

1. See Stephen T. Casper, "The Idioms of Practice: British Neurology, 1880–1960" (PhD diss., University College London, 2007), for the development of neurology and its practices; Janet Oppenheim, *Shattered Nerves: Doctors, Patients, and Depression in Victorian England* (Oxford: Oxford University Press, 1991), for a historical review of the meanings of nervous disorders; Mark S. Micale, "Jean-Martin Charcot and *les névroses traumatiques*: From Medicine and Culture in French Trauma Theory of the Late Nineteenth Century," in *Traumatic Pasts: History, Psychiatry, and Trauma in the Modern Age, 1870–1930*, ed. Mark S. Micale and Paul Lerner (Cambridge: Cambridge University Press, 2001), 115–39; and Mark S. Micale, "The Psychiatric Body," in *Companion to Medicine in the Twentieth Century*, ed. Roger Cooter and John Pickstone (London: Routledge, 2003), 323–46, for his consideration of the emergence of psychiatry at the turn of the twentieth century, and particularly the emergence of shell shock during the Great War and its treatment in institutional settings. See also Peter Leese, *Shell Shock: Traumatic Neurosis and the British Soldiers of the First World War* (Basingstoke: Palgrave Macmillan, 2002); and Ben Shephard, *A War of Nerves: Soldiers and Psychiatrists, 1914–1994* (London: Pimlico, 2002). For a much broader reading the relationships between emergent medical practices and the Great War, see *Medicine and Modern Warfare*, ed. Roger Cooter, Mark Harrison, and Steve Sturdy (Amsterdam: Rodopi, 1999).

2. Disseminated sclerosis, or multiple sclerosis (MS, as it has been termed since the 1950s), was and still is a disease claimed by neurologists. It is a disorder that is typically characterized by two or more lesions separated in both space and time in the central nervous system. It is a chronic condition in which multiple and variable symptoms wax and wane, making for an unpredictable prognosis of disability development. It generally occurs in early adulthood. It is a disease whose precise cause is unknown and there is no recognized cure.

3. Joanna Selborne and Lindsay Newman, *Gwen Raverat, Wood Engraver* (London: British Library; New Castle, DE: Oak Knoll Press, 2003), 14.

4. Charles E. Rosenberg, *The Care of Strangers: The Rise of America's Hospital System* (New York: Basic, 1987); *The Cultures of Caregiving: Conflict and Common Ground Among Families, Health Professionals, and Policy Makers*, ed. Carol Levine and Thomas H. Murray (Baltimore: John Hopkins University Press, 2004); Shelia Rothman, "Family Caregiving in New England: Nineteenth-Century Community Gives Way to Twentieth-Century Institutions," in Levine, *The Cultures of Caregiving*, 57–69. Anne Summers, "Hidden From History?: The Home Care of the Sick in the Nineteenth Century," *History of Nursing Society Journal* 4, no. 5 (1993): 227–43; and Joanna Bourke, "Effeminacy, Ethnicity, and the End of Trauma: The Sufferings of 'Shell-Shocked' Men in Great Britain and Ireland, 1914–1939," *Journal of Contemporary History* 35, no. 1 (2000): 57–69.

5. Emily K. Abel, *Hearts of Wisdom: American Women Caring for Kin, 1850–1940* (Cambridge: Harvard University Press, 2000), 2.

6. Jane Lewis, "Agents of Health Care: The Relationship between Family, Professionals, and the State in the Mixed Economy of Welfare in Twentieth-Century Britain," in *Coping With Sickness*, ed. J. Woodward and R. Jutte (Sheffield: European Association for the History of Medicine and Health, 1995), 163.

7. Abel, *Hearts of Wisdom*, 2.

8. Colin L. Talley, *A History of Multiple Sclerosis and Medicine in the United States, 1870–1960* (PhD diss., University of California, San Francisco, 1998); Jock T. Murray,

Multiple Sclerosis: The History of a Disease (New York: Demos Medical, 2004); Richard M. Swiderski, *Multiple Sclerosis Through History and Human Life* (Jefferson, NC: McFarland, 1998); and Colin L. Talley, *A History of Multiple Sclerosis* (Westport, CT: Praeger, 2008).

9. The Gwendolen Raverat (née Darwin) archive is held in the Department of Manuscripts and University Archives, Cambridge University Library, Cambridge. Letters cited from this archive carry the reference abbreviation CUL, with acknowledgment to the Syndics of the Cambridge University Library.

10. Jacques recorded his name as de Molins, although more commonly it is found as Demolins. Edmond Demolins (1852–1907) had made a study of the English public school system and published *A quoi tient la supériorité des Anglo-Saxons?* (1898) and *L'éducation nouvelle: L'école des Roches* (1903).

11. For details about Badley, the founder head master of Bedales, and his educational ethos, see John H. Badley, "Bedales School, Petersfield, England," *Elementary School Teacher* 5, no. 5 (1905): 257–66; and "Mr. J. H. Badley, Founder of Bedales," *Times* (Obituaries), March 7, 1967, 12.

12. Georges Pierre (1860–1938), and Helena Lorena Caron (18?–1906) married in 1884. Georges's father established Goyard and Raverat in 1870, after more than two decades working with his uncle-in-law, François Garnier, who had been the head of the public works department in Le Havre. Georges oversaw the fabrication business but focused upon wider maritime and commercial interests, in particular rice trading in the colonies. Helena bought a number of substantial properties to the marriage. For an account of Georges Raverat's role in developing Le Havre, see Claude Malon, *Le Havre colonial de 1880–1960* (Caen: Presses Universitaires de Caen, 2006), 25–29.

13. Estimates vary between 1.6 and 2 million for the number of British soldiers wounded in the Great War. See Joanna Bourke, "Wartime," in *Companion to Medicine in the Twentieth Century*, ed. Roger Cooter and John Pickstone (London: Routledge, 2000), 589–600. In Britain in 1920 there were 1,356 hospital places for neurotic ex-servicemen and 63,296 pension holders who were so labeled. See Leese, *Shell Shock*, 124.

14. Emily K. Abel, "Family Caregiving in the Nineteenth Century: Emily Hawley Gillespie and Sarah Gillespie, 1858–1888," *Bulletin of the History of Medicine* 68, no. 4 (1994): 576.

15. Geoffrey Keynes, *Gates of Memory* (Oxford: Oxford University Press, 1981), 87.

16. Gwen Darwin to Ruth & Nora, August 16, 1911, Gwen Raverat Archive (GRA), Add.MS.8904.1, 5372, CUL. Ruth and Nora were Gwen's first cousins.

17. George Darwin to Baron d'Estournelles de Constant de Rebecque, Newnham Grange, March 2, 1911, GRA, Add.MS.9209.1, 409, CUL. In this letter, Darwin uses the word "mondaines" to mean fashionable society.

18. Keynes, *Gates of Memory*, 87.

19. Christopher Hassall, *Rupert Brooke: A Biography* (London: Faber & Faber, 1964), 234.

20. Gwen Raverat to Lady Darwin, n.d. [January/February 1912], Lady Darwin's "Biography of Gwendolen Darwin," Unpublished Manuscripts, CUL.

21. Jacques Raverat, untitled manuscript, January 12, 1912, Sophie Gurney (née Raverat), cited by Frances Spalding, *Gwen Raverat: Friends, Family, and Affections* (London: The Harvill Press, 2001), 193.

22. Gwen Raverat to Lady Darwin, n.d. [spring 1914], Lady Darwin's "Biography of Gwendolen Darwin," Unpublished Manuscripts, CUL.

23. Gwen Raverat, *Period Piece*, 4th ed. (London: Faber & Faber, 1952), 122.

24. Gwen used both the words "real" and "proper" as adjectives for mostly physical illness and less so for nervous illness, although in both situations it was applied to aliments that they considered of a minor nature. See Gwen Raverat, "Aunt Etty," in *Period Piece*, 119–38, and Gwen Raverat to Nora Barlow [née Darwin], January 23, 1919, GRA, Add.MS.8904.1, 5311(61), CUL.

25. Jacques Raverat to Georges Raverat, January 3, 1915, GRA, Add.MS.9209.1, 1426, CUL. Mathilde was Georges' second wife.

26. Gwen Raverat to Lady Darwin, n.d. [summer 1915], Lady Darwin's "Biography of Gwendolen Darwin," Unpublished Manuscripts, CUL.

27. Gwen Raverat to Frances Cornford [née Darwin], n.d. [August 1914], Add.58398, vol. 26, Darwin and Cornford Papers, British Library, London.

28. Gwen Raverat to Nora Barlow [née] Darwin, January 23, 1919, GRA, Add. MS.8904.1, 5311(61), CUL; and Jacques Raverat to Virginia Woolf, n.d. [May 4, 1923], The Monks House Papers, University of Sussex.

29. Geoffrey Keynes to Jacques Raverat, No.10 Ambulance Train, Expeditionary Force, Boulogne, February 14, 1915, GRA, Add.9209.1, 968, CUL.

30. Gwen Raverat to Nora Barlow, [1918?], GRA, Add.MS.8904.1, 5306, CUL; Gwen Raverat to Nora Barlow, January 23, 1919, GRA, Add.MS.8904.1, 5311(61), CUL; and Nora Barlow to Gwen Raverat, n.d., GRA, Add. MS. 8904.1, 5317, CUL.

31. Gwen Raverat to Lady Darwin, n.d. [summer 1915], CUL; and Gwen Raverat to Nora Barlow, Villa Adèle, Vence, 25.5. [1922?], GRA, Add.MS.8904.1, 5325, CUL.

32. Gwen Raverat to Lady Darwin, n.d. [January/February 1912], Lady Darwin's "Biography of Gwendolen Darwin," CUL.

33. Geoffrey Keynes to Jacques Raverat, No.10 Ambulance Train, Expeditionary Force, Boulogne, February 14, 1915, GRA, Add.9209.1, 968, CUL.

34. J. S. R. Russell, "Disseminate Sclerosis," in *A System of Medicine*, ed. Thomas Clifford Allbutt (London: Macmillan, 1899), 90.

35. Ibid., 89.

36. Ibid., 90.

37. Ibid., 90.

38. Ibid., 91.

39. Olivier Gotch to Gwen Raverat, from MH M23, c/o GPO London, June 10, 1917, GRA, Add.MS.9209.1, 774, CUL.

40. Geoffrey Keynes to Jacques Raverat, No.10 Ambulance Train, Expeditionary Force, Boulogne, February 14, 1915, GRA, Add.MS.9209.1, 968, CUL.

41. Gwen Raverat to Nora Barlow, Villa Adèle, May 25 [1922?], GRA, Add. MS.8904.1, 5325, CUL.

42. Gwen Raverat to Nora Barlow, Villa Adèle, May 25 [1922?], GRA, Add. MS.8904.1, 5325, CUL.

43. Gwen Raverat to Nora Barlow, Vence, Wednesday, April 21 [?], GRA, Add. MS.8904.1, 5321(20), CUL.

44. Jacques Raverat to André Gide, April 2, 1915, Cahiers André Gide 8 (1979), Bibliothèque Doucet, Paris, cited by Spalding, *Gwen Raverat*, 239.

45. André Gide (1869–1951) had met Jacques through a mutual friend of his father's, the former professor of literature at Sèvres, Paul Desjardins. As a child Gide had long periods of illness, and his own father died when he was eleven. The family wealth enabled him to concentrate on writing. His work was first published in 1891, and in 1947 he received the Nobel Prize in Literature. In the 1920s he was chiefly known in avant-garde and literary circles. His writing reflected his personal tensions of discipline, puritanical moralism, religious faith, and sexuality. He had long and lively debates with Jacques in particular about the concept of the devil.

46. Gwen Raverat to Nora Barlow, Villa Adèle, May 25 [1922?], GRA, Add. MS.8904.1, 5325, CUL. The Raverats moved to Vence, southern France, in the late summer of 1920. It was an ambition that they had shared since before the war, and some thought it might help his illness.

47. Gwen Raverat to Tom Marshall, Villa Adèle, Vence, AM, n.d., GRA, Add. MS.9209.1, 1395, CUL.

48. Gwen Raverat to Nora Barlow, January 23, 1919, GRA, Add.MS. 8904.1, 5311(61), CUL.

49. Jacques Raverat to Stanley Spencer, January 20, 1914, Sophie Gurney, cited by Spalding, *Gwen Raverat*, 225.

50. George Darwin to Gwen Raverat, Newnham Grange, December 13, 1911, GRA, Add.MS.9209.1, 513, CUL; and Jacques Raverat to Cosmo Gordon, Newnham Grange, Sunday, GRA, Add.MS.9209.1, 1371, CUL.

51. Geoffrey Keynes to Jacques Raverat, November 4, 1916, GRA, Add.MS.9209.1, 983, CUL.

52. Jacques Raverat to Nora Barlow, [1918?], GRA, Add.MS.8904.1, 5303(29), CUL; Jacques Raverat to Cosmo Gordon, Weston, May 30, 1918, GRA, Add. MS.9209.1, 1373, CUL; and Geoffrey Keynes to Jacques and Gwen Raverat, Le Havre, December 30, 1914, GRA, Add.MS.9209.1, 967, CUL.

53. Gwen Raverat to Tom Marshall, Villa Adèle, Vence, AM, n.d., GRA, Add. MS.9209.1, 1395, CUL.

54. Gwen Raverat to Nora Barlow, Villa Adèle, AM Tuesday, GRA, Add.MS.89904.1, 5323(23), CUL.

55. Gwen Raverat to Nora Barlow, September 18, 1923, GRA, Add.MS.8904.1, 5334(44), CUL.

56. Gwen Raverat to Nora Barlow, April 19, 1924, GRA, Add.MS.8904.1, 5339(42), CUL.

57. Gwen Raverat to Nora Barlow, Peira Cava, July 9 [1924], GRA, Add.MS.8904.1, 5342, CUL.

58. Gwen Raverat to Nora Barlow, April 19, 1924, GRA, Add.MS.8904.1, 5339(42), CUL; Gwen Raverat to Nora Barlow, May 18, 1924, GRA, Add.MS.8904.1, 5340, CUL; Gwen Raverat to Tom Marshall, Villa Adèle, Vence, AM, n.d., GRA, Add.MS.9209.1, 1395, CUL; and Gwen Raverat to Nora Barlow, April [16?], 1921, GRA, Add. MS.8904.1.5322(21), CUL.

59. Gwen Raverat to Nora Barlow, Peira Cava, July 9 [1924], GRA, Add.MS.8904.1, 5342, CUL.

60. Gwen Raverat to Nora Barlow, April [16?], 1921, GRA, Add. MS.8904.1.5322(21), CUL.

61. Lindsay Newman and David A. Steel, *Gwen and Jacques Raverat: Paintings & Wood-Engravings: University of Lancaster Library, 1–23 June 1989*, Exhibition Catalogue, 2nd ed. (Lancaster: University of Lancaster), 16; Selborne, *Gwen Raverat, Wood Engraver*, 27; and John Gould Fletcher, "Woodcuts of Gwendolen Raverat," *Print Collector's Quarterly* 18 (1931): 337.

62. Gwen Raverat to Virginia Woolf, Vence, March 15 [1925], Letters from Virginia Woolf to Jacques and Gwen Raverat, Letter 30, Keynes.D.4.3, CUL; and Jacques Raverat to Gwen Raverat, n.d. [1924], Sophie Gurney, cited by Spalding, *Gwen Raverat*, 303.

63. Jean Marchand did, but Jacques thought he was being unduly kind and Gwen simply thought that Jacques had been late in maturing as an artist.

64. Gwen Raverat to Margaret Keynes, October 26 [1921], GRA, Add.MS.9209.6, 9, CUL.

65. Gwen Raverat to Margaret Keynes, added to Jacques Raverat to Margaret Keynes, November 11, 1919, GRA, Add.MS.9209.6, 9, CUL.

66. Gwen Raverat to Virginia Woolf, Vence, March 15 [1925], Letters from Virginia Woolf to Jacques and Gwen Raverat, Letter 30, Keynes.D.4.3, CUL.

67. Cited by Spalding, *Gwen Raverat*, 293, from a book review by Gwen Raverat at a later unspecified date.

68. Gwen Raverat to Nora Barlow, Vence, Saturday, December 1, 1924, GRA, Add. MS.8904.1, 5344(32), CUL.

69. See Gwen Raverat to Nora Barlow, Peira Cava, July 9 [1924], GRA, Add. MS.8904.1, 5342, CUL; and Jacques Raverat to Virginia Woolf, dictated to Gwen, February 1925, Letters from Virginia Woolf to Jacques and Gwen Raverat, Letter 26, Keynes.D.4.37, CUL.

70. Gwen had decided to visit England in October, following Aunt Etty's heart attack in September 1924.

71. P.S. from Gwen, Jacques Raverat to Virginia Woolf, dictated to Gwen, November 12 [1924], Letters from Virginia Woolf to Jacques and Gwen Raverat, Letter 19, Keynes.D.4.37, CUL.

72. The date of her drawing this untitled sketch (museum accession number: PD.66-1994, Fitzwilliam Museum, Cambridge) comes from the family. Sophie Gurney, telephone conversation with author, June 3, 2009. See also William Pryor, *Virginia Woolf and the Raverats: A Different Sort of Friendship* (Bath: Clear Books, 2003), 158; and Spalding, *Gwen Raverat*, 307.

73. Spalding, *Gwen Raverat*, 307.

74. Gwen Raverat to Virginia Woolf, Villa Adèle, Vence, April 22, 1925, AM, Letters from Virginia Woolf to Jacques and Gwen Raverat, Letter 33, Keynes.D.4.3, CUL. Gwen used her wood engravings to create series of prints. The print of Jacques reproduced above was one of forty. Similar portrait print runs numbered sixty.

75. Jacques Raverat to Virigina Woolf, November 12 [1924], Monks House Papers, Letters, University of Sussex; Gwen Raverat to Nora Barlow, July 9 [1924], GRA, Add. MS.8904.1, 5342, CUL; and Jacques Raverat to Virginia Woolf, dictated to Gwen, [January 1925], Letters from Virginia Woolf to Jacques and Gwen Raverat, Letter 25, Keynes.D.4.37, CUL.

76. Virginia Woolf to Jacques Raverat, Hogarth House, December 10, 1922, Keynes, D.4.37, Letter 2, CUL; and Jacques Raverat to Virginia Woolf, dictated to Gwen, Villa Adèle, Vence, AM, [December 1922], Keynes, D.4.37, Letter 3, CUL.

77. Gwen Raverat to Virginia Woolf, Villa Adèle, Vence, April 22, 1925, AM, Letters from Virginia Woolf to Jacques and Gwen Raverat, Letter 33, Keynes.D.4.3, CUL.

78. Jacques saw Edgar Adrian before he left for France in mid-1920, and wrote to him for help in July 1921. Jacques also wrote to Henry Head periodically: in June 1917, early 1920, August 1921, and in late 1921. Olivier Gotch to Gwen Raverat, from MH M23 c/o GPO London, June 10, 1917, GRA, Add.MS.9209.1, 774, CUL; Jacques Raverat to Tom Marshall, Nouvel Hotel, November 10, 1920, GRA, Add.MS.9209.1, 1384, CUL; Gwen Darwin to Nora Barlow, from Nouvel Hotel, Vence, [n.d.], GRA, Add.MS.8904.1, 5320, CUL; Jacques Raverat to Goldie, Vence, Sunday, August 17, 1921, GRA, Add.MS.9202.1, 1361, CUL; and Jacques Raverat, dictated to Gwen Raverat to Geoffrey Keynes, Nouvel Hotel, Vence, AM, [early 1920], GRA, Add. MS.9209.1, 1374, CUL.

79. Gwen Raverat to Margaret Keynes, added to Jacques Raverat to Margaret Keynes, November 11, 1921, GRA, Add.MS.9209.6, 9, CUL.

80. Frances Cornford to Jacques Raverat, January 16, 1915, GRA, Add.MS.9209.1, 328, CUL.

81. Jacques Raverat to Georges Raverat, GRA, Add.MS.9209.1, 1426, CUL.

82. Gwen Raverat to Margaret Keynes, [March 1925], Villa Adèle, in Pryor, *Virginia Woolf*, 157.

83. Gwen Raverat to Ka Arnold-Forster, n.d. [January 1925], Valerie Arnold-Forster, cited by Spalding, *Gwen Raverat*, 305.

84. See chapters 4 and 5 in L. Stephen Jacyna, *Medicine and Modernism: A Biography of Sir Henry Head* (London: Pickering & Chatto, 2008) for a discussion of Henry Head's artistic interests. Adrian and Jacques shared interests in art, hill walking, and mountaineering.

85. Jacques Raverat to Nora Barlow, Weston, August 16, 1918, GRA, Add. MS.8904.1, 5375, CUL.

86. Shortly after Jacques died Gwen wrote to Virginia Woolf of his last few days, which were a "mad nightmare" that she wished she could forget. Jacques could no longer swallow. Gwen Raverat to Virginia Woolf, Vence, March 15 [1925], Letters from Virginia Woolf to Jacques and Gwen Raverat, Letter 30, Keynes.D.4.37, CUL; See also Spalding, *Gwen Raverat*, 308.

87. Malcolm Nicolson and George W. Lowis, "The Early History of the Multiple Sclerosis Society of Great Britain and Northern Ireland: A Socio-Historical Study of Lay/Practitioner Interaction in the Context of a Medical Charity," *Medical History* 46, no. 2 (2002): 141–74.

88. Ibid., 172.

89. Ibid., 144.

Part Three

Patient Groups Construct the "Neurological Patient"

Chapter Five

Disappearing in Plain Sight

Public Roles of People with Dementia in the Meaning and Politics of Alzheimer's Disease

Jesse F. Ballenger

One of the most striking aspects of the rise of Alzheimer's disease (AD) since the 1970s has been the emergence of people with dementia publicly speaking for themselves about their illness and about the meaning of dementia. Of course, exemplary disease victims have been part of the modern cultural landscape throughout the twentieth century, both reflecting and shaping the development of medicine and the experience of illness.[1] But the nature of AD and other age-associated progressive dementias, which in the dominant trope of the AD advocacy movement destroyed the very selfhood of its victims, for a long time suggested that patients were not in a position to speak for themselves once their condition had been diagnosed. The victims of Alzheimer's disease, it seemed to the general public and even to most AD advocates, were destined ever to be spoken for rather than heard from.

By the end of the 1980s, autobiographical accounts by people diagnosed with AD and related disorders began to appear. By 2008, at least a dozen book-length memoirs by people diagnosed with AD and similar dementias had appeared in English. People with dementia were increasingly playing a visible role in advocacy efforts, including advisory roles and in one instance to the board of directors of the leading AD advocacy organizations; and people with dementia had formed Dementia Advocacy and Support Network International, an independent advocacy organization by and for people with dementia.

This chapter seeks to understand the rising public role of people with dementia and how it has shaped the meaning and politics of AD and related disorders, focusing mainly on the published autobiographical accounts of AD that have appeared in the United States. In part, this development follows a course similar to that of the broader history of disease, disability, and medicine. As with many other disorders, the public role of people with dementia began with explicit support for the goals of the medical research and policy establishment; revelations by prominent people that they have been diagnosed with AD became an important part of the campaign to raise public awareness and money for research. But as with disability more generally, people diagnosed with dementia also came to speak more critically about what they saw as the failures and limitations of mainstream research and policy, as well as about the burden of stigma associated with the disease—stigma that some argued doctors, researchers, care professionals, and policy activists too often exacerbated rather than relieved.

But if the public role of people with dementia has followed broader trends in the historical development of medicine, disease, and disability, their self-advocacy has been more challenging because the losses and limitations dementia does impose are not easily compensated for by adaptive technology or sheer willpower, as has been truer for some physical and mental disabilities. Moreover, in battling stigma and restoring a sense of self, people with dementia have not be able to ground their selfhood in the dominant values of modern culture—independence, self-control, and productivity. Thus the public testimony and activism of people with dementia potentially constitutes a profound challenge to some of the core values and accepted social arrangements of modernity.

Stereotypes and Silence: The Stigmatization of Senility and Aging in Modern American Culture

Prior to the 1970s, various forms of age-associated progressive dementia such as Alzheimer's disease, though recognized for decades in the psychiatric literature as having distinctive pathological and clinical features, were subsumed in most medical thinking and in popular discourse under the broad concept of senility. The concept of senility encompassed virtually the entire spectrum of aging experience, from noticeable but relatively benign lapses in memory to complete dementia—though it was the latter that drove growing cultural anxiety about aging. During this period, articles and books on the individual experience of aging written by aging people were commonplace. Often these books challenged the idea that all old people were or inevitably would develop dementia. Still, prior to the 1980s, no autobiographical account of the dementia experience or public testimony from a person with dementia had appeared.

Age-associated progressive dementia has been recognized in Western medicine since the ancients and has contributed significantly to the ongoing ambivalence about aging in Western societies, as expressed in one of Shakespeare's most quoted passages—the description of old age as "second childishness and mere oblivion, sans teeth, sans eyes, sans taste, sans everything"

(*As You Like It*). But the origins of the particularly intense fear in contemporary society of age-associated progressive dementia should be situated more recently and concretely in broader discourses about the fate of the aging body and mind in industrial society. Aging and dementia emerged as a significant public concern only in the modern era, with the industrial transformation of work and the emergence of a liberal social order.

In the United States, the period from roughly 1870 through the 1920s was a tumultuous one in which middle-class Americans were disturbed by the effects that the increasingly large-scale, impersonal organization of modern society had on traditional ideas about the moral agency of the individual and the individual's place in the community.[2] The problem of aging in a modern society was one source of this anxiety as a heated debate emerged about whether the aging body and mind could possibly keep up with the frenetic pace of change in the industrial workplace. This discourse was heavily gendered; commentators around the turn of the century focused on the problem of whether aging men needed to be removed from the workplace because, it was thought, their decrepit bodies and senile brains were hopelessly unable to keep up with the pace of modern life. Despite the emergence of private pension policy, social security to encourage retirement, and laws against mandatory retirement in most occupations, these issues have never been completely resolved and remains contested down to the present. Nonetheless a stereotype of senility took shape and solidified around the terms of this debate.[3]

A particularly vivid example of the stereotype of senility can be found in the of work of George Miller Beard, the New York neurologist best known by historians for his popularization of the diagnosis of neurasthenia—an ailment that many historians have seen as emblematic of late-nineteenth-century anxiety about the pace of modern industrial society.[4] In *Legal Responsibility in Old Age*, first published in 1874, and later incorporated into his much more popular book, *American Nervousness*, published in 1881, Beard claimed to have analyzed the biographies of 750 prominent individuals from every area of human endeavor to derive what he called the "law of the relation of age to work," which revealed, he claimed, that aging brought about a catastrophic decline in intellectual productivity. Beard concluded that the brain and the mental and moral faculties that depended on it were subject to the same deterioration as the rest of the body, and in fact would normally do so more rapidly.[5]

"Men die as trees die," he argued. "Slowly, and frequently at the top first. As the moral and reasoning faculties are the highest, most complex and most delicate development of human nature, they are the first to show signs of cerebral disease; when they begin to decay in advanced life we are generally safe in predicting that, if neglected, other faculties will sooner or later be impaired. When conscience is gone the constitution may soon follow."[6]

Beard argued that the loss of intellectual power made old men susceptible to a variety of moral failings as well. "One becomes peevish, another
avaricious, another misanthropic, another mean and tyrannical, another
exacting and querulous, another sensual, another cold and cruelly conserva-
tive, another vain and ambitious, and others simply lose their moral enthusiasm, or their moral courage, or their capacity of resisting temptation and
enduring disappointment."[7] Beard thus represented the senile man in a
number of characteristic guises—as miser, tyrant, fool, lecher—all of which
were characterized by the loss of self-control, which of course had become
the fundamental ordering principle of American culture as external authorities were eroded by the rise of liberal capitalism.

The stereotypical representation of the senile man as presented by Beard
remained dominant in medical and popular texts through the 1940s. It can be
clearly seen, for example, in William Osler's infamous "Fixed Period" address,
where he joked that having forfeited their productivity and creativity as they
aged, men over age sixty should be given mandatory retirement, and following a year of ease and reflection at a college established for the purpose, be
given an easy death by chloroform,[8] as well as in more formal medical texts
such as Ignatz Leo Nascher, *Geriatrics*, published in 1914—the first textbook
on the subject published in the United States.[9] And many gerontologists have
argued that it has persisted as a salient image of aging up to today.[10]

Representations of women appeared far less frequently in this discourse
on the fate of old age in modern society. And when women were described,
it was, not surprisingly, centered around domesticity rather than productivity and efficiency. For example, Osler followed up his joke about euthanizing
aging men by noting that "with a woman I would advise an entirely different
plan, since after sixty her influence on her sex may be most helpful, particularly if aided by those charming accessories, a cap and a fichu."[11] Osler did
not need to elaborate in his speech on the salutary influence this charming
old woman would exert, for in listing her props he summoned up one of the
most powerful images of domesticity in that era, a tug on the heartstrings
of young women that would cement their loyalty to hearth and home. This
image of the frail, bespectacled old grandmother, wrapped decorously in
her shawl, sitting by the fireside, absorbed in some old-fashioned devotion
to domesticity such as knitting or embroidery was a call to defend domestic
virtues that were supposedly threatened by the aggressive, competitive individualism of the public world. While the aged man's purported inability to
change with the times was a sign of pathology that marked him as useless,
the same inability in the aged woman was a sign of her virtue and the continued contribution she could make. This notion that women's domesticity
made them somehow less prone to senility persisted in popular and medical
representations of old age at least through the 1950s, though ironically by
the mid-1930s it had been reported in the medical literature that women

were in fact more likely to develop Alzheimer-type dementia than men—a finding that has been replicated many times since then but never satisfactorily explained.[12]

The construction of AD as a separate disease category by Emil Kraepelin, Alois Alzheimer, and their colleagues in the first decade of the twentieth century did not challenge this stereotype of senile decline. AD was defined by Kraepelin and Alzheimer as a presenile dementia occurring before the age of sixty-five. Although the brain pathology and clinical symptoms of AD were identical to that of the much more common senile dementia, to Alzheimer and Kraepelin it seemed to make no sense to call senile dementia a disease, for the pathological processes of old age were understood to be normal, while dementia, occurring at earlier ages even though associated with the same brain pathology, seemed to suggest a disease.[13] The widely held assumption that the deterioration of the body and brain were normal in old age was deeply embedded in medicine and Western culture more broadly; it seems to be the reason that the psychiatric literature maintained the distinction between AD as a rare disorder distinct from senile dementia through the 1970s, despite the fact that researchers were well aware of and puzzled by its apparent similarity to senile dementia from the outset.[14]

The idea that senility was an inevitable part of aging due to the deterioration of the brain was first challenged by professionals concerned with the problems of aging in the mid-1930s. Influence by the ascendancy of psychoanalysis and psychodynamic psychiatry and frustrated by the inability to solve the vexing conceptual problems of the Kraepelinian model of dementia, the relatively small group of psychiatrists writing about dementia developed a model that viewed it as the product of a dialectical interplay between biological, social, and psychological forces. Led by David Rothschild, clinical director of the Worcester State Hospital in Massachusetts, these psychiatrists observed that the correlation between the degree of brain pathology found at autopsy did not correlate perfectly with the degree of dementia observed in life. Some patients who had been labeled normal were found to have fairly high levels of Alzheimer-type brain pathology, and vice versa. Such discrepancies could best be accounted for, they argued, by looking outside of the brain to the psychosocial context of aging.[15]

By the 1940s and 1950s, virtually all American psychiatrists working on senile dementia, including Rothschild himself, who had developed his model on extensive postmortem evidence, stopped investigating brain pathology. Nor did they attempt to delineate various disease entities based on pathological lesions. Instead they folded Alzheimer-type dementia, cerebral arteriosclerosis, and functional mental disorders into a broad concept of senile mental deterioration whose pathological hallmarks were not brain deterioration but rather modern social relations. The locus of senile mental deterioration was no longer the aging brain, but rather a society that through mandatory retirement, social isolation, and the disintegration of traditional family ties stripped the elderly of their role in life. Bereft of any meaningful social role and suffering the effects of intense social stigma, it was not surprising that the elderly began to deteriorate mentally. As Rothschild argued, "in our present social set-up, with its loosening of family ties, unsettled living conditions and fast economic pace, there are many hazards for individuals who are growing old. Many of these persons have not had adequate psychological preparation for their inevitable loss of flexibility, restriction of outlets, and loss of friends or relatives; they are individuals who are facing the prospect of retirement from their life-long activities with few mental assets and perhaps meagre material resources."[16]

Other psychiatrists pushed the turn to the social much further than Rothschild, going so far as to argue that that social pathology should in fact be regarded as the *cause* of brain pathology. Maurice Linden and Douglas Courtney argued, for instance, that "senility as an isolable state is largely a cultural artifact and that senile organic deterioration may be consequent on attitudinal alterations," though the authors acknowledged that this hypothesis was difficult to prove.[17] David C. Wilson was less circumspect. He argued that the link between social pathology and brain deterioration was simply a matter of waiting for laboratory proof to support what was adequately demonstrated by clinical experience—that the "pathology of senility is found not only in the tissues of the body but also in the concepts of the individual and in the attitude of society." Wilson cited the usual evidence of pathological social relations in old age: the break-up of the traditional family, mandatory retirement, and social isolation. "Factors that narrow the individual's life also influence the occurrence of senility," he asserted. "Lonesomeness, lack of responsibility, and a feeling of not being wanted all increase the restricted view of life which in turn leads to restricted blood flow."[18]

Because it brought together cultural anxieties about the isolation, emptiness, and stigma of aging in modern society with the frightening symptoms of dementia, the broad concept of senile mental deterioration gained currency far beyond professional psychiatry. It figured especially in popular and professional discourse that sought to make retirement a meaningful and desirable stage of life by making it financially secure and emotionally satisfying. To the emerging profession of gerontology, the high prevalence of senile mental deterioration, as construed by psychiatrists like Rothschild, was an indictment of society's failure to meet the needs of the elderly. To the gerontologists and geriatricians who were shaping the aging field in post–World War II America, the assumption that physical and mental changes associated with aging rendered older people unfit for full participation in economic and social life no longer seemed acceptable. The aging of the population as a whole made such an attitude appear wasteful and inefficient, hardly the rightful outcome of progress.

Consigning the fastest growing segment of the population to "corner rock-ing chairs, to lifeless rooming houses, and even to mental hospitals" was increasingly seen as a major threat to the future prosperity of the nation.[19] Gerontologists and geriatricians set out quite literally to reverse negative assumptions that had dominated discourse about old age since the late nineteenth century, and in their view had produced much of what had been thought of as the inevitable physical and mental deterioration of senility. In their view, the aged were not so much stigmatized because they were senile, but rather more senile because they were stigmatized.

In the two decades following World War II, social gerontologists focused on developing a system of social support for aging individuals that would keep them from slipping into senility. By the early 1970s, this project had been largely realized, creating the socioeconomic policy framework for what historian Peter Laslett has called "the third age," and others have called the "young old."[20] Aging was made more economically secure through more generous pension and social security benefits, significant legal protections had been won against age discrimination, negative stereotypes in popular and professional discourse were increasingly challenged, and perhaps most important, the elderly themselves organized for effective political advocacy and action on their own behalf. All the problems of old age had not been solved, but older people and their advocates were in a much better position to stake claims.[21]

In this context of rising expectation for aging, the broad concept of senil-ity that conceived of dementia as merely the negative extreme of the same social and biological processes that all older people experienced began to seem less persuasive to a new generation of gerontologists. Psychiatrist and crusading gerontologist Robert Butler, who would become the found-ing director of the National Institute on Aging, made this argument a focal point in his Pulitzer Prize-winning book *Why Survive? Being Old in America* (1975). Butler and other gerontologist argued that virtually all of the physi-cal and mental deterioration commonly attributed to old age was more properly understood as the product of disease processes distinct from aging. Senility in this view was not a medical diagnosis, but rather a wastebasket term applied to any person over sixty with a problem. Worse, it rational-ized the neglect of those problems by assuming that they were inevitable and irreversible. "'Senility' is a popularized layman's term used by doctors and the public alike to categorize the behavior of the old," Butler argued. "Some of what is called senile is the result of brain damage. But anxiety and depression are also frequently lumped within the same category of senility, even though they are treatable and often reversible." Because both doctors and the public found it so "convenient to dismiss all these manifestations by lumping them together under an improper and inaccurate diagnostic label, the elderly often did not receive the benefits of decent diagnosis and treatment."[22] Gerontologists like Butler did not discount the reality of irreversible brain damage, as had an earlier generation of psychiatrists. Rather, they argued that the refusal to distinguish in any systematic way the various physical and mental disease processes from one another and from the process of aging itself was a manifestation of the ageism that kept society from taking the problems of older people seriously.

This reorientation shaped a new generation of clinical neurologists and psychiatrists, neuropathologists and biochemists—all of whom entered the field in the 1960s and 1970s and recast progressive age-associated dementia in old age as a number of disease entities distinct from the aging process (the most prevalent of them being AD).[23] But if laboratory research and biomedical discourse transformed senility into AD, it was the testimony of the people directly affected by it that elevated AD into public consciousness. Working together, interested researchers and family members made AD a funding priority for the federal government—a dread disease whose ravages made a monumental increase in federal funding a moral imperative.[24]

The redefinition of senility as AD and related conditions has been widely seen as de-stigmatizing aging by decoupling normal aging from pathological dementia, notwithstanding the fact that advancing age clearly remained the most salient risk factor. In fact, the impact of this shift was much more complicated. Much more an exercise in shifting stigma than in eliminating it, the AD construct fixed stigma more firmly and devastatingly than ever on people with dementia. If "senility" was an inevitable process of aging, it was also a nebulous process that ranged from mild forgetfulness to drooling idiocy, and the stigma associated with it seemed to be more malleable. AD by contrast seemed terribly concrete and final, its pathology made real by the authoritative technologies of biomedical science.

In the struggle to win federal support, AD advocates portrayed as vividly as possible the ravages of the disease. In testimony before Congress and interviews in the mass media, family members of AD victims recounted in harrowing detail the pain of watching the deterioration of a loved one and the burdens of caregiving, a topic upon which Katrina Gatley's chapter in this volume focuses. A stereotyped AD victim emerged—an empty shell, a zombie, the living remnant of a loved one who had really died years before. People with dementia were now at the very outer limit of stigma, regarded in the discourse on AD as no longer really being persons at all.

The Lost Selfhood and Last
Testaments of Exemplary AD Victims

AD advocates consistently aimed to reinforce two points when they described victims of the disease. First, they asserted that AD was an inexorable, relentless killer that caused intense suffering and anguish for its victims and the family members who cared for them. Second, they wanted to show that this was not simply a matter of going senile, for the disease struck victims in their prime, people who, whatever their age, were active and involved in life. These images obviously instantiated the reconceptualization of senility as Alzheimer's disease—a major killer that required the same level of public awareness and commitment as other dread diseases. The AD campaign described victims as intelligent, vigorous, and active before the disease struck. Most typically, they were at the pinnacle of, or retiring from, successful middle-class careers. If retiring, it was not to a bleak, boring life but to active leisure and involvement with the world. In 1980 testimony before Congress, psychiatrist Carl Eisdorfer complained of a widespread misconception concerning persons that the disease affected: "We have a classic notion of what the disease is, and unfortunately, we have a stereotype. It is—and I hate to be sexist, but because there are more older women than men, it is usually sort of a little old woman who is doddering around, sitting in a geriatric chair, not knowing time, place or person." He argued that "this is not the way we see the disease. We have the disease in one engineer [about sixty-two years old] who still, after two and a half years, shoots golf in the eighties and wins tennis cups."[25]

Although Eisdorfer's opposition between the victim as golf-playing engineer (AD as dread disease and hence a devastating personal and social tragedy) and the doddering old woman (AD as senility and hence less important a problem) suggests the continuation of the tendency to see dementia as essentially a problem of men, or at least an important problem to the degree that it affected men, this was in fact unusual in the discourse of the AD campaign. Women as much as men were clearly described as exemplary victims of the disease. In fact, the famous actress Rita Hayworth was the first real poster child for AD. Hayworth's tragic story appears to have captured perfectly the storyline that AD advocates were trying to tell. Although she rose to superstardom as a young woman in the 1940s on the basis of her erotic appeal and talent as a dancer, she was only in her early fifties and still turning in critically acclaimed film roles when she began to visibly suffer from cognitive deterioration. By the 1960s, Hayworth began to show signs of cognitive decline that would eventually be attributed to AD, and by the 1970s Hayworth's reputation began to be tarnished by reports that she could no longer work effectively because of an inability to remember her lines and that her personal behavior was becoming increasingly erratic. She was not diagnosed with AD until 1980, and throughout the 1970s her deterioration was widely attributed to alcoholism. Her talent and fame, her relatively young age, and the fact that the cause of her decline was overlooked so long perfectly embodied the points that the AD campaign was trying to make: AD was not just senility, it could strike down the most talented people in the prime of their lives, and it was far too little recognized and studied. By the time her diagnosis was made public in 1981, Hayworth could no longer make public appearances or statements, though she lived for six more years. She was never a spokesperson for AD, but she became the public face of it for millions of Americans. Her daughter, the Princess Yasmin Aga Khan, who gave up her singing career to care for her mother, became a leading AD advocate, raising tens of millions of dollars in her name.[26] Hayworth's lingering life of invisible dependence and deterioration through the 1980s dramatically illustrated the central trope of the AD campaign—that dementia destroys the selfhood of its victims while perversely allowing their bodies to live on and on.

This central theme of the AD campaign was also reinforced by two exemplary victims whose diagnoses were revealed in handwritten letters that received wide publicity. The first letter was written by Janet Adkins, who became well known as the first client whose suicide was facilitated by self-proclaimed "obitiatrist" Dr. Jack Kevorkian in 1990. She did not intend her note to be publicized, but it was revealed in the controversy about physician-assisted suicide that surrounded Kevorkian. The second letter was by former president Ronald Reagan, and stood as his final public message to the nation.

When Janet Adkins, a fifty-four-year-old former college instructor, was diagnosed with AD, she determined that she would end her life before crossing over into degrading dependency. Her short suicide note, which her husband, Ronald Adkins, and a close friend who had traveled with them signed as witnesses, reflected a calm determination to end her life before the ravages of AD could destroy it. "I have decided for the following reason to take my own life. This is a decision taken in a normal state of mind and is fully considered," she wrote, the slight lapses in grammar and punctuation perhaps indicating deterioration of her cognitive abilities. "I have alzheimers disease and do not want to let it progress any further. I dont choose to put my family or myself through the agony of this Terrible disease."[27]

Certainly, all accounts of how Janet Adkins arrived at her decision to end her life with Kevorkian's assistance suggest that these were her motivations and concerns. Ronald Adkins said that his wife had consistently expressed a desire to take her life from the time she was first diagnosed with AD and was told by the physician making the diagnosis that Ronald would have to care for her completely within a year. Her sons supported her right to make the decision, but disagreed with it and convinced her to enroll in a clinical trial of tacrine, which brought neither improvement nor delay in her deterioration. Although the medical team in Seattle that administered the trial told her that the course of her deterioration would be much more gradual than the initial doctor had indicated, and that she had at least two or three years, and possibly much longer, of relatively high-quality life before reaching the advanced stages of the disease, within a few months she made arrangement to travel to Michigan for Kevorkian's help, arguing that she needed to kill herself before the disease progressed to the point where she would be judged incompetent to decide her own fate.[28] "This was a very special woman," Ronald Adkins told reporters after her death. "She loved life. She was upset because she was losing her mind and her mind was everything to her."[29] Her sons, friends, and the minister with whom she planned her upbeat funeral service all confirmed that she knew exactly what she was doing, and that she "approached her death with the same zest and independence that she had shown during her life."[30] The picture that emerged of Adkins in newspaper accounts was the epitome of "successful aging"—a woman who embarked on the passage through middle age with confidence and vigor, taking on new challenges and new avenues for fulfillment. But she was also the epitome of someone keenly aware of the thin line between the pathological and the normal, between the mentally sound and the demented—a woman who could not countenance the prospect of losing it. As one journalist put it, "Janet Adkins knew what she wanted. She had played tennis, climbed the Himalayas, traveled around the world, hang glided, played Brahms duets with her husband, raised three sons, taught piano, taught English, learned T'ai Chi, studied reincarnation. Being addled and dependent was not her idea of living."[31]

Not surprisingly given Kevorkian's desire for publicity, the Adkins case drew a tremendous amount of attention in the popular media. Although Kevorkian's actions were all but universally condemned, few commentators found grounds to criticize the decision of Janet Adkins to end her life. "It is a Catch-22 situation," an expert on health law, quoted for an article in the *New York Times*, said. "You want to hang on as long as you are competent, but after you're incompetent and life is not worth living, it's too late, you can't do it anymore."[32] Somewhat paradoxically, Kevorkian's critics objected to his decision to assist Adkins's suicide both because she enjoyed a relatively high quality of life up to the time she pushed the button on his homemade suicide machine, *and* because the diagnosis of AD brought into question her competence to make the decision. On the one hand, virtually every report of her suicide in newspapers and the weekly news magazines emphasized her vigor and capacity for enjoyment of life by mentioning that only the week before she had beaten her thirty-two-year-old son in a tennis match, and in her last few days had been able to enjoy a romantic weekend with her husband. On the other hand, most of these accounts also raised the question of whether she was competent to make her decision. For example, *Time* noted that "one significant symptom [of AD] is sufficient mental deterioration to impair the ability to make decisions," and quoted an expert who noted that Kevorkian needed to claim that she made her decision competently, but that "the diagnosis of Alzheimer's is almost incompatible with that claim."[33]

Robert Butler came the closest to criticizing Adkins's decision, expressing concern about the impact of her suicide on the morale of the elderly:

"It's very demoralizing to hear of a 54-year-old giving up life when you're in your 80s and have heart disease and arthritis and some dementia and are still surviving, maybe working and taking care of your spouse."[34] This quote was unusual, however. More typically, commentators saw her either as a victim of Kevorkian's irresponsible behavior, or as someone dealing rationally if not heroically with her situation. An editorial in the *New York Times* compared her suicide to a death row execution. "One might . . . say that Mrs. Adkins had a choice whereas the condemned do not. But did she really? Janet Adkins had Alzheimer's disease. Her family was divided. Whether she was competent to make such a decision, as Dr. Kevorkian contends, is questionable. But whether Kevorkian is competent to decide on *her* behalf is not even questionable."[35] On the other hand, the editor of the *New England Journal of Medicine*, Marcia Angell, wrote in an op ed piece that patients with AD can expect their brains to be destroyed slowly over many years, during which they become increasingly dependent on and burdensome to their families. From this perspective, the decision to end life seemed rational. "The prospect for Janet Adkins was bleak. Moreover, modern medical care permits longer and longer survival under these circumstances, and patients are often subjected to the full panoply of aggressive treatment simply because it is available. What is someone like Janet Adkins, who valued her independence, to do?"[36] Thus to some Adkins might seem not a victim, but rather, in the words of one bioethicist, a "heroine for rational suicide."[37]

Ronald Reagan's farewell message to the nation revealed a much less disturbing form of heroism. Ronald and Nancy Reagan's decision to share his diagnosis was his last public action, taken with the conscious intention of greater awareness of this condition and clearer understanding of the individuals and families affected by it. Reagan had supported the AD campaign during his presidency, but his handwritten letter in 1994 telling the nation that he himself had been diagnosed with Alzheimer's marked a high point in public awareness that would be matched only when he died a decade later. Although Reagan was eighty-three years old at the time, his trademark physical vigor and sunny disposition remained intact, heightening the tragedy of the diagnosis. His farewell letter was both characteristically plainspoken and elegiac: "I now begin the journey that will lead me into the sunset of my life. I know that for America there will always be a bright dawn ahead."[38] Ronald and Nancy Reagan won widespread praise for courageously and generously sacrificing their privacy in order to advance awareness and support for increased funding of biomedical research into the disease. They and other members of the Reagan family ultimately did far more than lend the Reagan name to the fight against the disease. In 1995, the Reagans launched the Ronald and Nancy Reagan Research Institute of the Alzheimer's Association to raise and distribute private funds for the research. In addition, Nancy Reagan became an honorary member of the board of the Alzheimer's Association and an indefatigable advocate for research, and Ronald Reagan's daughter Maureen became an active member of the board.

Once Reagan's diagnosis was announced, Nancy was protective of their privacy and he virtually disappeared from public view. Occasional news reports of his condition described his progressive decline. For example, a 1997 story by Lawrence Altman in the *New York Times* noted that Reagan still appeared healthy and strong, but dwelled on the contrast between his vigorous years as president and the frailty and deterioration brought on by AD.[39] When news of Reagan's death broke in 2004, ten years after his AD had been revealed, one could be forgiven for being surprised to hear that he had in fact still been alive, having seemed to have read his obituary so many times before.

The three exemplary victims reinforced in very different ways the trope of the loss of self that was central to the AD campaign—Hayworth by suffering through a misdiagnosis that accounted, in retrospect, for much that had gone terribly wrong in her later life; Adkins by ending her life before the worst losses were endured; and Reagan by publicly revealing his fate before ebbing away in a long private fade to darkness. But paradoxically, though this loss of self trope seemed to preclude the possibility that people with dementia could speak for themselves, the successful campaign to make AD a household world made people with dementia more visible than ever before. Thus the AD movement, while stigmatizing dementia more deeply, ultimately encouraged people with dementia to step into the public and describe their experience.

Asserting Selfhood in the Liminal Space of AD

By the 1990s, the AD campaign had generated much greater awareness in both the general public and the medical community, with the result that people were being diagnosed earlier in the course of their dementia. This could be seen as a mixed blessing. On the one hand, fewer and fewer people would experience the anger and frustration of long years in which changes in cognition and behavior were misconstrued, as dramatized by the Rita Hayworth story. But on the other hand, people diagnosed with dementia had to adjust not only to the limitations imposed by the disease, which were often quite minimal when the disease was first diagnosed, but also to a radically uncertain future and to the heavy burden of stigma associated with the condition.

In this context, a new kind of exemplary person with dementia began to emerge in public view. In recent years, stories have begun to proliferate in the media of people who have publicly declared their dementia yet resolved not to disappear from sight. They are getting involved with advocacy work by speaking to groups of professionals and the general public, visiting their legislators, and playing a growing role within Alzheimer's Disease International and the Alzheimer's Association, which has established an early-stage advisory group that includes people with dementia; and additionally they have formed their own advocacy group—Dementia Advocacy and Support Network International. In many ways, their activism could be seen as supporting the AD advocates and medical authorities leading the AD campaign. But their activism can also be seen as challenge to the mainstream AD campaign, battling the stereotypes and baggage that well-meaning people have added to the experience of Alzheimer's disease and, more fundamentally, reasserting control over how their lives will be lived and how their experiences will be represented.

In trying to retain their identity in the face not only of their impairments but also of medicine's authority, the dementia memoirs seem to follow the course laid out by earlier narratives from the disability rights movement— summed up in the slogan "nothing about me without me." Historically, the disability rights movement was led by people with physical disabilities related mostly to mobility, sight, and hearing. In broad terms, the argument they developed was that people with disabilities—as fully competent and morally responsible persons—ought to be able to enjoy their rights and fulfill their responsibilities as citizens. Society's failure to make reasonable accommodation to their physical differences prevented people with disabilities from doing so. This basic idea of the disabled person as a fully competent and morally responsible person, to whom society owes a reasonable accommodation in order to allow them to fully enjoy their rights and responsibilities, is at the core of the 1990 Americans with Disabilities Act (ADA).

But the status of people with mental disabilities in this formula was somewhat ambiguous. The disability rights movement clearly recognized the right of people with mental disabilities to treatment and to educational opportunities—hence the ADA's mandate for special education programs and inclusion of students in public schools. But the broad disability rights movement did not immediately challenge our society's historical tendency to deny that people with serious mental disabilities were competent citizens and morally responsible people.

As people with dementia and other cognitive challenges are becoming more visible and speaking for themselves, they are challenging this narrow definition of competence and personhood. But there is at least one additional challenge. In the remainder of this chapter, I will discuss the emerging genre of book-length memoirs written by people diagnosed with AD and similar conditions, and how it challenges the idea of personhood that is fundamental to social and political relations in America.

To date, at least a dozen dementia autobiographies have appeared in English, all of them by people who were not well known as writers before.[40] On the surface at least, these books might contradict our notion of what a dementia narrative would be. All of the books were written by people with early onset dementia, and all but one while in the early stage of the disease, and all except that one take the form of conventional autobiography—so conventional in fact that one could be excused for wondering whether they are authentic dementia narratives, that is, whether the authors in fact do have AD, and if so, whether they received extensive editorial help to produce so coherent and focused a narrative, a question gently raised in a review of perhaps the most popular of them, Thomas DeBaggio's *Losing My Mind*.[41] This is less surprising when one thinks about the motivation of these authors in writing their lives. All of them are exemplary victims in the sense described above—solidly middle-class, responsible, productive, and successful people before the disease—and the stories they tell are of their struggle to maintain this identity in the face of both a radically uncertain future and a the potentially dehumanizing experience of being labeled with AD or some other form of dementia.

Discussing autopathographies in general, G. Thomas Couser argues that authors of these works can be seen as reasserting narrative control over their lives that is taken from them by their encounter with physicians. The process of diagnosing and treating any illness requires that doctor and patient engage in a kind of narrative collaboration; the patient offers up testimony about his or her experience of symptoms that the doctor interprets according to a system of medical knowledge generally unavailable to the patient. In the narrative work of diagnosis, patients turn their experience over to the physician, who renders an interpretation that may make sense of a baffling past, but gives doctors a measure of authority over the patient's life. From the diagnosis, the physician proceeds to prescription, treatment, and prognosis. "Thus doctors may both reinterpret patients' pasts and literally pre-script their futures. The process is collaborative but one-sided; patients submit their bodies to tests, their life histories to scrutiny, while doctors retain the authority to interpret these data." This process is not necessarily malign, and may be precisely what patients desire when they seek medical treatment. But it nonetheless involves surrendering control of one's body and, in the case of a diagnosis as serious as AD, one's future in a way that may seem a threatening objectification of the self. Thus, just as patients desire to vanquish or at least control the illness that alters their lives, "they may also wish to regain control of their life narratives, which they have yielded up to `objective' medical authority."[42]

Thus, it is not surprising that these authors do not employ narrative innovations to try to depict the dementia experience; they are trying in these works to reassert control and normality over lives that are threatened with radical uncertainty and contingency. The one exception to this is the book *Partial View* by Cary Smith Henderson, who was entering the middle stages of dementia and no longer capable of writing. He was however able to use a tape recorder to record brief observations about his experiences. The tapes were later edited by his family and the photographer who illustrated the book. As a result, the book appears as an unplotted collection of free-floating epigrams—what Henderson himself calls the "anecdotal career of an Alzheimer's patient."[43] Somewhat ironically then, although the less structured form of Henderson's book seems to capture the randomness and chaos that we might expect of a dementia narrative, it may be the least authentic since it is so much the product of editorial work by others. In any case, although Henderson's book lacks the conventional autobiographical structure of the others, his musings contain the same consistent and theme of coping with loss and deprivation that are more conventionally expressed in the other books.

The best way to briefly summarize these books is to point out that they all conform to a broader genre of patient narratives, what Arthur Frank in *The Wounded Storyteller* calls the quest narrative.[44] The titles of three of the books—*My Journey into Alzheimer's Disease, Living in the Labyrinth,* and *Show Me the Way to Go Home*—indicate immediately that the story of the author's illness is told in the shape of a journey, and the other books frequently employ metaphors of journey or spatial movement as well. As described by Frank, the quest narrative is the story of a long and difficult journey that ends with the hero receiving a boon. When an illness story takes the form of the quest narrative, the experience of illness is seen as a journey that is resolved when the narrator receives the boon of insight. Communicating that insight restores a sense of meaning and purpose for the author, and reconnects him or her to the world. All of the AD memoirs follow this basic structure, beginning when the diagnosis of Alzheimer's disease ruptures the expected flow of the author's life, followed by a chaotic period of denial, evasion, and isolation, and finally a resolution in which the author comes to accept his or her situation, restore vital connections to loved ones, and gain a renewed sense of life's potential and purpose through the very act of creating the narrative.

All of these authors confront the unsettling question of what remains of themselves when memory and language erode. "Am I anything without my memory and the simple skills of reading and writing I learned in childhood?" Thomas DeBaggio wonders in *Losing My Mind.*[45] In many passages he answers this question in the negative: "With failing memory, it is difficult to write long passages without getting lost in words. Where does the story go? Why does the pencil tremble? I see only the structure of words, their meaning elusive. I am often able to write only a sentence or two, enough to sketch what was to be brawny and complex. Do you understand I am not dying, just disappearing before your eyes?"[46] Yet in other passages, he sees his struggle as lending a dignity and purpose to his life that gives him joy despite these losses. "I have begun to adjust my life so each day has a structure to it, and a purpose; to enjoy every minute I can and to focus on the work I love. . . . I want to write the truest sentences I can in the hope my words give others the sense of struggle and joy I feel."[47] More important, DeBaggio recognizes in other passages that as his own memory fails, his existence will persist in the memory of others. "Although my memory is crumbling into obscurity, I am a memory for someone, living again in their recollection. . . . Our immortality, such as it may be, is not contained in what we dreamed or the secrets we kept; it is how our loved ones remember us."[48] But Alzheimer's provides no easy redemption for DeBaggio or any of these authors; in the final pages of the second volume of his memoirs he describes it as "a deadly hole in my life, a deep cistern in which I tripped unknowingly." As he waits for death, he longs only for a final farewell from his wife and son. But the very last words of the book trail into elegiac abstraction: "White gulls sweep from the sky. In a moment they soar to new heights on warm, familiar currents, as cars speed beneath them." He describes a solitary man walking along the sidewalk, just as he has for decades. Is it DeBaggio? His consciousness seems merged with the landscape, becoming perhaps someone else's memory. "As the walker comes to a turning point, he adjusts his cap low on his head, preparing to look into the bright rising sun. Balloons dance over electric lights high above the street."[49]

These authors find no easy answers to their questions, but ultimately resolve not to let these uncertainties paralyze them. In order to continue to understand themselves as intact persons, each of these authors had to radically redefine what it meant for them to be a person. They can no longer base their sense of self strictly on the values of independence, self-control, productivity, and self-fulfillment. Confronting AD, they must also find ways to value, or at least reconcile themselves to, dependency, contingency, and loss. In this way their narratives can be seen to constitute a challenge to our culture's dominant ideals of selfhood. In living lives that are of necessity free of the shackles of rationality, stable narratives, the illusions of independent agency, and the unity of experience, the person with dementia becomes, for better or worse, a prophet of some kind of postmodern selfhood.

There are certainly points in each of these narratives where the authors seem to speak to more general problems of selfhood. Diana Friel McGowin could be describing the general problem of anonymity and isolation that erodes a stable sense of self in modern society when she writes that "each one of us must feel they have worth as a living being—a person with the same rights and privileges as the people next door. I feel my lack of worth acutely when I am in large groups of people. Being in a crowd or even in a busy thoroughfare overwhelms me. All those people `of worth,' with places to go—who know where they are going."[50] Similarly, Cary Smith Henderson could be speaking of the general problem of the fragmentation and randomness of contemporary life when he says that "no two days and no two moments are the same. You can't build on experience. You can maybe guess what's going to happen a little while from now—minutes from now, hours from now—we don't know what to expect."[51]

If we accept this radically egalitarian reading of these narratives that at some level these authors are describing our experience as well as theirs, the implications are, I think, profound. As Arthur Frank has argued, the ethical challenge of illness is no less than reclaiming selfhood from the colonizing therapeutic discourse of modernity. Medical science at its most objective is nonetheless a set of values revolving around rationality and the desire for technical mastery of the world, and medical practices serve ideological purposes. The process of diagnosis itself—however objective the clinical and technological procedures may be—can also be understood as an effort to organize human experience according to these values, to get the patient to embrace the identity of disease victim, and to see this new identity as moral and appropriate. Narrative is a crucial resource in addressing the ethical challenge of medicine because, as these memoirs show, it can enrich the meaning of human experience in illness and reclaim the voice and perspective of the person from the discourse of diagnosis and therapy. These narratives provide grounds for optimism that a cultural space is being created where the sometimes conflicting imperatives of people and biomedicine can be held in creative tension. But these narratives also suggest that reclaiming the selfhood of the Alzheimer's patient, and perhaps reclaiming a viable concept of selfhood more generally, will require something more—a radical reconsideration of what we think it means to be a human being.

Notes

1. Barron H. Lerner, *When Illness Goes Public: Celebrity Patients and How We Look at Medicine* (Baltimore: Johns Hopkins University Press, 2006).

2. Robert H. Wiebe, *The Search for Order, 1877–1920* (New York: Hill & Wang, 1967); Jackson Lears, "The Ad Man and the Grand Inquisitor: Intimacy, Publicity, and the Managed Self in America, 1880–1940," in *Constructions of the Self*, ed. George Levine (New Brunswick: Rutgers University Press, 1992), 107–41; Wilfred M. McClay, *The Masterless: Self and Society in Modern America* (Chapel Hill: University of North Carolina Press, 1994); and Elizabeth Lunbeck, *The Psychiatric Persuasion: Knowledge, Gender, and Power in Modern America* (Princeton: Princeton University Press, 1996).

3. William Graebner, *A History of Retirement: The Meaning and Function of an American Institution, 1885–1978* (New Haven: Yale University Press, 1967); Carol Haber, *Beyond Sixty-Five: The Dilemma of Old Age in America's Past* (New York: Cambridge University Press, 1980); and Thomas R. Cole, *The Journey of Life: A Cultural History of Aging in America* (New York: Cambridge University Press, 1992).

4. Charles E. Rosenberg, "George M. Beard and American Nervousness," in *No Other Gods: On Science and American Social Thought*, ed. Charles Rosenberg (Baltimore: Johns Hopkins University Press, 1997), 98–108.

5. George Miller Beard, "Legal Responsibility in Old Age: Based On Researchers into the Relation of Age to Work," in *The "Fixed Period" Controversy*, ed. Gerald Gruman (New York: Arno Press, 1979), 4.

6. Ibid., 11.

7. Ibid.

8. William Osler, "The Fixed Period," in *Aequanimitas*, 2nd ed. (London: H. K. Lewis, 1906), 375–93.

9. Ignatz L. Nascher, *Geriatrics: The Diseases of Old Age and Their Treatment* (Philadelphia: P. Blakiston, 1914).

10. Dena Shenk and W. Andrew Achenbaum, *Changing Perceptions of Aging and the Aged* (New York: Springer, 1994).

11. Osler, "Fixed Period," 400.

12. Jesse F. Ballenger, *Self, Senility, and Alzheimer's Disease in Modern America: A History* (Baltimore: Johns Hopkins University Press, 2006), 25, 63–64.

13. Jesse F. Ballenger, "Progress in the History of Alzheimer's Disease: The Importance of Context," *Journal of Alzheimer's Disease* 9 (2006): 1–9.

14. Martha Holstein, "Alzheimer's Disease and Senile Dementia, 1885–1920: An Interpretive History of Disease Negotiation," *Journal of Aging Studies* 11 (1997): 1–13; and Martha Holstein, "Aging, Culture, and the Framing of Alzheimer Disease," in *Concepts of Alzheimer Disease: Biological, Clinical, and Cultural Perspectives*, ed. Peter J. Whitehouse, Konrad Maurer, and Jesse F. Ballenger (Baltimore: Johns Hopkins University Press, 2000).

15. Jesse F. Ballenger, "Beyond the Characteristic Plaques and Tangles: Mid-Twentieth-Century U.S. Psychiatry and the Fight against Senility," in Whitehouse, *Concepts of Alzheimer Disease*, 83–103.

16. David Rothschild, "The Practical Value of Research in the Psychoses of Later Life," *Diseases of the Nervous System* 8 (1947): 125.

17. Maurice Linden and Douglas Courtney, "The Human Life Cycle and Its Interruptions: A Psychologic Hypothesis," *American Journal of Psychiatry* 109 (1953): 912.

18. David C. Wilson, "The Pathology of Senility," *American Journal of Psychiatry* 111 (1955): 905.

19. Clark Tibbitts and Henry D. Sheldon, "Introduction: A Philosophy of Aging," *Annals of the American Academy of Political and Social Science* 279 (1952): 7.

20. Peter Laslett, *A Fresh Map of Life: The Emergence of the Third Age* (Cambridge: Harvard University Press, 1991).

21. Richard B. Calhoun, *In Search of the New Old: Redefining Old Age in America, 1945–1970* (New York: Elsevier, 1978); and Carole Haber and Brian Gratton, *Old Age and the Search for Security: An American Social History* (Bloomington: Indiana University Press, 1994).

22. Robert N. Butler, *Why Survive?: Being Old in America* (New York: Harper & Row, 1975), 9–10.

23. Ballenger, *Self, Senility, and Alzheimer's Disease*, chap. 4.

24. Ibid., chap. 5.

25. US Senate, Subcommittee on Aging, Committee on Labor and Human Resources, Ninety-Sixth Congress, Second Sessions, *Impact of Alzheimer's Disease on the Nation's Elderly* (Washington, DC: United States Government Printing Office, 1980), 98.

26. Lerner, *When Illness Goes Public*, chap. 8.

27. Jack Kevorkian, *Prescription Medicide: The Goodness of Planned Death* (Buffalo: Prometheus, 1991), 228.

28. Kirsten Rohde, Elaine R. Peskind, and Murray R. Raskind, "Suicide in Two Patients with Alzheimer's Disease," *Journal of the American Geriatrics Society* 43 (1995): 187–89.

29. Timothy Egan, "'Her Mind Was Everything,' Dead Woman's Husband Says," *New York Times*, June 6, 1990, B6.

30. Timothy Egan, "As Memory and Music Faded, Oregon Woman Chose Death," *New York Times*, June 7, 1990, A1.

31. Michael Betzold, *Appointment with Doctor Death* (Troy, MI: Momentum, 1993), 43.

32. Lawrence K. Altman, "Use of Suicide Device Sets in Motion Debate on a Disturbing Issue," *New York Times*, June 12, 1990, C3.

33. Nancy Gibbs, "Dr. Death's Suicide Machine," *Time*, June 18, 1990, 69–70. The expert was Dr. Joanne Lynn, professor at George Washington University, who was a prominent advocate of hospice care.

34. Melinda Beck et al., "The Doctor's Suicide Van," *Newsweek*, June 18, 1990, 46.

35. "Dying, Dr. Kevorkian's Way," *New York Times*, June 7, 1990, A22.

36. Marcia Angell, "Don't Criticize Dr. Death . . . ," *New York Times*, June 14, 1990, A27.

37. Laurence B. McCullough, "Ethical Challenges Posed by Injuries and Diseases of the Nervous System," *Medical Humanities Review* 10 (1996): 108–12.

38. From the complete text of the letter, found at http://www.americanpresidents.org/letters/39.asp (accessed February 2, 2005).

39. Lawrence K. Altman, "Reagan's Twilight—A Special Report: A President Fades Into a World Apart," *New York Times*, October 5, 1997, online at http://www.nytimes.com/1997/10/05/us/reagan-s-twilight-a-special-report-a-president-fades-into-a-world-apart.html?sec=&spon=&pagewanted=all (accessed May 17, 2010).

40. Thomas DeBaggio, author of two volumes of AD memoirs, could perhaps be considered an exception, as he was the author of a number of books on herbal gardening prior to being diagnosed with dementia.

41. Peter J. Whitehouse, review of *Losing My Mind: An Intimate Look at Life with Alzheimer's*, by Thomas DeBaggio, *New England Journal of Medicine* 347 (2002): 861.

42. G. Thomas Couser, *Recovering Bodies: Illness, Disability, and Life Writing* (Madison: University of Wisconsin Press, 1997), 10.

43. Cary S. Henderson, *Partial View: An Alzheimer's Journal* (Dallas: Southern Methodist University Press, 1998). 4.

44. Arthur W. Frank, *The Wounded Storyteller: Body, Illness, and Ethics* (Chicago: University of Chicago Press, 1995).

45. Thomas DeBaggio, *Losing My Mind: An Intimate Look at Life with Alzheimer's* (New York: Free Press, 2002), 43.

46. Ibid., 157.

47. Ibid., 29.

48. Ibid., 199–207.

49. Thomas DeBaggio, *When It Gets Dark: An Enlightened Reflection on Life with Alzheimer's* (New York: Free Press, 2003), 225–26.

50. Diana Friel McGowin, *Living in the Labyrinth* (Thorndike, ME: Thorndike Press, 1994), 112.

51. Henderson, *Partial View*, 47.

Chapter Six

The Cursing Patient

Neuropsychiatry Confronts Tourette's Syndrome, 1825–2008

Howard I. Kushner

Michael and Toby: An Introduction

I first met Michael (a pseudonym), a neighbor in his early teens, in 1980. Michael periodically would blurt out what sounded like barks and often ask inappropriate questions. He informed me that these behaviors were caused by an affliction called Tourette's syndrome (TS). When Michael was about eight years old he had developed uncontrolled eye blinking; soon after he developed more pronounced facial and body tics accompanied by vocalizations that at first sounded as if he was muttering to himself. When he approached his late teens he began to curse, regularly shouting out a series of obscenities, most often "fuck you!" His cursing was accompanied by uncontrollable blurting out of inappropriate remarks, which made it difficult for him to socialize with peers or with anyone unaware of the reason for his offensive behavior. At a public lecture he was apt to shout at the speaker, "Sit down, shut up!" Passing a noticeably obese woman he would blurt out, "fat pig!" Once, phoning an airline to make a reservation, he exclaimed, "There's a bomb on the plane!" The next day the FBI appeared at his door to question a suspected terrorist. When introduced to or passing by an African American, he could not stop himself from exclaiming, "Nigger!"

Like Michael, Toby (a pseudonym), a forty-something patient treated at our psychiatric clinic, developed tics and vocalizations when he was nine, and was diagnosed three years later with TS. Toby has mild obsessive-compulsive behavior (OCB). For instance, on his way to work, he feels compelled to touch every third car. He also has obsessive, repetitive thoughts of death and fears that his wife might leave him. Like Michael, Toby frequently blurts out the word "nigger" when he encounters an African American. Fat women evoke the comment, "you are so fucking fat"; a gay friend provokes the statement, "I want to suck your dick"; seeing large breasts, he proclaims, "you got big tits." At a synagogue service during the Jewish high holidays, Toby, who is Jewish, shouts out, "I love Jesus!" Toby attempts to cover up his embarrassing utterances by replacing the word "nigger" with "Nick," or "bitch" with "witch."[1]

In addition to cursing, which is clinically referred to as coprolalia, those afflicted with TS may display copropraxia, the acting out of explicitly sexual gestures or displays; echolalia, the repetition of one's own or others' words or phrases; and echopraxia, the imitation of others' behaviors or actions. Often, like Michael and Toby, TS sufferers seem to have a compulsion to articulate the most outrageous, if inappropriately appropriate, phrases and words for the occasion.

While Toby experiences a certain physical relief after his coprolalic utterance, his dominant emotion is embarrassment. "I love people," Toby insists. "I'm not prejudiced. . . . It's almost like the opposite." It is as if, explains the late Adam Ward Seligman, a Tourette's sufferer and author, someone comes to your door demanding, "don't think about monkeys." That command, of course, results in your thinking about nothing else. "Having Tourette syndrome," writes Seligman, "is a lot like not thinking about monkeys. The monkeys are the tics, vocalizations, urges, obsessions, behaviors and enactments that are with us constantly, overwhelming our daily lives. To live and function we have to keep the Tourette syndrome at bay—we have to try not to think about monkeys."[2]

Michael and Toby explain to those with whom they meet that their cursing and strange vocalizations are the result of TS. Nevertheless, the content and timing of these outbursts can be disturbing to anyone who is the target or for those who witness them. On the one hand, they are apt but painful characterizations, such as blurting out what may be obvious, but are tasteless or tactless. On the other hand, these unrestrained words and phrases can be threatening, as when Michael interjects the statement "I want to rape you" when talking to a woman. Finally, like Michael and Toby, TS sufferers can have difficulty controlling their tempers. Both Michael and Toby punch holes in walls. Toby regularly breaks the windshield of the family car, while Michael has been known to destroy his bathroom toilet.

Most persons diagnosed with TS have less florid behaviors than Michael and Toby; they neither curse nor display inappropriate sexual behavior. Typically, sufferers develop involuntary motor movements during early childhood (ages seven to nine). The motor tics, which occur frequently throughout the day, generally involve head and neck jerking, eye blinking, tongue protrusions, shoulder shrugs, and various torso and limb movements. A diagnosis of TS requires one or more vocal tics to have been present for some time. These may include barks, grunts, yelps, and coughs. Tics and vocalizations appear suddenly and characteristically are rapid, recurrent, nonrhythmic, and stereotyped. Often these signs and symptoms are coupled with obsessive and compulsive behaviors, such as a repeated series of actions that must be performed before entering or leaving a room. Tics wax and wane, often increasing in frequency and complexity; later tics replace earlier ones.[3] Motor movements, however, can be quite debilitating and painful. For instance, aside from the muscle strain caused by severe head jerking, tics can make reading an arduous if not impossible task.[4] Sometimes the tics disappear completely and never recur. Often, however, they merely remit, returning later in slightly different form with renewed force.

However, it is eruptive cursing and blurting out of inappropriate remarks that frame the lives of the most florid patients. Indeed, it is a rule that those with the most florid presentations, like Michael and Toby, are the least responsive to interventions and the most likely to suffer lifelong from TS.

The Patient's Voice in the Published Case

Explanations of what we label today as TS continue to rely on patients' narratives, such as those of Michael's and Toby's. Until recently, most of these stories have been collected and interpreted by clinicians. Diagnosing clinicians are influenced not only by a patient's narrative (often supplemented by reports from teachers, parents, and other family members), but also by the meanings given to it by the reports of referring physicians. Diagnosis and treatment of TS is complicated by the changing nature of its signs and symptoms and their tendency to wax and wane.

If clinicians face a daunting task interpreting the meaning of the signs and symptoms of a patient they have examined, it is even more difficult to judge a published case whose meaning has been interpreted in order to make a clinical argument about underlying causes or appropriate treatments. In its published form the clinical case becomes evidence for the author's conclusions. Even the most rigorous and honest reporters edit their presentations, often leaving out what previously might have been seen as a central element of the disorder (perhaps, familial conflict) or what later might become valuable (for instance, evidence of recurrent bacterial infection).[5]

As a result, the interpretation of clinical cases both influences and reflects clinicians' identification and treatment of TS. It also can frame the way individuals experience this affliction. For no matter what its underlying biology or psychology, how those with TS have experienced involuntary movements and unwelcome vocalizations has depended to a great extent upon culturally sanctioned expectations. A history of Tourette's patients must therefore simultaneously explore three distinct but overlapping narratives: the claims of medical knowledge, patients' experiences, and cultural expectations and assumptions.

These issues are most clearly illustrated by the multiple and competing readings of the most cited case of TS, that of the Marquise de Dampierre (1799–1884).[6] Even before the syndrome had a name, this cursing and tic-cing nineteenth-century noblewoman served as an emblematic example for a variety of competing theories about the mechanisms associated with humans' ability to self-consciously control their actions and behaviors. Her behavior served as Georges Gilles de la Tourette's classic example of the disorder that today bears his name.

The Emblematic Case of the Marquise de Dampierre

In 1885 the French neurologist Georges Gilles de la Tourette, working under the direction of the influential Salpêtrière neurologist Jean Martin Charcot, identified a combination of multiple motor tics and involuntary vocalizations as a distinct disorder he called Convulsive Tic Disease with Coprolalia.[7] Gilles de la Tourette based his claims primarily on the behavior of the eighty-five-year-old Marquise de Dampierre, who died in Paris in August 1884. The marquise was notorious for shouting out, in the middle of conversations, inappropriate or obscene words, especially "shit and fucking pig."[8] Her behavior had been reported sixty years earlier by Jean Marc Gaspard Itard (1775–1838) in an article about the twenty-six-year-old Madame de Dampierre he published in *Archives Générales de Médecine*.[9] "In the midst of a conversation that interests her extremely," Itard reported of Dampierre, "all of a sudden, without being able to prevent it, she interrupts what she is saying or what she is listening to with bizarre shouts and with words that are even more extraordinary and that make a deplorable contrast with her intellect and her distinguished manners. These words are for the most part gross swear words and obscene epithets and, something that is no less embarrassing for her than for the listeners, an extremely crude expression of a judgment or of an unfavorable opinion of someone in the group." The more she was revolted by a word's "grossness," explained Itard, "the more she is tormented by the fear that she will utter them, and this preoccupation is precisely what puts them at the tip of her tongue where she can no longer control it."[10]

Itard's account of the marquise's symptoms is extensive, but he examined her only briefly in her twenty-sixth year, eighteen years after the outbreak of her signs and symptoms.[11] Although Dampierre's bizarre behavior had been the subject of Parisian gossip for half a century, neither Gilles de la Tourette, his mentor Jean Martin Charcot, nor any physician since Itard had ever examined her.[12] Nevertheless, at Charcot's urging, Gilles de la Tourette selected Dampierre as his first example of the illness that he called "maladie des tics."[13] Based on Itard's description Gilles de la Tourette asserted that the illness began with childhood motor and vocal tics that over time increased in number and variety and the eventual appearance of coprolalia. This disease, he concluded, had a "degenerative" etiology in which the afflicted had inherited a nervous system weakened by the cumulative effects of the preceding generations' immoral behaviors. Although the tics might wax and wane they ultimately resisted all interventions. There was no hope, wrote Gilles de la Tourette, of "a complete cure," for "once a ticcer, always a ticcer."[14]

Although Gilles de la Tourette described eight other patients who either he or Charcot had examined, only the marquise fit his conclusions.[15] The story of the Marquise de Dampierre has become the conventional tale that appears in the opening paragraphs of almost every clinical overview of TS.[16] By the mid-1990s, the conventional citation of the case of the Marquise de Dampierre had evolved into an emblematic narrative, a sort of short-hand description of the onset and course of the disorder itself.[17] "Tourette's syndrome," wrote Stanley Finger in his encyclopedic *Origins of Neuroscience*, "can best be appreciated by looking directly at his [Gilles de la Tourette's] case of Madame de Dampierre."[18]

The Story of O.

The cursing Marquise de Dampierre served as an emblem of Gilles de la Tourette's tic disease, but it also reflected the frustration of clinicians, mainly neurologists, to treat actual cases of florid ticcing patients. Unable to cure their patients, many blamed their patients rather than the illness.[19] They constructed elaborate theories to explain why their interventions failed to cure or even ameliorate the ticcing behaviors they encountered.

This is evident in Henry Meige and Eduard Feindel's landmark study of 1902, *Les tics et leur traitement*, which was translated into English by the British neurologist S. A. Kinnier Wilson in 1907. The book would become the standard for diagnosis and treatment of motor and vocal tics for the next half century.[20] Meige and Feindel's view was compatible with the two strains of emerging explanations for a variety of seemingly psychopathological behaviors. On the one hand, it meshed with eugenics, which, as in Gilles de la Tourette's study, attributed behaviors like motor and vocal tics to degenerative inheritance. On the other hand, it segued into Freudian explanations of early childhood sexual repressive conflict. Thus *Tics and Their Treatment* framed the views and assumptions that European and American practitioners held about convulsive tics until the 1960s.

Les tics et leur traitement opens with "The Confessions of a Victim to Tic," an edited and annotated reproduction of a memoir written by a fifty-four-year-old businessman, referred to in the text only as O. O. suffered a lifelong affliction of facial, body, and vocal tics combined with an assortment of compulsive behaviors, which Meige and Feindel considered to be prototypical of the tic.[21] The text and conclusions of *Les tics et leur traitement* were actually completed before the authors discovered O.'s memoir. Meige and Feindel had difficulty locating an archetype of the behaviors they had described, but in 1901 they located an individual "who is a perfect compendium of almost all the varieties of tic, and whose story, remarkable alike for its lucidity and educative value, forms the most natural prelude for our study."[22] "The Confessions of a Victim to Tic" was edited and interpreted by Meige and Feindel to conform with and authenticate the authors' wider claims.

As clinicians' appropriation of the case of the Marquise de Dampierre demonstrated, such writing strategies are not unique in the history of the classification and treatment of tic behaviors. Emblematic cases are often recreated and interpreted *after*, rather than before, etiological theories have been generated. Like its predecessor case, "The Confessions of a Victim to Tic" would be appropriated and reconstructed by future theorists and writers as prototypes for their explanations of the causes for ticcing behaviors.

Meige and Feindel's reading of the case of O. is best understood in the context of their earlier research. It drew heavily on a series of articles that elaborated the view that in a susceptible population tics resulted from habits formed during childhood.[23] Framing their view of tics was a larger set of beliefs that implicated hereditary degeneration as a central feature in a variety of behavioral psychopathologies, a set of beliefs that Stephen Casper also notes in his study of the origins of the neurological exam in chapter 1 of this volume. Meige's 1893 doctoral thesis, *The Study of Certain Neuropathological Travelers: The Wandering Jew at the Salpêtrière*, described a putatively congenital illness that caused Jews to wander from place to place, making it impossible for them to form attachments to any place or nation.[24] Meige's analysis was based on his and Charcot's observations of Jewish patients at the Salpêtrière, supplemented by an assortment of popular writings on the topic of "wandering Jews," including notoriously anti-Semitic texts. Their Jewish patients, wrote Meige, were "constantly obsessed by the need to travel, going from city to city, from clinic to clinic, in search of a new treatment, of a yet unknown remedy. They try every medication that anyone suggests, greedy for novelties; but they quickly reject them, inventing a frivolous pretext for no longer continuing them, and the impulse reappears, when one fine day they run off entranced by a new delusion of a distant cure." The characteristics displayed by Jewish patients were, according to Meige, merely a reflection of a deeper "quality of their race." Jews are "first of all profoundly neuropathological. . . . And what's more they submit to irresistible impulses which trap them in a perpetual vagabondage. Their obsessive idea is not absurd to them; nothing is more legitimate than searching for lucrative work, or for an efficacious remedy."[25]

Similar observational methods informed Meige's claims of the congenital causes of ticcing behaviors. Persistent motor and vocal tics were evidence of a degenerative psychological disorder characterized by regression to infantile behavior. *All* tics, Meige insisted in a 1901 article, were psychological.[26] The patient's "mental state," he wrote in a 1902 article, "La genèse des tics," "played a central role in the genesis of the tic."[27] Even where the initial goal of tics was to react to or to avoid harm from some actual situation, the tic became habitual, after the cause and goal had disappeared, in those who had "a psychological predisposition that above all confirmed hereditary weakness of the will" (201).

Evidence for this hereditary weakness of the will was gleaned from an examination of a patient's familial pedigree, in which any of a number of conditions was portrayed as a hereditary cause of tics. O.'s family history, explained Meige and Feindel, confirmed "the existence of a grave neuropathic heredity, an unfailing feature of tic." His grandfather, who married a first cousin, was a stutterer and had facial and head tics; his brother also was a stutterer, while both his daughter and sister had facial tics, and a son was afflicted with asthma. Aside from his tics, O.'s general heath was excellent. He exercised regularly and he "maintain[ed] a vigor and agility above the average" and "his intellectual activity" was "keen" (1–2). Because, like O., many of their tic patients seemed to display extraordinary intelligence, Meige and Feindel adopted the view that these ticcers suffered from "superior degeneration," an inherited condition in which infantile regression was mixed with superior intellectual abilities (108).

Meige and Feindel explained that although most children eventually outgrew early ticcing behaviors, in a subset of children with a congenital predisposition like O.'s, motor and vocal tics as well as obsessive behaviors persisted. "Mimicry," wrote Meige and Feindel, "is strong in the child's nature, and bad habits are quickly contracted." If a child inherited "a nervous weakness" that child was especially susceptible to suggestion of all forms and therefore at great risk in developing tics (101). O. was a mimic. "A curious gesture or bizarre attitude affected by anyone," O. reported, "was the immediate signal for an attempt on my part at its reproduction." O. remembered that when he was thirteen he saw "a man with a droll grimace of eyes and mouth, and from that moment I gave myself no respite until I could imitate it accurately." Similarly, O. attributed his head tossing movements to his attempt to mimic two schoolmates who habitually tossed their long hair back by a shake of the head. Although O. reported that he had never experienced an irresistible urge to curse, Meige and Feindel claimed that O.'s impulse to use slang was "a sort of *fruste* [substitute] coprolalia" (2, 13).

Meige believed that the onset of tics could be connected to a response to an earlier pain or actual physiological event. The behavior persisted in those with congenitally weak self-control. O. reported that his eye and lip movements had their origins in reactions to actual stimulations, but they continued as if by habit long after initial stimulation ceased. Such admissions, noted Meige and Feindel, were evidence of O.'s "pathogenic" lack of will. When O. reported that his head and face movements were due to the annoyance caused by seeing the tip of his nose or his moustache, Meige and Feindel argued that it was O.'s "force of repetition" that "changes the voluntary act into an automatic habit, the initial motive for which is soon lost; and the patient shows the weakness of his character by making little or no effort at inhibition." O. insisted that he could not control these desires: "There seem to be two persons in me . . . I am at once the actor and the spectator; and the worst of it is, the exuberance of the one is not to be thwarted by the just recriminations of the other" (3–5).

O. related his ongoing and futile attempts to suppress and hide his tics but lamented that these strategies failed because they too "become so habitual that they are nothing less than fresh tics appended to the old. To dissemble one tic we fashion another." In an attempt to restrain his head tics, O. resorted to a series of failed and increasingly desperate contrivances, from resting his head on a cane, to wearing stiffly starched collars, to literally tying his head to his trousers. Nevertheless, Meige and Feindel discounted O.'s strategies and reasserted their view that O.'s behaviors revealed that psychological weakness always preceded the motor movements. O.'s explanations underlined Meige and Feindel's belief in the infantile nature of the man's behaviors (5–6).

Meige and Feindel found confirmation for their claims of a psychogenic pathology of O.'s tics in his ability to suppress his tics temporarily. "Should he find himself in the company of one from whom he would fain conceal his tics, he is able to suppress them for an hour or two, and similarly if he is deep in an interesting or serious conversation." Yet after a while, "he can refrain no longer," and "he will invent any pretext for leaving the room, abandoning himself in his moment of solitude to a veritable debauch of absurd gesticulations, a wild muscular carnival, from which he returns comforted, to resume sedately the thread of the interrupted dialogue." As further evidence of O.'s ability to control his tics if he set his mind to it, Meige and Feindel pointed out that O. managed to cycle, and that "his devotion to billiards, or to such exercises as fencing or rowing, is never interfered with by an unruly tic. He is a great fisher, and . . . he will remain motionless indefinitely." If "interest in his prospective catch fade[d]," however, O.'s tics immediately returned (10–11).

O. reported that his uncontrollable tics were like a "desire for forbidden fruit. It is when we are required to keep quiet that we are tempted to restlessness." When instructed to be silent in school, O. remarked that he sought "to evade the galling interdict by giving vent to some inarticulate sound. In this fashion did my 'cluck' come into being." Such statements confirmed

Meige and Feindel's view that O.'s account of the origin of his tics supplied further evidence of a "mental infantilism" that prompted children to do exactly what they were forbidden to do. "They seem animated by a spirit of contrariness and of resistance; and if in normal individuals reason and reflection prevail with the approach of maturity, in these 'big babies' many traces of childhood persist, in spite of the march of years" (12–13).

What is extraordinary about their judgments, as Meige and Feindel admitted, was that O. "has managed and still manages important commercial undertakings, demanding initiative and decision, and so far from sparing himself in any way, he has exhibited a combination of caution and audacity that has stood him in good stead." Instead of recognizing this as an adaptive strategy by which O. was able to channel his compulsive tics in the service of his vocation, Meige and Feindel cited O.'s successful business career as evidence that O. could selectively control his tic behaviors whenever he chose. O.'s failure to do so at other times, they insisted, proved that his tic behaviors were the result of willful bad habits and of a "mobile and impulsive temperament" (16–17). Meige and Feindel were so attached to their assumptions about the psychopathology of ticcers that they failed to appreciate the pain and hopelessness that O. attempted to convey. "In regard to my tics," O. wrote, "what I find most insupportable is the thought that I am making myself ridiculous and that everyone is laughing at me. I seem to notice in each person I pass in the street a curious look of scorn or pity that is either humiliating or irritating." Most of all O. wished to be inconspicuous and to hide his tics by any means available. But, he lamented, "nine times out of ten our efforts are abortive simply because we invent a tic to hide a tic and so add to the ridicule and the disease" (17).

Focusing on their preconception that heredity had combined with habit and weakness of will, Meige and Feindel denigrated the very source they drew upon. "Alike in speaking and in writing," wrote Meige and Feindel, "O. betrays an advanced degree of mental instability." Although they based their theoretical claims on O.'s written memoir and their subsequent interviews with him, Meige and Feindel characterized O.'s conversation as "a tissue of disconnected thoughts and uncompleted sentences." When O. reported that he had several times entertained thoughts of suicide, Meige and Feindel made light of the matter, informing their readers that "the suicidal tendencies of some sufferers from tic are seldom full-blown" (17–19).

O.'s treatment lasted only a few months and combined physical restraints and breathing exercises.[28] "The patient," wrote Meige and Feindel, "has recovered his self-confidence, and the compliments of his friends prove an additional restorative." O.'s physicians admitted that "the tics still recur, but their number is less, their duration shorter, their severity considerably diminished." O. added that he "very much doubted whether I shall ever have the necessary perseverance to master all my tics, and I am too prone to imagine fresh ones; yet the thought no longer alarms me. Experience has shown the possibility of control, my tics have lost their terror."[29] Although the case of O. framed Meige and Feindel's text, their treatment of him lasted less than a year. They continued to write about tics and their treatments, but O. never reappeared in their articles. Thus, it remains impossible to learn to what extent O.'s reported improvement was permanent or merely another episode in a life filled with waxing and waning tics.

Wilson's translation of *Les tics et leur traitement* made Meige and Feindel's views available to a wide cross-section of the Anglo-American medical community. Anglo-North American and continental clinicians drew on as well as adapted Meige and Feindel's work to construct a physiopsychological set of explanations that connected bad habits with motor and vocal tics and obsessive behaviors.[30] Most often, as with Meige and Feindel, these symptoms were also tied to nonspecific hereditary factors.[31] Some physicians, particularly in North America, relied on the all-purpose diagnosis of neurasthenia (nervous exhaustion) as a vehicle for incorporating Meige and Feindel's explanations with emerging psychoanalytic claims about the origins of tics.[32]

Enter Psychoanalysis

In 1921 the Hungarian neurologist and psychoanalyst Sandor Ferenczi (1873–1933) outlined the first purely psychoanalytic analysis of tics.[33] Ferenczi's paper, "Psycho-Analytical Observation on Tic," would become the sanctioned psychoanalytic statement on tics.[34] Yet Ferenczi reached his conclusions without ever examining a single ticcing patient. Instead he relied entirely on the reports in Meige and Feindel's *Les tics et leur traitement* (1902), particularly on their description, reproduction, and discussion of O.'s "Confessions of a Ticqueur." Ferenczi sought to justify his omission of actual clinical cases by claiming that he had few opportunities to personally observe ticcing patients in his private practice. By relying on Meige and Feindel, Ferenczi claimed, oddly for a psychoanalyst, that he could not be accused of biased observations or of making suggestions to a patient.[35]

Although all medical researchers tend to shore up their claims by referencing the work of important predecessors, with psychoanalysis this practice required turning to Freud for validation. Ironically, Freud himself had said little explicitly about tics.[36] Thus Ferenczi and later psychoanalysts were forced to interpret the few contradictory hints that Freud had offered in passing conversation in a way that was congruent with psychoanalytic categories. "When I incidentally discussed the meaning and significance of Tic with Prof. Freud," wrote Ferenczi in 1921, "he mentioned that apparently there was an organic factor in the question."[37] Ferenczi reinterpreted Freud's remark to mean that tics were psychological: Freud, explained

Ferenczi, should be understood as suggesting that particular organs serve a "psychical representative" of a repressed conflict rather than as a physiological site for tic production. Tics were psychogenic conflicts that manifested themselves physiologically, as body movements and vocalizations.[38] Having demonstrated his allegiance to the master's insight, Ferenczi drew on Meige and Feindel's arguments and examples, translating them into a psychoanalytic vocabulary.

Ferenczi concluded that tics were "stereotyped equivalents of Onanism [masturbation]" and that the connection of tics with eruptive cursing (coprolalia)[39] was "nothing else than the uttered expression of the same erotic emotion usually abreacted [released by acting out] in symbolic movements."[40] A number of earlier observers, including J. C. Wilson (1897) and Otto Lerch (1901), had connected masturbation with tics and coprolalia, *but* they had argued that ticcers were *actual* masturbators.[41] Turning this notion on its head, Ferenczi and his followers argued that tics resulted from *repressed* masturbatory desires. According to Ferenczi, tics were best understood as a form of "*constitutional narcissism,*" where "*the smallest injury to a part of the body strikes the whole ego.*" Ticcers were overly sensitive and their tics were the "motor expressions" of this hypersensitivity to external stimulation. The "hyperaesthesia" [hyperkinetic movements] were an "expression of narcissism, the strong attachment of the subject to himself, his body, or a part of his body," which Ferenczi tied to Freud's notion of "the damming-up of organ libido [energy associated with instinctual drives]." That is, these patients had repressed their wishes for sensual bodily pleasures, especially, but not only, those attached to their genitalia. Coprolalic outbursts and the inability to restrain a thought were, for Ferenczi, a substitute release of energy in those incapable of enduring a stimulus to their body without an immediate defense reaction. Involuntary cursing and blurting out other inappropriate speech were motor reactions through which these repressed emotions toward organ stimulation were released.[42]

A physical illness, such as an eye infection, in patients with dammed-up libido led to a subsequent eye tic because of the unconscious defense against the infection's stimulation of the eyelids. The resultant tic was the psychic reaction to the physical stimulation caused by the infection: The tics displayed by these patients could be "traced back to the 'traumatic' displacement of libido and, . . . the motor expression of Tic arises from defence reactions against the stimulation of such parts of the body."[43]

Whatever else it did, Ferenczi's explanation transformed Gilles de la Tourette's classification into a psychoanalytic category in which motor tics and involuntary vocalizations were only one set of possible outcomes of a repressed narcissistic childhood injury. Quoting O.'s statement that "I must admit that I am full of self-love and am particularly sensitive to blame or praise," Ferenczi found that this confession "show[s] tic patients as of a mentally infantile character, narcissistically fixated, from which the healthy developed part of the personality can with difficulty free itself." The fact that the vocal outbursts of these patients often had a sexual or "organ-erotic (perverse)" content was further confirmation for Ferenczi of their narcissism. He endorsed Meige and Feindel's conclusion that "every tic patient has the mind of a child." They are "big, badly brought-up children accustomed to give way to their moods[,] never having learned to discipline their wills."[44]

However, Ferenczi rejected Meige and Feindel's explanation that these behaviors resulted from a predisposition or from degeneration. In particular, Ferenczi claimed, Meige and Feindel neglected the unconscious sexual component that underlay all tics.[45]

Ferenczi's explanations formed the bedrock of all future psychoanalytic claims about the causes of tics and involuntary cursing. Like Ferenczi's attempt to find legitimation in Freud, others returned to Ferenczi's 1921 statements with a reverence generally reserved for the master himself.[46] Yet, ironically, Ferenczi's claims were based on the cases and writings of Charcot's descendants, Meige and Feindel, rather than Freud. Like Gilles de la Tourette, Ferenczi erected his typology and conclusions on a patient he had never examined. Following Ferenczi, a generation of psychoanalysts would frame their diagnosis and treatment of actual patients on an emblematic patient whose psychoanalytic diagnosis was based on textual interpretation rather than on clinical interaction.

Freddie and Pete Encounter Margaret Mahler

The most important of Ferenczi's interpreters was his student, Hungarian-born pediatrician and neurologist Margaret Schoenberger Mahler (1897–1985). From 1943 to 1949 Mahler produced a series of articles that reintroduced the designation "Gilles de la Tourette's Disease," remolding it into a psychoanalytic frame as "tic syndrome." Although Mahler adopted Gilles de la Tourette's description of the symptom course, she parted company with his explanation of the underlying causes of these behaviors. If the signs and symptoms of Tourette's disease were identifiable, the cause of the condition, wrote Mahler, was obscure. Mahler believed that convulsive tics most often had an organic substrate, but that tic behaviors manifested themselves only in those susceptible children who had experienced severe, repressed familial psychological conflicts. That is, the organic factors were necessary, but not sufficient by themselves to produce tics. "There is quite likely a substratum of organic disease," wrote Mahler and neurologist Leo Rangell in 1943. "The important fact, however, is that this factor in itself would be insufficient to bring on the syndrome, but that it renders the individual defenseless against overwhelming emotional and psychodynamic forces." Therefore, like Ferenczi, Mahler emphasized the need for intervention on the psychic rather than the somatic level.[47]

Coauthored with Rangell, who focused on the neurological issues, the paper discussed the ticcing behaviors of an eleven-year-old boy named Freddie. Freddie's case became the focus for discussion of a number of other psychoanalytic studies and an exemplar for psychosomatic tic syndrome.[48] Freddie was seven years old when his first eye blinking began. This was soon followed by head twitching, arm shaking, lip puckering, and tongue protrusions. At night, Freddie's body shook as he attempted to fall asleep. His mother often had to take him out walking in the middle of the night to relieve his restlessness. Then Freddie began making involuntary noises that resembled a dog or cat, which caused him great difficulty at school. When agitated or excited, Freddie imitated others' words and actions. Although his symptoms briefly lessened in intensity, they always returned with renewed force and additional involuntary movements and behaviors.[49]

Mahler and Rangell observed Freddie for more than two and a half years. Although they wrote that it was likely that Freddie evidenced a "constitutional inferiority of the subcortical structures producing physiological dysfunction," they insisted that this in itself was insufficient to account for his symptoms. Rather, the organic component "renders the individual defenseless against overwhelming emotional and psychodynamic forces." Freddie's motor and vocal tics were a "psychiatrically determined . . . pathological attempt to solve a conflict situation."[50]

Freddie's medical history revealed a number of striking and puzzling organic features. Mahler and Rangell suspected, but could not verify, an earlier encephalitis, which given Mahler's view should have excluded her diagnosis of tic syndrome. Tonsillitis, resulting in a tonsillectomy at age four, and frequent ear infections suggested a history of streptococcal infections. Most interesting was that when examined for a month in 1941 after an episode of severe tics, Freddie's temperature daily rose to between 100 and 101 degrees without any evident cause. This was accompanied by an increase in his pulse rate to 110. The temperature generally elevated at midday, and once it reached 103. Freddie sweated excessively. He was obese, which his examiners attributed to his insatiable appetite. A Rorschach test was interpreted as indicating that Freddie suffered from a mild neurophysiological disorder and that his tics might be due to an epileptic condition.[51]

Unable to explain Freddie's peculiar somatic symptoms, Mahler and Rangell focused their analysis and treatment on the psychological. They attributed Freddie's obesity to his mother's having overindulged him with food, "compensating for her conscious as well as unconscious guilt feelings" because "Freddie was an unplanned, unwanted child" who the mother had attempted to abort during pregnancy. Freddie's nausea with occasional vomiting was attributed to hysteria.[52]

The onset of Freddie's tics was connected to his ambivalent feelings toward his older brother Gilbert. In seeking to obtain approval from Gilbert, wrote Mahler and Rangell, Freddie imitated the eye blinks of Gilbert's close friend and play companion. This, the therapists explained, satisfied an unconscious wish that Gilbert would view his younger sibling as a substitute for the blinking companion. When Gilbert ignored his younger brother in favor of others, Freddie's involuntary movements exacerbated. Freddie was also angry at Gilbert for abandoning him and developed night restlessness, which, according to his psychiatrists, was an attempt to seek revenge against Gilbert, with whom he shared a room. Simultaneously, this provoked guilt in Freddie, which only intensified his involuntary movements. "Gilbert can't study because of my movements," Freddie admitted, "and might even fail in school."[53]

Freddie displayed no coprolalia. Yet this very lack of obscenity—Freddie "kept his own vocabulary spotlessly free of any dubious words and shunned and avoided such expressions by others"—convinced Mahler and Rangell that he was "defending himself against the latent existence of 'mental coprolalia.'" Finally, according to his therapists, Freddie was addicted to excitement. He went to the movies as often as possible and "devoured" comic books and action stories. It was in these instances that Freddie's imitative tendencies (echolalia and echopraxia) manifested themselves most persistently.[54]

Having identified the centrality of psychological mechanisms to Freddie's behavior, Mahler and Rangell, nevertheless, were not sanguine about the long-term efficacy of psychotherapy. Reporting that Freddie's symptoms had improved during psychotherapy, the two therapists did "not wish to convey the impression that they believe the course of the disease has been checked, or that any permanent or basic changes have taken place." *Maladie des tics* was a relentless disease and Freddie's prognosis, they concluded, was "unfavorable" because of "a substratum of organic disease or deficiency, the dominance of and lack of control over the subcortical system of expressional motility, and the inability to retain inner stimuli without discharge."[55]

On the one hand, Mahler and Rangell insisted that organic factors merely provided the soil in which childhood conflict might manifest itself in vocal and motor tics. On the other hand, the failure of psychoanalytic therapies to eradicate these symptoms was laid at the feet of their organic cause, which Mahler and Rangell argued was insufficient, in the absence of psychic conflicts, to bring on the condition in the first place. As contradictory as this reasoning may seem in retrospect, it appears to have not lessened the enthusiasm for psychoanalytic interventions in cases of convulsive tics. For whatever limitations psychoanalytic therapeutics displayed in terms of curing these conditions, it was, at least, a fully elucidated system that could be called upon to explain each symptom displayed by those diagnosed with convulsive tics. With its self-proclaimed psychosomatism, psychoanalytic interventions appeared to be integrating whatever organic elements contributed to tics. From that perspective, psychoanalysts were able to lay claim to both the psychic and somatic traditions.

In July 1945, Mahler edited a collection of articles she had solicited for the journal the *Nervous Child*, which she conceived as serving as an overview and for psychiatric diagnosis and treatment of pediatric tic syndrome.[56] The collection elaborated and endorsed Mahler's psychosomatic theory of tics; most of the contributors drew directly on Mahler's published diagnoses and treatment of patients. To these "typical cases" Mahler and her colleague Irma Gross added the case of Pete.[57]

Pete was an eleven-and-a-half-year-old boy whom Mahler and Gross had selected as a patient with a typical example of tic syndrome.[58] Pete's case, along with Mahler and Rangell's 1943 case study of Freddie, would become emblematic touchstones for psychoanalysts as they wrestled with the diagnosis and treatment of tics for the next quarter century.

Pete's initial symptoms—throat clearing, rolling his eyes, mouth twitching, yawning, and stretching his neck—appeared when he was three or four. These continued, waxing and waning, even disappearing entirely for a year, until Pete was ten. Then the symptoms reappeared with increased intensity and with frequent vocalizations. This combination of tics and uncontrolled vocalizations expressed themselves on Pete's entire body, including his face, diaphragm, trunk, and extremities, and incapacitated him. Pete was admitted to Mahler's care at the Psychiatric Institute and Hospital in January 1945.[59]

Mahler and Gross's psychoanalytic examination convinced them that Pete's behaviors resulted from his anxious grandmother and his mother having "overindulged and infantalized the boy." This served as evidence for Mahler's main thesis that conflict over Pete's motor freedom by his caregivers was typical of children with tic syndrome. Mahler and Gross uncovered three other typical factors in Pete's case—phobic fears, frequent occurrence and discussion about accidents, and overattention to his body.[60]

Initially Pete was allowed to introduce any subject for discussion, but eventually Mahler moved the focus to what she believed to be Pete's "basic problems," which were sexual in nature. Mahler and Gross interpreted Pete's initial nonchalance and putative disinterest about sexual issues as a signal of his repressed concerns with sexuality:

> In discussing sexual material Pete adopted an attitude of objective matter-of-fact interest and inquisitiveness. For instance, he asked a series of questions of a scientific nature, starting with the structure of snow flakes, which were then falling, going over the crystallography in general, and ending with his statement: "The more you know of this stuff, the more interesting it is. It is not like sex. My cousin used to tease me because I didn't know about sex . . . so now I know it, and there is nothing much to it. It's not so interesting." In

fact, we may assume that Pete really meant that sex *is* the subject which seems inexhaustibly interesting to him.[61]

As with the noncursing Freddie, Mahler uncovered repressed coprolalia in Pete. His sexual fantasies and preoccupations, according to Mahler and Gross, were both forerunners of and the "noncrystallized equivalents" of involuntary cursing.[62] Pete grew depressed and discouraged because his tics did not abate and complained to his mother that psychiatry was "witchcraft and superstition." When questioned by his therapist about these attitudes, Pete responded, "It's silly that's all. All this talk. How can it help me? It's like the Middle Ages. Those faith healers. That's just like this business."[63] Mahler attributed Pete's outburst to the therapy's success in exposing the unconscious sexual issues that had enabled Pete's tics and the boy's fear of his own sexuality. To prove the point, Mahler asked Pete if he knew how condoms worked. "Because they have no holes, they keep the germs from getting in or out," Pete replied. Pete's use of the term "germs," which the therapists had introduced in the first place, revealed their patient's fears and preoccupations. Their evidence for this was Pete's question about what type of germs caused elephantiasis and dropsy, diseases he had read about in *Life* magazine. His query was interpreted by Mahler and Gross as reflecting Pete's obsession with masturbation: "Pete worried about his swellings, and the probability of his awareness that during mumps [which he recently had] the testes may become involved was interpreted as the motivation for his present preoccupation with such 'swellings' as elephantiasis and dropsy. He admitted knowing that his testes could have been affected while denying any concern with his characteristic defense: 'I didn't have to watch them; I figured that if they got it they'd swell up and hurt just the way my face did.'" Pete's refusal to acknowledge his fear that mumps could cause his testes to swell protected him from discussing other swellings of his genitals—erections. When Mahler connected these issues, Pete "characteristically felt like dropping the disquieting subject, and went on in the next interviews with minute reports on his tics."[64] Mahler and Gross saw this reaction as proof of Pete's fear of his own erections.

During his free associations Pete had connected putting his hands on dangerous places with having discovered condoms in his parents' dresser drawers.[65] Pete's therapists believed that this association again pointed to the issue of masturbation. First, they pointed to Pete's conspicuous preoccupation with his body, moving from concerns about swelling to his hands. Second, Pete's report of his mother's statement that it was "too late" for her to get pregnant revealed his own displaced anxieties about using up his reproductive energy through masturbation. Third, Pete tended to turn all discussions toward sexual matters. Next, Pete was ambivalent toward adult authority, which restrained his freedom while protecting him from unwanted sexual impulses. Finally, Pete's dream of his arm moving back to touch a warm radiator was, for Mahler and Gross, clearly symbolic of masturbatory ambivalence.[66]

Succeeding interviews more explicitly elicited questions from Pete about erections and, finally, after much prodding, masturbation itself. Pete was also informed that his conflicted feelings about masturbation could have led to his tics. He remained skeptical: "You told me the tics came because of the mixed-up feelings and lots of those feelings have to do with the sex business. Well," Pete reminded his doctors, "I've had tics since I was about 3 years old. How does that fit in?"

At this point, reported Mahler and Gross, Pete's tics had abated with only residual eye deviations and eyebrow elevations. Several weeks later, Pete's facial tics returned. His therapists attributed this exacerbation to their treatment of a new patient, resulting in a sibling rivalry as Pete and the new patient competed for psychiatric attention. In the end, by the summer of 1945, Pete was less satisfied than his caretakers, who pronounced him cured.[67]

In May 1946 Mahler and her colleague Jean Luke coauthored a follow-up of ten pediatric ticcing patients that was published in the *Journal of Nervous and Mental Diseases*. While in an earlier follow-up study the team had examined the charts of eighteen ticcing children, Mahler and Luke reduced the number to ten, excluding all girls from the sample. Although Freddie had been part of the earlier follow-up study, he was dropped from this study. Mahler and Luke explained that they had discarded many cases of proven organic involvement or psychosis in which tic syndrome was only a complicating factor. Thus Freddie and Pete, whose cases already were and would continue to serve as exemplars of Mahler's tic syndrome, were eliminated from her most detailed examination of the outcome of psychotherapy. She had decided that, strictly speaking, neither fit her criteria for tic syndrome in the first place.[68]

Mahler and Luke's most sobering finding was that psychotherapy often failed to remove or even ameliorate a patient's tics (435, 440–41). Mahler and Luke, however, did not conclude that psychoanalysis should be jettisoned in cases of tic. To the contrary, psychotherapy retained its central role, once that role was clearly understood. The disappearance of ticcing symptoms was not the chief aim of therapy because "disappearance of the tics was not always accompanied by improvements in the total personality." In fact, in some cases, overall adjustment was reached even though a few tics persisted, whereas in other cases where the tics disappeared, the patient remained psychologically disabled. This confirmed the wisdom of the psychoanalytic concept that the "symptoms serve the purpose of discharging dammed-up instinctual impulses in a pathologic way. Thus, the tics represent a kind of morbid release, a safety valve for release of tension" (42–43).

From this perspective Mahler had reconstructed the apparent failure of her method to relieve vocal and motor tics as a success, whereby the goal of treatment was no longer merely symptomatic relief, but rather avoidance of a greater psychopathology that might follow if the patient's need for release from dammed-up libido was restrained by removing the ticcing behaviors. Early intervention was essential; doing nothing was dangerous because, Mahler warned, even when tic syndrome seemed to disappear, it was usually replaced by a severe personality disorder (445).

In 1949 Mahler wrote about tic syndrome for the last time. Reviewing sixty cases of children diagnosed with tic, Mahler reaffirmed her belief that tic syndrome resulted when overprotective mothers infantilized their (overwhelmingly male) children who already had a constitutional tendency toward hypermotility. Mahler sought to refine her earlier findings, confirming again in this study that psychotherapy appeared to have little impact on ticcing symptoms. Attempting to separate the therapeutic successes from the failures, Mahler, who initially had segregated infectious causes of tics to establish a psychogenic type she called tic syndrome, drew a further distinction between "tic disease" and "impulsive tiqueurs." Tic disease, according to Mahler, was a psychosomatic "organ neurosis of the neuromuscular apparatus" in which the tics "in themselves represent the central and essential disturbance." Impulsive ticcers, by contrast, were those whose tics were a sign or symptom of other psychopathologies. Although the grounds for such a distinction among her patients were far from overwhelming, Mahler erected the categories to help explain, ex post facto, why some ticcers got better and others did not. Surprisingly, she claimed that the prognosis was "relatively favorable" for those with tic disease in contrast with those for whom tics were merely a symptom of a deeper disorder. Like her predecessors, Mahler constructed a self-evident solution—those who were cured suffered from a different disorder from those who were not.[69]

Although the aim of Mahler's typological distinction was to alert therapists about the types of children who might experience the best clinical outcomes, Mahler's discussion of her patients betrayed extreme frustration. In fact, one might read her language as an indictment of the afflicted. Mahler declared that those children with tic disease were the most rigid and resistive to giving up defensive mechanisms. They "lack spontaneity and initiative" and "defend themselves by overcompliance." By doing so, children with tic disease "have complied with their mother's wish for their remaining vegetative creatures, with no will and intention of their own." By contrast, the "impulsive tiqueur, . . . like a delinquent, is artful in evading therapeutic interference by 'acting out' and projection mechanisms."[70] It seemed that Mahler had concluded that the greatest obstacles to effective treatment of tics were the patients and their mothers, rather than the disorder itself.

"Twitchy": Emblem of a New Paradigm

TS first came to wide contemporary public knowledge in 1972 when a group of New York City area parents of afflicted children launched The Tourette Syndrome Association (TSA). The leaders of the TSA were most intent on replacing the dominant psychoanalytic framework that tied TS to bad parenting and early childhood sexual conflict. They were spurred on by the work of New York psychiatrist Arthur K. Shapiro, associate clinical professor at New York Hospital, Cornell Medical Center, and his wife, clinical psychologist Elaine Shapiro.

In April 1965 a twenty-four-year-old woman was referred to the Shapiros for psychotherapy. They reported that the woman's "symptoms were striking and bizarre: spasmodic jerking of the head, neck, shoulders, arms, and torso; various facial grimaces; odd barking and grunting sounds; frequent throat clearing; and periodic and forceful protrusion of the tongue."[71] Although she displayed no coprolalia during the initial visit, the woman reported that at other times she could not restrain herself from occasionally shouting out the word "cocksucker." When the patient was ten, sometime after she had begun biweekly injections of an unnamed medication for hay fever, her arms began to twitch, "shortly followed by twitching and jerking of the head and neck." Her signs and symptoms increased and by high school her movements had led her classmates to refer to her as "Twitchy." Although they waxed and waned over the years, the twitching and jerking always returned, "insidiously worsened." At age twenty-two, "short, loud screams began," followed six months later by "throat-clearing, rasping and barking noises, and coprolalia." Although the woman managed to confine her screaming and cursing to when she was home, when out in public "other symptoms increased, such as throat-clearing, barking noises, and tongue-protrusion." Social tensions, wrote the Shapiros, exacerbated her tics. "A representative sample of symptoms occurring during one minute would include twenty jerks of the head, neck, and torso, two tongue-protrusions, and two grunts or barks."[72]

Both her mother and the patient attributed these behaviors to psychological factors. Noticing that the patient could control her tics and vocalizations for brief periods of time, the mother assumed that her daughter's problem was definitely not organic, a view shared by the referring psychiatrist, whose diagnosis was "habit tic with hysterical personality." The patient herself admitted that when she "occasionally saw someone twitching and jerking, her immediate reaction was that the person was crazy."[73]

Elaine Shapiro recalled when "this first patient" walked into Arthur Shapiro's office. "I know that Arthur was absolutely convinced," she said, "that the cause of the patient's disorder was organic, not psychological."[74] Hospitalizing the woman for the next several months, Shapiro administered thirty-six neuroleptics and antidepressants and combinations of drugs,[75] settling finally on the major neuroleptic tranquilizer haloperidol (a dopamine antagonist) "because marked improvement had been reported [in medical journals] in five patients." For the succeeding eleven months he treated the young woman with dosages ranging from 1.5 to 10 milligrams per day. "From the first day of treatment," wrote Shapiro, the "symptoms disappeared." At the higher dosages there were, however, severe Parkinson-like side effects. Shapiro finally settled on 3 milligrams per day as the most effective treatment.[76]

In their 1968 article reporting successful treatment of the young woman with haloperidol, Arthur and Elaine Shapiro not only argued that the etiology of these symptoms was an "organic pathology of the central nervous system," but also, at Arthur's insistence, presented their findings as evidence of the therapeutic and intellectual paucity of psychoanalytic psychiatry.[77]

The Shapiros' article laid out a sort of master narrative for all the media stories and testimonials that would follow. This patient's symptoms began at age ten and for the next fourteen years the many physicians who treated her "communicated to the patient and her family that emotional illnesses caused the symptoms." Although psychotherapy did nothing to relieve the woman's symptoms, it did have "a harmful effect on her fantasies and character formation." The woman's earlier diagnosis of "personality disorder with inadequate and passive dependent character traits" was, the Shapiros told their readers, "based on psychiatric impression."[78] From the Shapiros' perspective, psychoanalytic treatment most likely "contributed to the patient's shyness, inhibited aggression, passivity, and fantasies of insanity."[79] The Shapiros decried (in a sentence that they would repeat in several articles) "the fashion in medicine to attribute symptoms and diseases without demonstrable organic pathology to a psychological wastebasket diagnosis." And, with an obvious reference to Mahler's patients, the Shapiros warned that psychoanalytic treatment of these symptoms "may result in iatrogenic [physician-induced] psychopathology. Physicians should be sensitive and cautious about the possible harm to patients of premature psychological diagnosis."[80]

In 1972 a group of New York City area parents, most of whose children were being treated by the Shapiros, organized a support group. The parents, who would soon incorporate and settle on the name The Tourette Syndrome Association (TSA), published personal notices in the *New York Times* inviting those who displayed ticcing symptoms, or whose family members displayed ticcing symptoms, to contact the association.[81]

DO YOU HAVE MULTIPLE TICS?

Involuntary muscular actions, verbal noises, facial tics, repeating actions, or obscene words, foot stamping, head and shoulder jerking, occurring in combination and changing from time to time. For additional information please write to The Gilles de la Tourette Syndrome Association, Inc. Box 3519, Grand Central Station, New York, New York, 10017.[82]

The Shapiros played a central role in the formative years of the association. After 1972, as each of the Shapiros' new studies appeared or a paper was delivered at a professional meeting, it would be presented simultaneously in association meetings and its conclusions would appear in the TSA newsletter. As I discuss more fully below, this collaboration between lay and medical personnel would play a crucial role in shaping the understanding of the Tourette's sufferer. Often the TSA would reprint and distribute these studies to its membership, to those inquiring about Tourette's, and to physicians requesting assistance and information.[83]

Unfortunately, haloperidol did not work for most of Shapiros' patients over the long run.[84] In fact, Arthur Shapiro saw haloperidol as a gross antipsychotic agent whose action could tell us very little about the etiology of the illness.[85] The Shapiros' insistence on an organic etiology of TS essentially rested on their clinical experience and on their profound mistrust of psychoanalysis.

As early as 1972 Arthur Shapiro had concluded that although "haloperidol . . . gives almost complete relief to most Tourette's victims . . . about one-fifth of them get only around 80 percent relief."[86] Most problematic were haloperidol's many side effects even among those patients whose tics it controlled. As a 1972 *Wall Street Journal* article reported, "There is a major drawback to the drug. Since it has to be given in large dosages, Tourette's patients starting treatment usually undergo extremely unpleasant side effects, ranging from frightening muscle contractions in the upper body to restlessness to lethargy. During the first months of treatment, while the dosage is being adjusted, to give maximum relief of symptoms with minimum side effects, patients often have to be coaxed to take the medication."[87]

Interviews with the Shapiros' patients and their families revealed the limitations of haloperidol over time. Even those patients who did not experience Parkinson-like side effects often reported that haloperidol, in the words of one of Shapiro's early patients, turned them into "zombies."[88]

University of Oregon psychiatry professor Paul H. Blachly, whose coauthored 1966 study had reported amazing success with haloperidol,[89] revised his views a decade later in a letter to TSA leader Sheldon Novick. Blachly wrote that even though haloperidol had "decreased the frequency and intensity" of motor and vocal tics his patient "preferred his symptoms to the dysphoric effect [anxiety] induced by the droperidol (intravenous haloperidol)."[90] Abbey Meyers, the New York City TSA coordinator, whose eldest son was under Shapiro's care, reported that although "Haldol controlled his tics, it had turned him into a zombie."[91]

Another patient, "Tommy," who had begun treatment with the drug when he was nine and whose mother's testimonial to Shapiro's treatment appeared in *Good Housekeeping* in 1976,[92] revealed a different story over time. Over the next three years Tommy's symptoms worsened. Shapiro reacted by increasing the dosage of haloperidol. "Paradoxically," his mother reported, Tommy's "TS symptoms seemed to increase as we increased his medication. His side effects were now more alarming because he was experiencing school phobias (even though he maintained an A average), suicidal thoughts," and slow, atypical ticlike movements (possibly tardive dyskinesia) that she feared may have been brought on by the medication. Tommy's parents had him hospitalized at the Yale Child Study Center under the supervision of Dr. Donald Cohen. "Amazingly," the mother remembers, "as they detoxified him and took him off all drugs, his TS symptoms became milder and milder. Also, his suicidal thoughts vanished and he said he was looking forward to returning to school."[93]

In fact, the TSA had been receiving letters since the late 1970s from its members complaining about the deadening effects of haloperidol. One mother, an officer of the San Diego chapter, wondered whether "squelching a child's tics completely, to make it possible for *us* to deny he had a problem, or for him to stay in public school or be on a team or in a club, is as ghastly as child-beating—it's only more subtle and more sophisticated." The decision of whether to continue her child on haloperidol was "sort of like being asked which leg we would like to have cut off. Do we want to have our child ostracized from school, sports, and friendships because of tics—or do we want him to be taken places with oatmeal between his gears instead of oil, deprived of the only tools he can really develop to create his own life out of the raw material nature has given him?"[94] As a result of these letters and her own child's experience, Meyers, the New York TSA coordinator, alerted the membership in July 1980 that "since the majority of children [diagnosed with Tourette's] are treated with Haldol, parents and teachers must be aware that this medication can add to their child's problems by blunting cognitive processes."[95]

In October 1980 Elaine Shapiro moderated a panel of six young adults diagnosed with TS. Only two were still using haloperidol. One of them, twenty-year-old Phyllis, had been diagnosed only the previous year when she was put on Haldol. Two others had switched to the norepinephrine enhancer clonidine (Catapres), a drug approved only for use to control high blood pressure. Orrin Palmer, who had been Shapiro's patient since 1965, had recently graduated from college and would soon enter medical school. He reported, contrary to the emblematic story that had appeared about him in 1975 in *Today's Health*, that he had "not been helped by any medication."[96]

By 1981, although numerous medical and popular articles hailed haloperidol as a miracle drug for the treatment of TS, patients, their families, and physicians increasingly expressed reservations about the drug's side effects. One of the leaders of the TSA revealed in 1981 that in 1975 when Shapiro had placed his seven-year-old child "on a low dosage of haloperidol, the symptoms improved remarkably. However several months later the symptoms returned and were more severe and the medication dosage was increased [to] 20 mgs. of haloperidol per day. Not only did this prove to be ineffective, but our child developed side effects, not completely recognized at the time." The parent reported that his child's problems included "difficulty in concentrating on school work, restlessness and marked problems with hand-writing. This child, who is still remembered by her first grade teacher as one of the most intellectually gifted students she had, was intellectually impaired in the second and third grades." The effects of haloperidol were so devastating that the child "had to be transferred to a private school so that there would be less pressure . . . by the teacher, who couldn't deal with her problems of restlessness and difficulty in concentrating." And, the father added, these side effects "brought ostracism socially, making for a most painful childhood."[97]

Concerns like these had become so numerous by 1983 that the new TSA medical committee chair, Ruth Bruun, wrote a column in the newsletter asking patients and their families not to overreact to reports about the potential side effects of haloperidol. Bruun was convinced that "though well intentioned, this negative information may have been overemphasized, and may actually be preventing some patients from receiving treatment which otherwise might be helpful to them." The problem, Bruun implied, may be that insufficiently experienced practitioners were unaware that "the accepted treatment methods for both Haldol and Catapres involve a very slow and cautious increase of medications and much attention to the development of side effects."[98]

Unfortunately, things have not improved for florid patients in the last thirty years. Like the Shapiros' patients in the 1980s, our patient Toby was treated with Haldol when in his twenties, but like so many others, he could not tolerate the side effects. In fact, Toby's reaction to the drug resulted in psychosis: "I started to hit my face and [bite my] nails" and I "locked myself in the room because I didn't [want] people to find me." Rushed to a hospital, Toby was sedated and put in a straightjacket. His caretakers increased the Haldol dose, but Toby remembered, "I got worse and worse because they were raising up the Haldol, and I got to a point where they had to take me out a lot of time on hand cuffs. . . . I could not think straight . . . I was beating the shit out of myself. I was tired. I just wanted to close my eyes and not wake up anymore." Toby gained 130 pounds while on Haldol and had pulled out almost all his teeth. "I was hurting, the whole body was hurting. It was almost like, and I don't believe in the devil or anything, it was almost like my body was taken over by evil spirits." Finally taken off the drug, Toby's psychosis remitted, but his TS remained. Today Toby is on a combination of neuroleptics, but he is convinced that what best relieves his tics is daily use of marijuana. "If I take a joint of three or four inches of it, it goes away for a few hours. . . . It's illegal [but] it's the only thing that takes the tics away."[99]

The New Confinement of the Florid Patient

The goal of the initial founders of the TSA, all of whose children exhibited florid cases of TS, was to persuade the public that the bizarre behaviors associated with patients like my neighbor Michael, our patient Toby, and their own children was an organic illness rather than a result of defective parenting or of ill-behaved children. They also wished to move the medical research community to adopt a sustained research program aimed at finding an organic etiology for TS. More than forty years later, funded research has increased exponentially, but, despite periodic announcements of breakthroughs, the etiology of TS remains elusive. Meanwhile, due to increased diagnoses, enabled by heightened awareness and by a broadened case definition, the TS population has grown significantly. Along the way, the disorder's most familiar and devastating marker, the cursing patient, has become increasingly marginalized. As in the days before the Shapiros' groundbreaking work, florid patients are in danger of being consigned almost to invisibility. It is as if the continued presence of the cursing patient threatens the claims of therapeutic success, including the dominant paradigmatic assumption that the cause of TS can yet be found in the genome. But florid patients do live on, now as adults, often without support networks or robust health care. Some of them drift in and out of our adult psychiatry clinic at Emory University. There are, however, few clinics for adult TS patients or even psychiatrists trained to treat them. In the worst, but unfortunately not untypical scenario, florid TS sufferers turn to self-medicating agents ranging from nicotine and marijuana to alcohol and illicit substances. Often they wander isolated and lonely on the fringes of society.

Despite efforts, florid sufferers remain objects rather than subjects. "I often wish doctors and researchers would leave the comfort of their laboratories and offices to spend time at a local TSA support group meeting," writes Susan Hughes, a mother of an afflicted child. "I believe they would gain more knowledge from listening to parents and hearing the family histories than they would learn from drawing another tube of blood, ordering another EEG or completing another questionnaire."[100] Reporting on his experience at the First International Tourette Syndrome Symposium held in 1981, neurologist Oliver Sacks noted that the "ninety-odd papers . . . while presenting a vast amount of new and exciting information, gave no feel whatsoever of what it was like to have Tourette's." As a Tourette-afflicted friend of Sacks reacted, "I don't know what they are talking about, they are not talking about me. They don't put across what Tourette's is really like."[101]

More than any other individual, Sacks has made a concerted effort to listen to what patients reveal about their experience with TS. Encouraged In 1974 by Sheldon Novick, the first TSA medical director,[102] Sacks, reluctant at first, would soon become the most well-known and influential translator of the patient experience to a wide lay audience. Sacks humanized the TS patient experience through a series of individual portraits that in combination suggested that those who embraced rather than fought their neurological challenges might find hidden talents or, at least, positive strategies to engage their TS in the service of their work and life. His famous 1985 collection, *The Man Who Mistook His Wife for a Hat,* included the essay "Witty, Ticcy Ray." Ray, according to Sacks, had transformed his otherwise debilitating tic into the service of his talent as a drummer. Faced with the hypothetical choice of losing his tics and musical skills if his TS were suddenly cured, Ray, according to Sacks, chose his Tourettic personality.[103] Writing in the *New York Review of Books* in 1987, Sacks pleaded with his fellow neuropsychiatrists to "listen minutely to our patients, and observe them, everything about them, with a comprehensive eye."[104] His 1992 *New Yorker* article describing the life of a surgeon who, despite his florid TS, not only performed surgery but also flew small airplanes, argued that florid TS need not lead to a life in isolation.[105]

As Sacks has shown us, practitioners and researchers can gain much from listening to what florid patients and their families tell them. But the history of TS tells a different story. Rather than listening to the Marquise de Dampierre, her medical commentators appropriated her symptoms to shore up their preconceived theories. As a result, subsequent physicians concentrated on the patient's will, ignoring the repeated testimony by the afflicted that they were unable to control their symptoms (at least for more than a brief period). Meige and Feindel's influential twentieth-century text appropriated the "confessions" of O. to demonstrate that ticcers could not be trusted.[106] Throughout the twentieth century, those who treated ticcers (by whatever method was in vogue) rarely heeded their patients' complaints that their problem was their tics. Ironically, it was the psychoanalysts who appeared to pay the least attention to their patients' words. Thus Mahler's eleven-year-old patient Pete, frustrated that his therapist refused to see his tics as his central problem, proclaimed that psychoanalysis was "witchcraft."

Today, influenced by the success of pharmacological agents for symptom control and theories that suggest we focus on the patient's affect rather than the content of their words, practitioners often neglect to listen carefully to the particular experiences that patients and their families report. For instance, our patient Toby attributes his successful life (teaching children with disabilities, being married, and having a child) to the ongoing support of his parents, who expected from him as a child as much as they did from his non-TS brother, but were totally supportive at his darkest moments. Toby finds a similar balance from his "strict" but loving wife.

Even if more is learned about how genetic and postinfectious factors may combine to produce involuntary tics and eruptive vocalizations, patients and their families will still require the empathetic skills of their practitioners. "The medical and mental health communities are venturing to make sense of Tourette syndrome," wrote Adam Ward Seligman and John H. Hilkevich in their 1992 collection of essays. "For those of us afflicted with it and those who live and work with us, making sense of it may be less important than finding ways to use it, even to be empowered by it."[107] TS, writes photojournalist and florid sufferer Lowell Handler, "is a rhythm I am stuck with, which will continue for my lifetime and for the lifetime of everyone it affects."[108]

Seligman, Hilkevich, and Handler suffer from florid cases of Tourette's; they blurt out words and phrases despite their attempts to suppress them. TS is most debilitating when its persistent symptoms include echolalia, shouting out inappropriate phrases, compulsive touching, and, most of all, eruptive cursing. Of course, tics and vocalizations alone can be extraordinarily troublesome and debilitating. But patient histories going back almost two centuries, when combined with clinical experience, observations at TS support groups, and interactions with TS sufferers, reinforce the reality that the greatest distress and debility come with the most persistent and florid symptoms, especially those that include coprolalia. In part, this is because the florid afflicted suffer from the greatest public and private humiliation and thus the most social isolation.

Befriended and encouraged by Oliver Sacks, a number of florid Touretters including Adam Seligman and Lowell Handler have attempted to use their life histories as exemplars of florid TS. Unfortunately these efforts have had mixed results. Seligman's life and tragic death at age thirty-seven in 1999 serves as a reminder of the price exacted from the marginalization of the adult florid patient. At eighteen, Seligman like so many other patients was unable to tolerate haloperidol. However, another dopamine antagonist, Orap (pimozide), seemed to provide relief. Unavailable in the United States, Seligman transported Orap (illegally) from Canada. When US customs agents seized Seligman's drugs at the Canadian border, he appealed to his congressman for assistance. That congressman, Henry Waxman, happened also to be chair of the House Subcommittee on Health and Environment.

At an FDA hearing in Washington, DC, on June 26, 1980, Seligman, Handler, and TSA leader Abbey Meyers gave impassioned testimony about Tourette's and the need for federal support for "orphan drugs" like pimozide.[109] The hearing received national press coverage, including major stories in both the *New York Times* and the *Los Angeles Times*. These accounts, particularly of young Seligman's testimony, caught the attention of Maurice

Klugman, producer of the popular weekly television series *Quincy*, starring Maurice's brother Jack Klugman. Maurice decided to devote an episode (March 4, 1981) to Tourette's and the problems that patients like Seligman faced in obtaining potentially effective drugs like pimozide. *Quincy* not only educated the American public about Tourette's as an organic disorder, but also helped get the then stalled Orphan Drug Bill passed by the House of Representatives and eventually, in January 1983, signed into legislation that made it much easier for pharmaceutical firms to undertake the development of so-called orphan drugs.[110]

Seligman's action was lauded at national and local TSA meetings where he retold his story. However, Orap, as with other drugs Seligman tried, would prove ineffective. Unable to control his florid TS, Seligman embraced it and dedicated himself to serving as a living example of the difficulty and possibility of living with TS. By the late 1980s, Seligman was a fixture at national TSA meetings, a symbol of the victories possible through patient activism. However, as so often is the case among those for whom dopamine antagonists (and their combinations) fail, Seligman turned to other substances for self-medication, in his case alcohol. By 1992, thanks to a twelve-step program, Seligman had weaned himself off alcohol. In 1991 he published a novel, *Echolalia: An Adult's Story of Tourette Syndrome*,[111] and in 1993 he published, with fellow TS sufferer John Hilkevich, *Don't Think About Monkeys*, with a foreword by Oliver Sacks. That year Seligman married a young woman, also afflicted with TS.

Seligman, with his florid symptoms unabated, also served as a reminder of the failure of antipsychotics to alter emblematic TS.[112] Though embracing his illness, Seligman was no longer asked to participate on national TSA panels. The more he attempted to reinsert himself into the professional dialogue, the more he suffered rejection. By the mid-1990s Seligman could be found at national and regional TSA meetings, sitting behind a table hawking his poetry and books.[113] Excluded from participation in the conversation about the illness that had become his identity, Seligman died literally of a broken heart in 1999.

Like Seligman, Lowell Handler, twenty-seven at the time of his testimony at the orphan drug bill hearings, would find no long-term solution to his florid tics with Orap. Like Seligman, Handler turned to self-medication, in his case to marijuana. His addiction cost him his marriage. Like Seligman, Handler, befriended in his twenties by Oliver Sacks, concluded that his salvation rested in embracing his TS rather than, like O. and so many others, trying to cure it. In contrast to Seligman, Handler's strategy seems to have proven more successful, but the story he tells is all too familiar. His widely acclaimed 1998 documentary, *Twitch and Shout: A Touretter's Tale*, and the book of the same title, are powerful portrayals of the isolation and humiliation that accompanies adults with florid TS. Although Handler provides a narrative of triumph over adversity, he reminds his viewers and readers that his victories are tentative because "Tourette is unpredictable [and it] . . . is part of my life, not always good, but . . . an integral facet of an ever-evolving personality."[114] And the sad truth is that few adults with florid TS can point to even modest victories.[115]

By *DSM-IV* criteria, those who curse represent a statistical minority. In addition, recent studies have suggested that mild TS may be a common developmental disorder in young children. Weary of the association of TS as a cursing disease, patient support groups have increasingly attempted to distance the public portrayal of TS from its most florid symptoms.

As the TS phenotype has been broadened, we run the risk of sanitizing TS and, in the process, unintentionally, characterizing its most florid victims as "other" and "exceptions." In short, we run the risk of stigmatizing those who, through no fault of their own, are compelled by a brain malfunction to curse because they constitute a minority and no longer represent the "real" problem. Yet, without the stories of these cursing ticcers, from the Marquise de Dampierre in the 1820s to the late twentieth-century articles and books by Oliver Sacks, Adam Seligman, and Lowell Handler, the world never would have been educated about TS in the first place.

With the exception of *Twitch and Shout*, recent documentaries about TS aimed at the general public and worried parents rarely focus on the florid patient. The 2005 TSA film, *I Have Tourette but Tourette Doesn't Have Me*, highlights a group of exceedingly gifted young people, most of whom have relatively mild presentations.[116] But TS afflicts a wide spectrum of the pediatric population, most of whom have ordinary talents and a number of whom have florid presentation that, unfortunately, places them at great risk of having experiences as adults similar to those of Seligman, Handler, Michael, and Toby. Indeed, without the stories of adult florid sufferers, psychiatrists, neurologists, and researchers never would have been authorized (or funded) to investigate this disorder, and they never would have been able to treat the less florid majority. It would be a tragedy if now those who are the most afflicted become reclassified as "abnormal" cases of TS and, as a result, resegregated. In widening the TS phenotype to include more children, those with florid TS represent a minority. But a well-meaning attempt to reassure parents that their diagnosed children will neither curse nor display other florid symptoms should not authorize us to neglect those who do. This would serve as a gothic reenactment of times past when the afflicted were blamed for our failure to ameliorate their suffering.

Notes

I thank Shlomit Ritz Finkelstein, PhD, and Jorge Juncos, MD, for our many conversations and for supplying me with the transcripts of "Toby" and other patients as part of our larger study, Shlomit Ritz Finkelstein, Howard I. Kushner, and Jorge Juncos, "Adult Patients with Tourette Syndrome." The study was approved by a full board committee of the Emory University Institutional Review Board on June 19, 2007, IRB00002397. Thanks to Roger Freeman, MD, for his many midcourse corrections of my work and to Carol R. Kushner for her editorial assistance. Financial Disclosure Statement: No Industry Funding. Research supported by: National Institutes of Health, National Institute on Drug Abuse, 1RO1 DA015707-01A2, "Current Smokers: A Phenomenological Inquiry," 2004–8; National Institutes of Health, National Library of Medicine, G13LM007855, "Public Education and Communication on Improving Health Care Delivery for Kawasaki Disease," 2004–8; and Engelhard Foundation, "Sophomore Year at Emory, Living and Learning Experience: An Interdisciplinary Seminar Course/Internship in Addiction and Depression," 2005–8. All translations in this article are my own.

1. Shlomit Ritz Finkelstein, Jorge L. Juncos, Rob Poh, and Howard I. Kushner, unpublished interview with "Toby," August 6, 2007, TQA. Emory University, Department of Psychiatry.

2. Adam Ward Seligman and John S. Hilkevich, eds., *Don't Think About Monkeys* (Duarte, CA: Hope Press, 1992), 1–2.

3. For an informative overview see Ruth Dowling Bruun and Bertel Bruun, *A Mind of Its Own: Tourette's Syndrome: A Story and a Guide* (New York: Oxford University Press, 1994).

4. For accounts written by those diagnosed with Tourette's syndrome, see Seligman and Hilkevich, *Don't Think About Monkeys*; and Lowell Handler, *Twitch and Shout: A Touretter's Tale* (New York: Penguin Press, 1998).

5. As Kathryn Montgomery has recently argued, despite its reliance on scientific knowledge and its use of technology, medicine is not a science. Rather, it is a science-using practice whose goals are to prevent illness and care for the sick. See Kathryn Montgomery, *How Doctors Think: Clinical Judgment and the Practice of Medicine* (New York: Oxford University Press, 2006), viii.

6. Howard I. Kushner, "Medical Fictions: The Case of the Cursing Marquise and the (Re)Construction of Gilles de la Tourette's Syndrome," *Bulletin of the History of Medicine* 69 (1995): 224–54.

7. Georges Gilles de la Tourette, "Étude sur une affection nerveuse caractérisée par de l'incoordination motrice accompagnée d'écholalie et de coprolalie (jumping, latah, myriachit)," *Archives de Neurologie* 9 (1885): 26, 180.

8. Her words in French were "merde" and "foutu cochon," which literally translates into "shit" and "filthy pig," but the more accurate colloquial meaning of "foutu cochon" is "fucking pig." Her obituaries included descriptions of her "notorious" cursing.

9. Chief physician at l'Institution Royale des Sourds-Muets in Paris, Itard had gained worldwide notice twenty-five years earlier as the physician charged with educating Victor, the so-called Wild Child of Aveyron. Lucien Malson, *Wolf Children* (followed by *The Wild Boy of Aveyron* by Jean Itard), trans. Peter Ayrton, Joan White, and Edmund Fawcett (New York: Monthly Review Press, 1972), 91–178. See also Harlan Lane, *The Wild Boy of Aveyron* (Cambridge: Harvard University Press, 1979).

10. Jean M. G. Itard, "Mémoire sur quelques fonctions involontaires des appareils de la locomotion, de la préhension, et de la voix," *Archives Générales de Médecine* 8 (1825): 405.

11. For a detailed discussion of Itard's article, see Kushner, "Medical Fictions, 224–54, esp. 232–36.

12. For a more detailed discussion, see Howard I. Kushner, *A Cursing Brain?: The Histories of Tourette Syndrome* (Cambridge: Harvard University Press, 1999), 19–21.

13. Gilles de la Tourette, "Étude sur une affection nerveuse," 21.

14. Georges Gilles de la Tourette, "La maladie des tics convulsifs," *La Semaine Médicale* 19 (1899): 155–56; and Gilles de la Tourette, "Étude sur une affection nerveuse," 188.

15. See Kushner, *Cursing Brain*, 22–25.

16. See Harold Stevens, "Gilles de la Tourette and his Syndrome by Serendipity," *American Journal of Psychiatry* 128 (1971): 489–91; Arthur K. Shapiro et al., *Gilles de la Tourette Syndrome* (New York: Raven Press, 1978), 15–18; Paul Guilly, "Gilles de la Tourette," in *Historical Aspects of the Neurosciences*, ed. F. C. Rose and W. F. Bynum (New York: Raven Press, 1982), 397–415; A. J. Lees, "Georges Gilles de la Tourette: The Man and his Times," *Revue Neurologique* 142 (1986): 808–16; Michel Dugas, "La maladie des tics: D'Itard aux neuroleptiques," *Revue Neurologique* 142 (1986): 817–23; Arnold J. Friedhoff and Thomas N. Chase, eds., *Gilles de la Tourette Syndrome* (New York: Raven Press, 1982); Mary M. Robertson, "The Gilles de la Tourette Syndrome: The Current Status," *British Journal of Psychiatry* 154 (1989): 147–69; David E. Comings, *Tourette Syndrome and Human Behavior* (Duarte, CA: Hope Press, 1990); and Paul Sandor, "Gilles de la Tourette Syndrome: The Current Status," *Journal of Psychosomatic Research* 37 (1993): 211–26.

17. See Bruun and Bruun, *A Mind of Its Own*, 8–10; and Peter G. Como, "Obsessive-Compulsive Disorder in Tourette's Syndrome," in *Behavioral Neurology of Movement Disorders*, ed. W. J. Weiner and A. E. Lang (New York: Raven Press, 1995), 281.

18. Stanley Finger, *Origins of Neuroscience: A History of Explorations into Brain Function* (New York: Oxford University Press, 1994), 233–34.

19. For a discussion of this phenomenon, see Jerome E. Groopman, *How Doctors Think* (Boston: Houghton Mifflin, 2007), 23–25.

20. Henry Meige and Eduard Feindel, *Tics and Their Treatment*, with a preface by Professor Brissaud [revised and updated version of *Les tics et leur traitement* (1902)], trans. and ed. S. A. Kinnier Wilson (New York: William Wood, 1907), 13.

21. Ibid., 1.

22. Ibid. Meige and Feindel's search for an "ideal" ticceur is reminiscent of Charcot's standard procedure of seeking a typical, exemplary patient that would serve for a model in a variety of syndromes.

23. Henry Meige and Eduard Feindel, "L'état mental des tiqueurs," *Progrès Médical* (September 7, 1900): 146–49; and Meige and Feindel, "Sur la curabilité des tics," *Gazette des Hôpitaux* (June 20, 1901): 673–77.

24. Henry Meige, "Étude sur cértaines névropathes voyageurs: Le juif-errant à la Salpêtrière," *Nouvelle Iconographie de la Salpêtrière* 6 (1893): 191–204, 277–91, 333–58. Meige's text was reprinted and edited with a preface by the French psychoanalyst Lucien Israël, *Le juif-errant à la Salpêtrière* (Paris: Collection Grands Textes, Nouvelle Objet, 1993).

25. Israël, *Le juif-errant à la Salpêtrière*, 22–23, 27, 109.

26. Henry Meige, "Tics variables, tics d'attitude," *Société du Neurologie de Paris (Bulletins officiels)* (July 4, 1901): 249.

27. Henry Meige, "La genèse des tics," *Journal de Neurologie* (June 5, 1902): 201.

28. Meige and Feindel, *Tics and Their Treatment*, 21–22, 328–30, 319–24. Also see Henry Meige and Eduard Feindel, "Traitement des tics," *Presse Médicale* (March 16, 1900): 125–27; Edouard Brissaud and Eduard Feindel, "Sur le traitement du torticolis mental et des tics similaires," *Journal de Neurologie* (April 15, 1899): 141–49; Jean-René Cruchet, "Le tic convulsif et son traitement gymnastique (Mèthode de Brissaud et Mèthode de Pitres)," Thèse pour le Doctorat en Médecine (Bordeaux: G. Gounouilhou, Imprimeur de la Faculté de Médecine, Bordeaux, 1902), 96–97.

29. Meige and Feindel, *Tics and Their Treatment*, 229–30, 22.

30. Citing Meige and Feindel, a British physician wrote in 1907 that "the mental state of [ticcing] patients is frequently not quite normal, the will may be feeble, the power of concentration lacking, and the character in other ways unstable." Eric D. Macnamara, "Habit Spasm," *Westminster Hospital Reports* (1907): 53.

31. E. W. Scripture, "Tics and Their Treatment," *Archives of Pediatrics* 26 (1909): 10–11.

32. A San Francisco physician explained in 1911 that childhood tics developed because "the fatigued mind is stimulated at a time when it should be rested." The treatment of tic was "definitely and intimately connected with the etiology and symptomology [*sic*]" of neurasthenia and "its prevention" was "inherently a part of the prophylaxis of all pediatric nervous states." E. C. Fleischner, "The Treatment of Tic in Childhood," *California State Journal of Medicine*, no. 9 (1911): 379. For a discussion of neurasthenia, see Barbara Sicherman, "The Use of a Diagnosis: Doctors, Patients, and Neurasthenia," *Journal of the History of Medicine* 32 (1977): 33–54.

33. For a discussion of Ferenczi's relationship with Freud, see Peter Gay, *Freud: A Life for Our Time* (New York: Norton, 1988), 187–89, 576–87; and Paul Roazen, *Freud and His Followers* (New York: Knopf, 1974), 355–71.

34. Sandor Ferenczi, "Psycho-Analytical Observation on Tic," *International Journal of Psycho-Analysis* 2 (1921): 10.

35. Ibid., 7.

36. Howard I. Kushner, "Freud and the Diagnosis of Gilles de la Tourette's Illness," *History of Psychiatry* 9 (1998): 1–25.

37. "The circumstance of the Tic being peculiar among neurotic phenomena gives strong support to the idea of Freud regarding the heterogeneous (organic) nature of the symptom." Ferenczi, "Psycho-Analytical Observations on Tic," 2–3.

38. Ibid., 4–5, 10, italics in original.

39. Throughout, Ferenczi spelled "coprolalia" as "copralalia."

40. Ferenczi, "Psycho-Analytical Observations on Tic," 1.

41. J. C. Wilson, "A Case of Tic Convulsif," *Archives of Pediatrics* 14 (1897): 885; and Otto Lerch, "Convulsive Tics," *American Medicine* (November 2, 1901), 695.

42. Ferenczi, "Psycho-Analytical Observations on Tic," 5–10 (italics in the original).

43. Ibid., 6.

44. Ibid., 9–10, 22, quoting Meige and Feindel, *Les tics et leur traitement*, 88–89.

45. Tics, for Ferenczi, increased in power during early puberty, pregnancy, and childhood, at the time "of increased stimulation of the genital regions." This explained why vocal outbursts often developed "into anal-erotic obscenities." For Ferenczi, these behaviors were a "displacement from below upwards"; repressed sexuality, especially repressed masturbatory urges, manifested themselves as a tic. The

"excitability" of ticcers and their "tendency to rhythmical rubbing" was further evidence of the "genitalisation" of tics, which in some cases included "definite orgasm." Ferenczi, "Psycho-Analytical Observations on Tic," 27–28.

46. There were a few exceptions. In 1925 Melanie Klein, one of the founders of the object relations approach to psychoanalysis, wrote that she was in "essential disagreement" with Ferenczi's claim that "the tic is a primary narcissistic symptom having a common source with the narcissistic psychoses." Although Klein endorsed the view "that tic is an equivalent of masturbation," she was convinced that "the tic is not accessible to therapeutic influence so long as the analysis has not succeeded in uncovering the object relations on which it is based." Melanie Klein, "Zur Genese des Tics," *Internationale Zeitschrift für Psychoanalyse* 11 (1925): 332–49; reprinted and translated as "Contribution to the Psychogenesis of Tics," in Melanie Klein, *Contributions to Psychoanalysis, 1921–1945* (London: Hogarth Press, 1968), 117–39; quotation, 133.

47. Klein, "Zur Genese des Tics," 593; and Klein, *Contributions to Psychoanalysis*. Mahler not only had read Gilles de la Tourette, but also was familiar with Charcot's, Guinon's, and Meige and Feindel's views.

48. Psychoanalyst Louise J. Kaplan remembered in 1976 that "Mahler's 1943 [her first] paper on the tic syndrome was instantly recognized as a classic." Louise J. Kaplan, *Oneness and Separateness: From Infant to Individual* (New York: Simon & Schuster, 1978), 15.

49. Margaret Schoenberger Mahler and Leo Rangell, "A Psychosomatic Study of Maladie des Tics (Gilles de la Tourette's Syndrome)," *Psychiatric Quarterly* 17 (1943): 582.

50. Ibid., 592–93.

51. Ibid., 581, 583–84, 593. Mahler and Rangell decided to omit fully reporting the psychological analysis of Freddie's inkblot test. The conclusions were published two years later by Margaret Naumburg, an art therapist hired to work with Freddie. Margaret Naumburg, "The Psychodynamics of the Art Expression of a Boy Patient with Tic Syndrome," *Nervous Child* 4 (1945): 374–409; see 378–79. Naumburg's essay, along with one including Freddie's Rorschach, appeared later in a volume edited by Mahler.

52. Mahler and Rangell, "Psychosomatic Study of Maladie des Tics," 581, 588.

53. Ibid., 585, 587.

54. Ibid., 586–88.

55. Ibid., 600. Part of Freddie's treatment included art therapy with Margaret Naumburg, who published an extensive article on Freddie's therapy including thirty samples of his drawings in Mahler's edited 1945 volume. Naumburg, "Psychodynamics of the Art Expression," 407–8.

56. Margaret Schoenberger Mahler, ed., "Tics in Children," special issue, *Nervous Child* 4 (1945): 306–419.

57. Margaret Schoenberger Mahler and Irma L. Gross, "Psychotherapeutic Study of a Typical Case with Tic Syndrome," *Nervous Child* 4 (1945): 359–73.

58. Ibid., 359.

59. Ibid., 363. Laboratory and neurological examinations revealed no organic problems. Pete was sedated during his seven-and-a-half-week hospital stay, but the sedatives had no effect on his tics. His doctors also attempted to interview Pete under hypnosis induced by sodium amytal. This procedure only caused Pete to fall asleep.

60. Mahler and Gross, "Psychotherapeutic Study," 361–62.

61. Ibid., 364.

62. Ibid.

63. Ibid., 365.

64. Ibid., 365.

65. Ibid., 367. When Pete complained, "As long as you don't give me any 'real' treatment with medicine, it [the tics] will always get better in the hospital and worse again as soon as I go home," Mahler and Gross believed that they had hit psychological pay dirt: "Using his own statement that the tics were bound to increase at home, it was pointed out to him that something in the home environment must have to do with the tics' exacerbation" (366).

66. Ibid., 369.

67. "The little movements are back again. But, the big ones that annoyed me, are still all gone. If those could be cured, why shouldn't these?" (ibid., 371–72). Pete was also the main subject of Zygmunt Piotrowski's essay on Rorschach, which concluded that Pete's "Rorschach record reveals many tensions and conflicting tendencies which might be responsible for the tics." Zygmunt A. Piotrowski, "Rorschach Records of Children With a Tic Syndrome," *Nervous Child* 4 (1945): 350–51.

68. Margaret S. Mahler and Jean A. Luke, "Outcome of the Tic Syndrome," *Journal of Nervous and Mental Diseases* 103 (May 1946): 433–45.

69. Margaret Schoenberger Mahler, "A Psychoanalytic Evaluation of Tic in the Psychopathology of Children: Symptomatic and Tic Syndrome," *Psychoanalytic Study of the Child* (1949): 279–310.

70. Ibid., 307.

71. The original report of this case appeared in Arthur K. Shapiro and Elaine Shapiro, "Treatment of Gilles de la Tourette's Syndrome with Haloperidol," *British Journal of Psychiatry* 114 (1968): 345–50. A more accessible version is in the introductory chapter of Arthur K. Shapiro, Elaine S. Shapiro, Ruth D. Bruun, and Richard D. Sweet, *Gilles de la Tourette Syndrome* (New York: Raven Press, 1978), 1–9; quotation, 1.

72. Shapiro and Shapiro, "Treatment of Gilles de la Tourette's Syndrome with Haloperidol," 345.

73. Ibid., 345–50.

74. Interview with Elaine S. Shapiro, June 13, 1996. Elaine Shapiro sees herself as having played a secondary role to Arthur in the work on Tourette's syndrome. Arthur "was really doing the major work and I was ancillary, but I wasn't thinking about some of the issues as deeply as he was," Elaine asserted in our interview. However, an examination of the record and numerous interviews with those who worked with both during these years suggests that her role ultimately was equal to his. Arthur would discuss every aspect of his work with Elaine and in almost every publication they were joint authors; Elaine took the primary authorship of articles on education and testing.

75. "Each drug was repeated two or three times," including placebos, "pentobarbitone, 90 mg., chlorpromazine, 50 mg., meprobamate, 200–800 mg., diazepam 5 to 10 mg.," with no results. "Slight effect on symptoms was noted with diazepam 20–40 mg., imipramine and amitriptyline 25 to 50 mg." The "best" results were achieved with amitriptyline 75 mg. q.i.d. [four times per day or 300 mg.] and diazepam 10 mg. q.i.d., but this dosage had to be discontinued because of severe mydriasis."

"Improvements had been reported for a combination of drugs which were tried on this patient in the following dosages: trimethadione 300 mg. b.i.d. [twice a day] thioridazine 25 to 100 mg. q.i.d., and trifluoperazine 20 to 50 mg. t.i.d. [three times a day]." Responses were good at even higher dosages, but, reported the Shapiros, "drowsiness, akathisia and mydriasis were severe." Shapiro and Shapiro, "Treatment of Gilles de la Tourette's Syndrome with Haloperidol," 347.

76. "Akathisia [restlessness, a need to walk or pace, or the inability to sit for a long period] and akinesia [muscle weakness, fatigue, and, in extreme cases, the inability to move muscles] occurred at dosages over 4 mg. per day, and Parkinsonism occurred at 10 mg. per day" (ibid., 347).

77. In retrospect it is not surprising, given the dominance of psychoanalysts on the editorial boards of American psychiatric journals in the 1960s, that the Shapiros' article was rejected for publication by every major American psychiatric journal, finding a home only in 1968 in the *British Journal of Psychiatry*.

78. Shapiro and Shapiro, "Treatment of Gilles de la Tourette's Syndrome with Haloperidol," 347.

79. Ibid., 349.

80. Ibid., 349.

81. Interview with Sy Goldis, Jericho, New York, October 10, 1997.

82. This one is taken from Public and Commercial Notices, *New York Times*, October 6, 1974, but it first appeared in 1972. These notices resulted in more than one hundred responses by 1974 (TSA NL, fall 1974).

83. Among those articles were: Arthur K. Shapiro, Elaine S. Shapiro, and H. Wayne, "Treatment of Tourette's Syndrome with Haloperidol, Review of 34 Cases," *Archives of General Psychiatry* 28 (1973): 92–97; Elaine S. Shapiro, Arthur K. Shapiro, Richard D. Sweet, and Ruth D. Bruun, "The Diagnosis, Etiology, and Treatment of Gilles de la Tourette's Syndrome," in *Mental Health in Children*, vol. 1, *Genetics, Family, and Community Studies*, ed. D. V. Siva Sankar (Westbury, NY: PJD, 1975): 167–73; and Arthur K. Shapiro and Elaine S. Shapiro, *Tic Syndrome and Other Movement Disorders: A Pediatricians Guide*, pamphlet produced for the TSA and funded by the Laura B. Vogler Foundation, Inc., Bayside, New York, 1980.

84. When he first used haloperidol, Arthur Shapiro had no explanation for its probable pharmacologic action. In fact, as late as 1994 he still had no idea how haloperidol actually worked—except that it "poisons" the system. Of course, by the mid-1970s Shapiro was aware of the consensus that haloperidol reduced transmission of dopamine and what that implied about the role of the basal ganglia in Tourette's. Arthur Shapiro, interview, September 21, 1994.

85. Ibid.

86. Shapiro quoted by Barry Kramer, "Rare Illness Reduces Its Victims to Shouts, Grunts—and Swearing," *Wall Street Journal*, June 20, 1972, 1, 15.

87. Kramer, "Rare Illness," 5.

88. John Teltscher, interview, May 14, 1997, New York City. Despite the fact that Teltscher stopped taking haloperiodol at age twelve, he believes that the side effects adversely affected him well into adolescence.

89. Janice R. Stevens and Paul H. Blachly, "Successful Treatment of the Maladie des Tics, Gilles de la Tourette's Syndrome," *American Journal of Diseases in Children* 112 (1966): 541–45.

90. "I have treated but four patients with Tourette's syndrome. The first was the subject of a paper by Dr. Janice Stevens. . . . Two others were children and I lost track of them several years ago." Paul H. Blachly to Sheldon Novick, April 7, 1975, Novick correspondence, Emory University, Atlanta, Georgia.

91. Interview with Abbey Meyers, May 21, 1997. Sy Goldis, an early president of the TSA, remembers a parallel experience for his daughter, also a Shapiro patient. Interview with Sy Goldis, October 10, 1997.

92. Claire Gold (a pseudonym), "Something Terrible Was Happening to Our Son," *Good Housekeeping*, September 1976, reprint 4 pages, no page numbers; and taped interview with "Claire Gold" (who has asked to remain anonymous), New York City, May 12, 1997.

93. Claire Gold to author, June 19 1997; Mrs. Gold's letter went on: "At the time, Dr. Cohen did not believe that Tommy's school phobia was due to Haldol©, but rather to family dynamics. However, as Dr. Cohen began to treat more and more children like Tommy, he recognized the pattern of higher doses of Haldol© causing school phobia in some children, and subsequently wrote a paper on it. Fortunately for Tommy, there is a happy ending to his story. Much to Dr. Cohen's objection, we allowed Tommy to resume Haldol (1/2 mg) once he returned home, and to monitor his own dose, under our supervision. We explained to Tommy that there appeared to be a narrow window, within which his symptoms would respond to Haldol©, and beyond that, his symptoms would increase, rather than decrease, when he raised the medication. By the time Tommy was 14, he gradually weaned himself off Haldol© and has not needed any medication since."

94. Peggy Harmon to TSA, November 15, 1976, TSA NL, January 4, 1977, 4.

95. Abbey Meyers, "Education and the Tourette Child," TSA NL 7, no. 3, July 1980, 2.

96. When the "panelists were asked about the value of psychotherapy in accepting the diagnosis of T.S., Mark [a twenty-three year old] felt it was important to have a good friend who is unbiased. Another panelist felt that it is important to have someone around to talk to and help build up your confidence." "Discussion of Tourette Syndrome in Young Adulthood," TSA NL 8, no. 1, January 1981, 1–2.

97. Sheldon Novick, "The Role of the Medical Director of the Tourette Syndrome Association," draft ms. prepared for presentation at the First International Symposium on Gilles de la Tourette's Syndrome and Related Dysfunctions of the Central Nervous System, New York City, May 28, 1981. Novick sent this draft to Arnold Friedhoff on May 20, 1981, for comments. Original in TSA archives.

98. Ruth D. Bruun, "Side Effects and Haloperidol," TSA NL, spring 1983, 5.

99. Finkelstein et al., unpublished interview with "Toby," 2007.

100. Susan Hughes, *What Makes Ryan Tick?: A Family's Triumph over Tourette Syndrome and Attention Deficit Hyperactivity Disorder* (Duarte, CA: Hope Press, 1996), 5.

101. Oliver Sacks, "Tics," *New York Review of Books*, January 29, 1987, 40.

102. Kushner, *Cursing Brain*, 178, 181; TSA NL, January 1975; and Oliver W. Sacks to Sheldon Novick, July 25, 1974, Novick correspondence, Emory University, Atlanta, Georgia.

103. Oliver W. Sacks, "Witty, Ticcy, Ray," in *The Man That Mistook His Wife for a Hat and Other Clinical Tales* (New York: Vintage, 1985).

104. Sacks, "Tics," 40.

105. Oliver W. Sacks, "A Sugeon's Life," *New Yorker*, March 16, 1992, 85–94; reprinted in Oliver W. Sacks, "A Surgeons Life: L-DOPA, Haloperidol, Tourettic," in *An Anthropologist on Mars* (New York: Vintage Press, 1995).

106. Given his views, Sacks's statement that Meige and Feindel's discussion of the case of O. is "one of the finest examples of . . . collaboration I know" is puzzling. It reflects, writes Sacks, "a time in which patients and physicians still spoke the same language—and it was still possible for both to collaborate, producing between them a perfect balance of description and comment." See Sacks, "Tics," 38. Sacks repeats this argument almost verbatim in Jonathan Mueller, "Neuropsychiatry and Tourette's," in *Neurology and Psychiatry: A Meeting of the Minds*, ed. Jonathan Mueller (Basel: Karger, 1989), 160–62.

107. Seligman and Hilkevich, *Don't Think About Monkeys*, 199.

108. Handler, *Twitch and Shout*, xxvii. Similarly, see Nick Van Bloss, *Busy Body: My Life with Tourette's Syndrome* (London: Fusion Press, 2006).

109. Handler, *Twitch and Shout*, 53–63.

110. The bill provided subsidies for liability insurance for users of these drugs, support for researchers, and funds for studies to determine future needs for orphan drugs. Also, if no private company could be persuaded to produce these drugs, a federal agency created by the legislation was authorized to do so. TSA NL 8 (2), April 1982, 2; TSA NL 9 (2), Spring 1982, 2; TSA NL 9 (3), Summer 1981, 6–7; TSA NL, Spring 1983, 9. The hearings also helped to launch a career for Abbey Meyers, who is executive director of NORD, the National Organization for Rare Disorders.

111. Adam Ward Seligman, *Echolalia: An Adult's Story of Tourette Syndrome* (Duarte, CA: Hope Press, 1991).

112. I first met Seligman in 1993 when he was the featured speaker at a San Diego TSA chapter meeting. Turning his head almost rhythmically, first to the left and then to the right, each time forming his lips as if to spit without actually expectorating, Adam told us about his life with TS. During the question period following the talk a woman sitting in the front row asked him a question, which Seligman answered, but in the middle of his response he blurted out "douche bag!" and then continued speaking. Another hand was raised in the audience and for half an hour Adam deftly handled the questions, always punctuating his responses with parenthetical foul language or remarks that seem so particularly inappropriate as to be purposeful.

113. In 1995 Seligman and his wife Julie published poetry focusing on their joint experiences with TS. Julie Ann Furger and Adam Ward Seligman, *The Marriage Vow: Poetry and Reflections Celebrating the Married Life* (Mt. Shasta, CA: Echolalia Press, 1995).

114. Handler, *Twitch and Shout*, xxvii.

115. There are of course others who have and continue to write about their experiences with florid TS. However, these writings rarely find broad audiences and are often published by obscure presses with limited circulation. See Brad Cohen and Lisa Wyscocky, *Front of the Class: How Tourette Syndrome Made Me the Teacher I Never Had* (Acton, MA: Vander Wyk & Burnham, 2005).

116. Ellen Goosenberg Kent (director), *I Have Tourette's But Tourette's Doesn't Have Me* (produced in association with TSA, 2005).

Part Four

The Patient Constructs the "Neurological Patient"

Chapter Seven

The Psychasthenic Poet

Robert Nichols and His Neurologists

L. Stephen Jacyna

This chapter is concerned with a particular neurological patient, the poet, dramatist, and self-confessed neurasthenic Robert Nichols (1893–1944).[1] Nichols can be seen as representative of the functional cases that still fell within the purview of British neurologists in the early decades of the twentieth century.[2] Because Nichols's first contacts with these neurologists came in the aftermath of his experience of modern warfare, his case may be seen as an aspect of the history of traumatic neurosis.[3] Above all, however, Nichols provides a particularly rich instance of how an immersion in the language and practice of psychology provided the means to contrive new forms of identity. The resources through which Nichols achieved this new sense of self were not entirely textual in nature. They also flowed from a series of interpersonal transactions that included, yet transcended, the clinical encounter. Through a study of the bodily performances, as well as the words, of his doctors, Nichols sought to remake himself in their image.

The main source for exploring these interactions are the copious letters Nichols sent to Henry Head (1861–1940), the chief of his neurologists.[4] This correspondence began during World War I and continued into the 1930s. In contrast, relatively few of Head's letters to Nichols have survived. For most of the period covered by this correspondence, Head was unable to write because he had succumbed to Parkinson's disease. Numerous letters to Nichols from his wife, Ruth, do however exist and give some indication of how Head responded to the outpourings of his erstwhile patient.

Nichols first met Head in 1915 in a "dismal attic" at the Palace Green Hospital in London—an institution dedicated to the care of officers evacuated from the front for some form of shell shock. Head had evidently been "bearded" by a female acquaintance who "told him he must go and see a young friend of hers who was eating his heart out and getting no good from his doctors."[5] Some ten years later, Nichols reported this encounter as, in his words, "on the whole the most important event in my life to date."[6] It was indeed an epiphany that was to alter his identity.

Nichols gave a vivid representation of his first impression of the neurologist who was to figure so prominently in this later life: "Dr Henry Head F.R.S. [Fellow of the Royal Society], a plump, bland, slightly Mephistophelian figure pushed open the door in the hospital cell & sat down & asked me if I liked [Joseph] Conrad—the first sensible & honest question that had been put to me since I came out of France."[7] Nichols was thus taken by the unexpected gambit with which Head opened their first conversation. But a vivid image of this new doctor's bodily presence was also imprinted on his memory:

> You know, Henry, I took to you from the very moment you sat down. It was your way of putting your bag on the ground & settling into your seat. You set down that bag with such care—evidently you were 'on the job': I spotted the craftsman. You settled yourself down with such an air of relish & of not being hurried—of guarding yourself against any possibility of being rushed—for all the world as if you descried something in me at once & felt I might be worth not a cure, but a chat. The immense & subtle flattery of that![8]

Ruth Head was moved to exclaim, "It is so wonderful that you noticed his every gesture and what they meant."[9] She thus recognized Nichols's sensitivity to the nonverbal repertoire whereby Head manifested his clinical persona. In later life, Nichols was often to dwell on these gestures—on Head's habitual movements, poses, expressions, and turns of phrase; on occasion, he even sought to mimic them.

Nichols had come to Palace Green after suffering what his commanding officer called a "slight nervous breakdown" following a particularly heavy bombardment in September 1915.[10] In 1930 Nichols provided his own, more extensive, account of what had led to this breakdown. He told the Heads that he had become a soldier through a mixture of vainglory and genuine outrage occasioned by German aggression:

> You see that I had very definite ideas and these ideas I kept pretty well all through the war—but then I had my little war. When things were at their worst—they culminated at a rest station after being evacuated completely exhausted. . . . I fell back on pride. You see I got to the pitch when I no longer really cared about England when all that was left me was my individual soul. The truth is I had my little war—just enough to break me physically (you know that) & to make me indifferent psychically to (a) Belgium (b) England, but not enough to knock the Soldier idea out, or rather not so much the Soldier as the idea of an 'experiencing being.' I had thought I was going to suffer a lot in France & I had suffered very little & quite differently from what I had supposed. On the hilltop at the rest station I concluded that my little sacrifices . . . [were] useless & my future ones likely to be equally so . . . & that nobody cared two pence (why should they? I was only

one soldier among millions) Nonetheless I had the pride of having chosen as a free person. I still thought I should be killed or die before the close of the war. . . . In a word the war had become a private affair.[11]

There is remarkably little here of the horror of war. A sense of existential crisis that antedated the outbreak of hostilities is much more prominent. The war indeed offered an escape from these dilemmas. The collapse that Nichols had experienced was chiefly significant for what it revealed of the inherent weaknesses of his mental constitution. He regarded these psychic flaws to be hereditary in origin. Initially, Nichols blamed his tendency to neurasthenia upon his maternal ancestry: his mother had spent the last years of her life in a lunatic asylum. As his self-analysis became more tutored and profound, however, he came to see the true root of his problems in his father's personality.

Although sufficiently recovered to be discharged from Palace Green, Nichols continued to be plagued by a range of symptoms. Thus in May 1917 he wrote: "Dear Headlet, I go on fairly well. Bad night last night. Kept on waking up. Slight fever. Bad dreams—dreamed that man took a bet to kiss a corpse—problem for Freud. Cannot say it was an inhibited impulse eh? Shall use the idea in a ghastly playlet."[12] While Nichols was sometimes able to make light of his condition, on other occasions he threatened to be overwhelmed by feelings of desolation: "I'm done for. I see nothing, I feel nothing, I can record nothing. All is ashes. God has taken away the desire of life from mine eyes. Let me go somewhere where I shall never see any of you again—I write this letter in helpless, chilly tears—'I was a man and now I am a ghost.'"[13]

This psychic suffering formed part of a wider range of afflictions. Nichols lamented in February 1918: "At intervals my right arm is full of pain. The veins all swell & the hand becomes cold & cramped. If it is rheumatism only it's damn cruel for it prevents me writing for first the pen is difficult to wield & secondly the pain & the worry of it prevents me bending my mind to the subject."[14]

Such laments were conjoined by pleas for help from a neurologist on whom Nichols professed himself to be ever more dependent. Thus in July 1917, he pleaded: "If only I could be with you for days together—although I am so weak that I rebel against you—for in you I touch a man, a real man."[15] Head's significance to his patient thus went well beyond his purely clinical persona. His patient found some therapeutic benefit in his doctor's moral character and indeed in his physical presence. Nichols continued to call on Head for support and advice even after the latter was obliged to retire from practice. These appeals were especially insistent, and sometimes desperate, during the extended periods that Nichols spent in Japan and the United States.

Thus while en route to Japan, Nichols complained: "I feel the strain on all my nerves. When I get to work things may be a little better—but I am working hard on the boat: if the strain continues in this sort for two months in Japan I shall ignominiously crack up & what is my final terror is the fear that the doctors may not see my case as you see it." Fear of separation from his neurologist had itself become a source of acute anxiety. "If I could only see you sometimes!" he told Head, "without you I have no more <u>lastingness</u> in courage than the poorest stager who ever entered a race."[16] In the event, Nichols did find a European doctor in Tokyo who was able to meet some of his needs. But he doubted whether this practitioner (a surgeon) "really knows about neurasthenia."[17]

In the following months, Nichols's condition deteriorated. He found most aspects of Japanese society and culture repugnant and prone to exacerbate his condition; indeed, he viewed the Japanese character as inherently pathological in nature and his sojourn in their country as a form of incarceration. "Whatever you do," he lamented, "they [the Japanese] laugh. Whatever happens they always laugh. You, Henry, find a lunatic asylum sometimes trying in spite of your training. Imagine what this one is for me."[18] The problem, he later concluded, was that the natives possessed "no psychology. The Japanese don't appear to know what the word means."[19]

Even the physical environment was deleterious to his health. "The climate," he lamented, "is awful for neurasthenia—the climate is never the same for two minutes together & the atmospheric tension passes from that of a stale tepid & nerveless hot bath to that of the interior of a Leyden jar charged with the highest potency of electricity. Gods! I am on the rack. My nerves stretch & burn."[20]

Nichols suffered a variety of somatic symptoms, including what he called a "muffled burning pain just beneath my ribs." But Nichols was more alarmed by a sense that "I seem to have lost myself. . . . Am I getting over something or am I breaking down?" He became subject to hallucinations, some of which recalled the symptoms of his original breakdown. One such "phantasy" involved "a return of the figure of Dick Pinsent[21]—as in hospital Autumn 1915—standing in the right hand corner of the room (where he used to stand)." Nichols feared that the local surgeon he was consulting was out of his depth: "Will he see if I get or am already gaga?" In Nichols's view, no other doctor could take the place of Head: "O Henry, Henry, Henry if I could only see you!"[22]

Because of Head's growing incapacity, Nichols was upon his return to England nonetheless obliged to seek help from another neurologist. George Riddoch (1888–1947) had been a protégé of Head and continued to practice in London after his mentor retired. By 1927 Nichols had begun to consult Riddoch about his nervous complaints. Even so, he continued to report to Head on what transpired at these meetings. Thus in August of that year

Nichols confided to Head that Riddoch "went over [him] very thoroughly."
Riddoch had assured his patient:

> All's well & that it is only my tummy—that the nervous system is in perfectly
> good order & that I have nothing to worry about, that I'm too anxious to get
> well & over my work etc. He didn't explain the sudden attacks of terror but
> seemed to think they were entirely to do with my tummy & the sudden appre-
> hensiveness I suffer from when my leg gets really bad.

Riddoch had advised his patient to "take it as easy as possible."[23]

But Nichols was as much taken by the persona of his new neurologist as
by the assessment of his condition. He described Riddoch as "extremely
sympathetic—an extraordinarily sympathetic person. His voice is beautiful
& he has a nice Scotch accent. . . . I felt much comforted by him."[24] Nichols's stress upon the importance of Riddoch's personal qualities in constitut-
ing the neurologist's professional persona is echoed in other sources. His
obituarist noted that while Riddoch was "a distinguished neurologist and an
able teacher," "his pupils and his patients will think of him first as a person
and as a friend." Much of what Riddoch taught, the obituary continued, was
"remembered because he said it, and because of the way he said it."[25]

Riddoch's congeniality, as much as his professional acumen, figured
prominently in accounts of subsequent consultations. Thus in October 1930,
Nichols wrote that he had "rolled off to Riddoch," who "was just as nice as
could be & bucked me up no end by telling me that for a pronounced neurotic who has been told that he has tuberculosis I was really doing very well
& could pat myself on the back for it." Riddoch however offered no prospect
of a cure; he advised Nichols that he "should probably never be wholly like
other people & without some anxiety neuroses." This offered Nichols a new
perspective on his condition. Riddoch further "astonished" his patient by
telling him that he "could drink a little sherry."[26]

Riddoch felt competent to range over the full gamut of Nichols's complaints: he had been diagnosed as suffering from TB and was eventually to
require a nephrectomy. When Nichols was unable to obtain satisfactory advice
about the state of his health from another physician, "that angel Riddoch"
relieved his anxiety "in two ticks." Riddoch "made it plain—which [Frank]
Kidd didn't sufficiently—at least not to my muddled & nervous brain—that
there was a definite negative on tubercle bacilli & a positive on coli." But Riddoch then proceeded to provide his patient with a further service; he placed
the particular anxiety that Nichols had felt about the results of these tests in
the larger context of his patient's psychopathology. Nichols writes,

> [Riddoch] tentatively put forward that perhaps the 'I am slowly going under'
> idée fixe of mine is really the birth of an unconscious wish fulfilment in my
> mind because I find life so difficult & always have ever since I was destroyed at

school. . . . In the presence of tubercle infection the subconscious longing for solution-of-all-problems finds an excellent anchorage, it pitches on this sets up house & gnaws at the will to live.[27]

Nichols found this analysis "extremely good sense" and wished that Riddoch had gone further. Riddoch, however, took the view that "psychological treatment, while it might do a lot of good, might also be dangerous—in a word [Nichols] was a tricky sort of watch with lots of . . . 'springs' to take to pieces, oil & reassemble." Although frustrating, Nichols found such "caution" an endearing trait in Riddoch. He saw it as Riddoch replicating an aspect of Head's style of practice: "I felt the presence of Henry & his caution & nearly laughed outright." Riddoch was not yet as wily a psychologist as his mentor; he was, nonetheless, in Nichols's opinion,

awfully good at his job. I know he gave me suggestion but I don't know when it was. I rather think it was when he made me touch my nose first with one finger & then another. And he lulled me beautifully with parallels from Schubert etc. But the froth of flattery on the beer of psychological fact was spread so deftly that the beer went down oh deliciously. I came out feeling braced.[28]

As well as employing psychological methods and advising therapeutic foreign trips, Riddoch on at least one occasion also prescribed the barbiturate Luminal in order to "calm down" his patient. Although the drug achieved its effect, it also made Nichols uneasy. He confided to Head: "I'm getting scared of it. I suppose it's all right, but it makes me feel terribly safe, alarmingly safe. What a strange life people with equable temperament must lead. I am every now & then coming to realise how very different most lives—most I suppose—are from mine. It must be <u>odd</u> to be stable, not to have the beam tilting all the time."[29] There was more than a hint that Nichols had come to regard his supposed abnormality as central to his sense of identity; the prospect of a "cure" alarmed him.

Nichols evidently developed strong emotional bonds with the neurologists who treated him. His admiration for them sometimes verged on adulation. More generally, he professed, "I love doctors. They are the only profession that were ever consistently merciful to me & that understood what hell this world is."[30] In Nichols's eyes the doctor had indeed come to displace the priest. In a somewhat analogous fashion, Marjorie Lorch has in chapter 3 of this volume discussed the challenge that medicine posed to the traditional role and authority of the legal profession.

Nichols had some knowledge of the scope of the practice of his neurologists. Much of their time was occupied with organic cases—for which little, if anything, could be done beyond palliative measures. In contrast, however, Nichols ascribed an extraordinary potency to what a neurologist such as Head could achieve on the "purely psychological side"[31] of his practice.

When dealing with functional cases, the neurologist could in effect create new personalities.

In his letters Nichols articulated the view of the self as a malleable and indeterminate entity. Thus in June 1918, when asked of "news of myself," he declared: "I seem to have fifty selves in me at present and half of them are demoniac."[32] Nichols maintained that this sense of personal indeterminacy was central to his pathology:

> When one's neurasthenic one as it were unconsciously tries on different selves only to become conscious that none of them fit & to become more frantic as this self drags round the shoulders & that one flops round one's feet. . . . There is a definite feeling that none of one's clothes fit—hypaesthesia of the skin I suppose: that of course I know they have investigated. . . . To get back to the selves. I'm coming to think that we live through a definite cycle of selves— or rather that isn't quite it. There is as-it-were a wardrobe of selves.[33]

The neurasthenic might on this markedly postmodern view of the self experiment endlessly with various forms of identity. The process did not, however, occur in isolation. Nichols acknowledged that certain key figures in his life—such as the novelists Arnold Bennett and Aldous Huxley—had played a role in modulating his identity at different times in his life. But none had been a more effective shaper of the self than Head. Indeed in June 1925 Nichols declared, "The modern me in so far as it is useful is your creation."[34]

This ability to fashion new, more "useful," more viable selves from the neurotic wrecks Head encountered was, Nichols wrote to Ruth Head, at the heart of his genius as a clinician: "It isn't only that he cured bodies & mended minds astray. He has fortified hundreds in spirit & some, such as myself, he has made—physically, morally, philosophically, intellectually, even aesthetically. I am a changed man since I knew him."[35] On this view, an exceptional doctor such as Head took on the role of an artist who refashions his clinical materials into a new form according to aesthetic as well as functional principles.

But although this was a medical accomplishment, Nichols ascribed much of this ability to fashion new selves to Head's extraclinical activities. Head was himself a poet as well as devoted to music and the plastic arts. Nichols attributed Head's success on the "the purely psychological" side of his practice "quite as much as to your existence as an artist as to your existence as a scientist. These individuals were your medium & the creation of this new stance was your work of art."[36]

The image of the patient as the medium upon which his neurologist worked might suggest a passive notion of what it was to be a neurasthenic. But in fact Nichols adopted a more active role in the negotiation of his condition. In particular, he took it upon himself to gain some competence in current psychological theory—a proficiency that both enabled him to be an informed interlocutor in his exchanges with his doctors and to gain a more refined understanding of his condition. Soon after his discharge from Palace Green, Nichols had begun to speculate about the nature of psychological processes. Thus in a letter of October 1916 he took as his "Subject": "To account for knowledge that an inspiration is correct." The "Process" that he proposed to explain this mental state was that "Rationality, baffled, gives up Problem A but cogs of sub-conscious mentality continue in revolution: dragging up experiences as on an endless chain from the well of the unconscious." This led him to consider the nature of the "Unconscious," which Nichols suggested comprised "the accumulated visual images, forefathers. Conservation of energy: conservation of thought (thought & process unconscious of themselves): thought itself a mode of energy." Although he found such speculations irresistible, Nichols frankly admitted that he was ill equipped to pursue them with any rigor: "Must get a book on psychology—that can be taken in by pure perception. I've no brains."[37]

In the coming years, Nichols acquired many such books, as well as collecting works dealing with other aspects of science. When, in the summer of 1927, he decided to rearrange his library—"so that one subject runs into another in 'an interesting' manner"—he gave an indication of the range of his reading:

> Biology—Evolution—Primitive Man—Social Evolution—Physical Basis of Society—Sciences & Life—Utopian Thought—Socialism—Various types of Social Thought—Bolchevism [sic]—Fascism etc—& underneath these Social Psychology—Individual Psychology—Pedagogics or for another series I was mainly (more or less) trying to put today what is science? (Metaphysical Foundations) astronomy—Modern Physics—Matter & Mind—Mysticism & Logic—Philosophy.[38]

The more particularly psychological aspect of Nichols's attempts to educate himself in the rudiments of science acquainted him with the work of Freud and Carl Jung. He also had at least a passing acquaintance with the ideas of the Gestalt school and of the American behaviorists. Indeed he felt competent to judge the merits of various accounts of the mind.

Thus, seeing the "Freud film <u>Secrets of the Soul</u>,"[39] led Nichols to reflect: "The fact is Freud made a wonderful discovery & then botched it. I feel [William Halse Rivers] Rivers was much more on the track. Fears are more important than desires if only for the reason that obligation is more powerful than impulse in most 'civilized' men & women & obligations become ever more & more complicated as the social heritage becomes more complex."

Moreover, there were at least "two bad holes in Freud." As far as "sex is concerned," Freud had made "the big mistake of tending to think that the tendency is <u>not</u> to indulge in whereas the fact is that it is indulged but is surrounded by an atmosphere of <u>fear</u> & shame & it is the suppression of the fear & shame that causes the odd quirks & exaggerations." Nichols ended by wondering: "Has anyone ever psycho analysed Freud on the evidence of his own work?"[40]

A reading of William James's *Principles of Psychology*, on the other hand, provided Nichols with valuable information about the mental processes involved in artistic creativity.[41] The same book, moreover, provided a valuable insight into Nichols's own morbidity. While leafing through James's pages, he found "an account of my cloudiness & depression & good work has always been my best tonic. But W. James has given me a good tip—simulate sleepfulness, go through the actions & it will perhaps appear."[42]

But the work of the French psychologist, Pierre Janet, was to prove of most use to Nichols in the understanding and management of his pathology. In the spring of 1932, following the failure of his play *Wings over Europe*, he felt his condition worsen to an alarming extent. In May, he told Head: "My nerves are in a rotten state & I cry at the slightest thing. . . . I play Schubert (Quintet in C Major) and Bach incessantly on the gramophone trying to lift the weight off my chest." By the following month he was "in a despondent condition & my brain seems overlaid with mud." Nichols felt he was suffering "some sort of, I hope, temporary dissolution of the will." He longed for the conversations he had enjoyed when Head was still in practice. He had considered consulting Riddoch—"But I simply can't afford it these days." Nichols was therefore forced to rely on his own therapeutic resources. These included listening to music and reading the works of Goethe, an author to whom Head had introduced him. However, Nichols complained, "The usual aids—Beethoven, Goethe etc. don't seem to work. . . . There's an inner collapse of some sort. It's as if I'd been living beyond my moral means. . . . I wish I could find some way to get integrated again."[43] Nichols's casual use of the technical physiological term "integration" to characterize his psychic processes is itself an indication of how his sense of self was shaped by biomedical discourse.

In desperation, Nichols turned to Pierre Janet's *Psychological Healing*. He had read the book some time before and it gave him "some hope one time." Nichols was, in particular, taken with Janet's concept of "psychasthenia."[44] Janet had, drawing upon a range of case studies, described the symptomatology of this condition, which he saw as related to but distinguishable from neurasthenia. Psychasthenics were, above all, characterized by "an enfeeblement of their mental powers."[45] This was manifested in a sense of lassitude, an inability to complete tasks, along with a range of obsessions and phobias. Psychasthenics were tormented by a sense of "incomplétude"—a feeling of inadequacy that characterized their "psychological phenomena."[46] Nichols considered this clinical picture to be a more accurate representation of his own mind than any of the other psychological systems with which he had previously been acquainted.

In his letters to Head, Nichols sought to explain how the concept of psychasthenia had enabled him to grasp the roots and nature of his condition. He confessed that "reading of Janet has been a great shock to me"—a shock of recognition. Janet had, for instance, helped him to understand why the death of his friend, the novelist Arnold Bennett, had such a profound influence on his mental state: "This was a typical symptom of psychasthenia—leaning on somebody else." He felt, however,

> Janet I think goes wrong & is a little cynical when he says that the psychasthenic always wants "to be loved for his own sake" meaning irresponsibly without having to make any return. What has comforted me in these relations has been being allowed to love. That the guidance I have been given by great people like you & Arnold & John Jay Chapman, all this guidance would have been nothing had I not been able to love for that was the only return I could make. . . . I feel alive—typical psychasthenic!—when I love somebody. . . . When I am in the psychasthenic condition, I am exhausted & can love nothing. I can for instance look at my favourite flower the sea poppy & it means nothing to me. But directly this queer capacity to love comes back I can see it.[47]

Nichols seemed intent on expanding Janet's concept to make it include not merely lassitude—or "accidie" as he called it—but also a state of existential despair. "In the psychasthenic condition," he declared, "there is no meaning in things—there are only stones. I cannot reconcile myself to meaninglessness. And this is one of the things I hold against the progress of science—that it has latterly provided us with so much heterogeneous information that we have been utterly incapable of coping with it. It does not deny meaning but has no concern for it." Such mental anguish was superimposed upon a medley of physical symptoms, including headaches and sluggishness.[48]

Nichols became aware of these ideas through his reading of *Psychological Healing*, the English translation of one of Janet's works. Janet had coupled his system of psychodynamics with a therapeutic regime. In the depths of the crisis that he suffered in the spring and summer of 1932, it was this practical aspect that was of most immediate concern to Nichols. He concluded that Janet appeared to suggest two modes of treatment for the psychasthenic: "(a) to find something outside, some sort of relaxation possibly & then refreshed to tackle the work [?] & chance the subsidence of disturbing factors (b) to track backwards subjectively & face the factors."[49]

Nichols experimented with various techniques that might fall under the first of these rubrics. On June 25, he informed Head that "I have discovered a way of dealing with my nerves when out of tune. I have taken to arranging flowers." (This was despite the fact that he suffered from hay fever.) He also found painting of some therapeutic value. Nichols combined the two activities by sending his former neurologist a watercolor of one of his flower arrangements.[50]

But the chief value that Nichols derived from his reading of Janet involved an attempt "to track backwards subjectively & face the factors" that underlay his psychasthenia. Janet, he told Head, "gives me a lot to think about." He quoted a passage from *Psychological Healing* that embodied the "best thing" he had thus far found in the book: "It is undesirable to retain a large quantity of energy when the tension has been lowered, for this gives rise to agitation & disorder. When the tension is low, it may be well to dissipate in one way or another a considerable amount of energy, so that a proper balance may be re-established between the quantity of energy & the psychological tension."[51]

Nichols perceived in Janet's claim that "in persons who are well balanced, . . . there must be a definite relationship between the amount of available energy and the psychological tension" the key to an understanding of his own mental dynamics. He told Head that "I see now that half my mistakes in life have been due to the agitation & disorder existent when energy is plus & tension minus." This imbalance between the psychic energy available to Nichols and his ability to direct it in productive and meaningful ways explained his "extraordinary impulses undertaken, though I knew it not, to equilibrate the two." In his recognition that the true root of this impulse to indulge in frenetic yet futile activity lay in a sense of "incompleteness," Janet had "got hold of something enormously important to all neurotics."[52]

His appreciation of Janet's writings was, moreover, at least partly aesthetic in character. Whereas "Freud & Co irritate me and are perhaps dangerous to my structure as poet," Nichols declared that "I like Janet. His temperament suits me." More important, reading Janet's text had achieved an important therapeutic effect: "Since beginning Janet yesterday I haven't seen either Hughie [Kingsmill?]'s face or taken a reverie ride in the sports car." He was treating the state of despondency into which he had fallen by a mixture of rest and "the interest of Janet, without which I relapse into indifference. Yesterday I managed a little work. I am now waiting a favourable opportunity to recommence, for I feel if I attempt it & fail I shall be worse off than ever."[53]

Nichols was not, however, content to apply the psychological insights he had gained only to his own case. He advised Head that "several people— including [Arthur] Bliss—have remarked that I am quite a good intuitive psychologist & that I have ideas of technique that are useful to them. I should really like to master the subject of depression & its treatment in order to be useful to myself & to my friends."[54]

Although this alleged psychological intuition was to some extent an inherent—perhaps even a hereditary—disposition, Nichols maintained that "damn it all, Henry is largely responsible." He maintained that what attracted psychologically needy people to him was "something that Henry put there—a sort of patience & compassion and some gleams of that rare element, unknown to the physicists, called gumption. But it means giving out!"[55] The psychologist in Nichols was thus one aspect of the remodeling he had undergone under Head's care. It was a capacity with which his therapeutic encounters had *endowed* him.

As early as 1919, Nichols had claimed that "I too, Henry, have, alas! some small modicum of the clinical eye I rag in you."[56] During the war, Nichols had used this supposed clinical acumen to identify the symptoms of neurosis in others. Thus in May 1917 Nichols wrote to Head concerning a Royal Flying Corps officer he had encountered. In a quasi-clinical report he recorded:

> It is easy to see that the strain of continued fighting on three fronts & of— more particularly—flying & fighting is beginning to tell on him. He is slow of speech now (which I don't think he always was), a little contracted about the eyes which fall into a dead stare at intervals—which again I don't think they always did. But you will see the symptoms. I send him to you because you seem to specialise in flying men & you will do him justice: he has a fine record.[57]

This pattern was to be repeated over the coming years. Nichols in effect took on the persona of a junior doctor referring cases to his chief. On one occasion during the war he tried to persuade the novelist D. H. Lawrence to consult Head; Lawrence, alas, "wouldn't hear of it."[58]

After Head's retirement from practice, Nichols began to send neurotics he had diagnosed to Riddoch. Increasingly, however, he was not content merely to act as a kind of neurological procurer for those with formal medical qualifications. Instead he assumed a therapeutic role himself. On an individual basis, he anticipated aspects of the more confident, proactive neurological patient that Jesse Ballenger, among others, has documented acting collectively later in the twentieth century.

Thus in September 1929 Nichols took it upon himself to try to help an uncle who was severely depressed following a stroke. Nichols clearly saw himself in this instance as a proxy for Head: "Some voice beyond myself seemed to come into me—some of that voice was my darling old Henry's—& in a quiet way I think I gave him just a finger (no more alas) to hang onto."[59]

In the following spring Nichols undertook a more sustained effort to help a troubled friend named Leslie "Anzie" Wylde.[60] Anzie had lost a leg at Gallipoli and still suffered from the effects of an enteric infection he had contracted in the army. Moreover, "there are several psychological tangles." Anzie was tormented by "war memories—bayoneted Turks & himself lying out in the blazing sun." Anzie had "become convinced of his own nothingness." The heavy drinking to which he had resorted to escape from this state of depression had merely made Anzie's condition worse.[61]

Because his existing medical advisers seemed unable to appreciate the psychological dimension to the case, Nichols tried to persuade Anzie to consult Riddoch. When his friend refused, Nichols felt obliged to intervene himself:

I did all I could for Anzie. Two or three times he got in a fearful funk & started whispering to himself & it was only next day that I understood what he'd been whispering was "spiders—spiders—spiders." Poor old Anzie clung to me & cried & cursed & boasted & every now & then sort of collapsed. I love Anzie— he's one of the best friends I ever had & dead straight & a brave man—so I wrestled with him psychologically for all I was worth & got him quiet & quite sober at last. . . . He kept on saying, "I'm slipping, I'm slipping," but I couldn't get him to go.

Nichols tried to convince Anzie's wife that "the basis was psychological but she only sort of shrugged it off so-to-speak & said it wasn't any good." Nichols conceded that the case was beyond his capacity and begged Head for advice: "Now, Henry, how are we to get him to Riddoch?"[62]

In a later letter, Nichols reflected upon his efforts in this as well as in other cases. He described his attempts to help Anzie and another friend named Philip Heseltine as akin to moving around their mental "furniture." In Heseltine's case, Nichols's status as a fellow sufferer facilitated this process: "The fact that I was feeling very ill helped for he felt drawn to me, felt that I too was near the end of my tether & could smell death in the air." Nichols had proceeded with caution; he "moved it gently" until he

at last got to the big move ie when you place the mirror in front of the man. He didn't for an instant deny that he drank too much. I shall never forget the way he said "You see that's the only time I'm happy & one can't live without some moments of happiness now & then." (This is quite true. I learned it in Japan. Usually this happiness takes the form of indulgence in the phantasies that hope projects from her ~~magic lantern~~ cinema machine.) But poor Phil had no hope. Drunkards—or perhaps pseudo drunkards seldom have.

Anzie, in Nichols's view, held forth more hope of improvement. But he conceded that his own endeavors were of limited value; Anzie's best hope lay in admission to an "institution."[63]

By the following year, Nichols, however, had come to feel himself capable of diagnosing and even helping complete strangers after only the briefest of acquaintances. Nichols recounted how in the course of a train journey in January 1931, he

ran into a case . . . a gentle, finely cut young face with forlorn eyes & a weak mouth. He ordered a whisky & soda & somehow almost instantly I knew he was a drunkard or well on the way to becoming one. Usual story of course in the case of young gentlemen with finely cut features who are only sons. . . . I diagnosed from a certain wistfulness a mother in the case. In about half an hour—he wasn't tight nor an egoist but simply an affectionate nature developed & repressed—I had it all—or most of it—out of him & spent the rest of the journey to Ashford trying—quite vainly—to straighten things up a bit.

Nichols conceded that his own talents as a psychotherapist were of limited value; if Head were still in practice, "I'm convinced he both would & could cure him."[64] Nonetheless, he seemed unable to resist the impulse to seek to emulate the neurologist who had seemingly also assumed the role of mentor.

By 1933 Nichols was sufficiently assured of his grasp of psychological technique to offer to interpret one of Ruth Head's dreams. Her husband had previously declined to essay the task. "But the reading," he warned, "is sad. (Wait till the servants are gone before reading it.)" Indeed Nichols suggested that the "painful" nature of the true meaning of the dream was the reason that Henry had refused to interpret it. Nichols nonetheless expressed a wish "to know whether Henry by & large approves the analysis of his friend." He signed the letter "Robert Nichols, M.D."[65]

Something of the clinical identity to which he aspired had evidently transferred to Nichols's bodily presence. During a stay in Salzburg that had been prescribed by Riddoch as a means of working off "unspent psychic energy," Nichols's attention was drawn to the local prostitutes who "came round in groups of three calling me 'Herr Doktor' (why, I wonder?)."[66] Nor did the medicalized Nichols confine himself to the treatment of psychological disorders. While in Vienna in early 1933 some of his friends succumbed to influenza, and Nichols assumed responsibility for their treatment. The roles of patient and caretaker were thus not mutually exclusive. He noted with interest the psychic states that accompanied this exercise: "I did enjoy playing the doctor. There was a queer feeling pitting myself against something & of combining knowledge of what to do with how to do it. Also I liked dominating (sinister thought!), liked saying 'you will do so & so.'"[67]

Robert Nichols's case provides a particularly richly documented insight into the experience of one variety of neurological patient in the early decades of the twentieth century. He was obliged to assume that role due to the exigencies of a war that left him prostrate and open to definition as a victim of shell shock. This diagnosis took him from a dressing station on the western front to the Palace Green Hospital in London. Here he encountered a neurologist whose practice encompassed such functional cases as well as patients who had suffered physical injury to the brain and nerves.

Nichols was thus defined and consigned according to the categories of the ruling medical discourse. What is notable, however, is the enthusiasm with which he assumed this status. He proceeded to reconstitute his identity around playing the role of Henry Head's "Pet Neurasthenic."[68] He immersed himself in the literature of contemporary psychology, sifting through the various competing schools until he found in Pierre Janet a voice that seemed to speak directly to Nichols's need for a scientific framing of his own nature. Nichols's case may be seen as symptomatic of the role of the discourses of medical psychology in shaping the twentieth-century self.[69]

What is no less striking is that Nichols was not content to seek merely a theoretical psychological understanding. He did not aspire just to converse about the nature of neurosis with his neurologists in an informed way; he also aspired to master some of their clinical skills. In a sense, he sought to *become* his doctors.

His case therefore bears on some of the principal themes concerning the patient. It shows how inadequate it is to view the patient either as an essentialist category or as the mere by-product of a dominant discourse. Nichols saw himself as the product and victim of his times: of his class, heredity, and his war. But at the same time he demonstrated agency in dealing with his destiny. He shaped his identity, but in doing so he relied on the discursive resources available to him, notably those provided by psychological medicine. As well as being a son, husband, soldier, and poet he was indeed a "neurological patient," a condition that became central to his sense of self. But that status stood in an unstable and constantly renegotiated relationship with the other selves that also constituted Robert Nichols.

Notes

1. For a biography of Nichols, see Anne Charlton and William Charlton, *Putting Poetry First: A Life of Robert Nichols, 1893–1944* (Norwich: Michael Russell, 2003).

2. See Janet Oppenheim, *Shattered Nerves: Doctors, Patients, and Depression in Victorian England* (New York: Oxford University Press, 1991), 29–31.

3. For an overview, see Allan Young, *The Harmony of Illusions: Inventing Post-Traumatic Stress Disorder* (Princeton: Princeton University Press, 1995).

4. On Head, see L. Stephen Jacyna, *Medicine and Modernism: A Biography of Sir Henry Head* (London: Pickering & Chatto, 2008).

5. Ruth Head to Robert Nichols, February 11, 1925, Nichols papers, uncatalogued, British Library, London (hereafter NP).

6. Robert Nichols to Henry Head, June 26, 1925, NP.

7. Ibid.

8. Ibid.

9. Ruth Head to Robert Nichols, February 11, 1925, NP.

10. Charlton, *Putting Poetry First*, 51.

11. Robert Nichols to Henry and Ruth Head, August 26, 1930, NP.

12. Robert Nichols to Henry Head, May 3, 1917, NP.

13. Robert Nichols to Henry Head, August 3, 1918, NP.

14. Robert Nichols to Henry Head, February 6, 1918, NP.

15. Robert Nichols to Henry Head, July 17, 1917, NP.

16. Robert Nichols to Henry Head, February 16, 1921, NP.

17. Robert Nichols to Henry Head, March 30, 1921, NP.

18. Robert Nichols to Henry Head, June 6, 1921, NP.

19. Robert Nichols to Henry Head, April 6, 1923, NP.

20. Robert Nichols to Henry Head, May 9, 1921, NP.

21. A friend of Nichols who had been killed at the Battle of Loos in September 1915.

22. Robert Nichols to Henry Head, March 30, 1921, NP.

23. Robert Nichols to Henry Head, August 16, 1927, NP.

24. Ibid.

25. W[alter]. R[ussell]. B[rain]., "Obituary," *Lancet* 1 (1947): 672.

26. Robert Nichols to Henry Head, October 26, 1930, NP.

27. Robert Nichols to Henry Head, May 10, 1931, NP.

28. Ibid.

29. Robert Nichols to Henry Head, February 24, 1932, NP.

30. Robert Nichols to Henry Head, March 30, 1921, NP.

31. Robert Nichols to Henry Head, July 7, 1927, NP.

32. Robert Nichols to Henry Head, June 21, 1918, NP.

33. Robert Nichols to Henry Head, August 25, 1929, NP.

34. Robert Nichols Henry Head, June 26, 1925, NP.

35. Robert Nichols to Henry Head, September 1924, NP.

36. Robert Nichols to Henry Head, July 7, 1927, NP.

37. Robert Nichols to Henry Head, October 9, 1916, NP.

38. Robert Nichols to Henry Head, [Summer 1927], NP.

39. A film by the German director, Georg Wilhelm Pabst, which made extensive use of Freudian imagery, especially in its dream sequences.

40. Robert Nichols to Henry Head, July 18, 1927, NP.

41. Robert Nichols to Henry Head, August 2, 1927, NP.

42. Robert Nichols to Henry Head, August 7, 1927, NP.

43. Robert Nichols to Henry Head, June 4, 1932, NP.

44. See Sonu Shamdasani, "Claire, Lise, Jean, Nadia, and Gisèle: Preliminary Notes Towards a Characterisation of Pierre Janet's Psychasthenia," in *Cultures of Neurasthenia: From Beard to the First World War*, ed. Marijke Gijswijt-Hofstra and Roy Porter (Amsterdam: Rodopi, 2001), 363–85.

45. Pierre Janet, *Les obsessions et la psychasthénie*, 2nd ed. (Paris: Félix Alcan, 1908), 1:ix.

46. Ibid., 1:270.

47. Robert Nichols to Henry Head, June 12, 1932, NP.

48. Ibid.

49. Robert Nichols to Henry Head, June 4, 1932, NP.

50. Robert Nichols to Henry Head, June 25, 1932, NP.

51. Pierre Janet, *Psychological Healing: A Historical and Clinical Study*, 2 vols., trans. Eden and Cedar Paul (London: George Allen & Unwin, 1925), 2:938.

52. Robert Nichols to Henry Head, July 3, 1932, NP.

53. Ibid.

54. Ibid.

55. Robert Nichols to Henry Head, January 14, 1933, NP.

56. Robert Nichols to Henry Head, July 21, 1919, NP.

57. Robert Nichols to Henry Head, May 14, 1917, NP.

58. Robert Nichols to Henry Head, January 23, 1933, NP.

59. Robert Nichols to Henry Head, September 8, 1929, NP.

60. See Jean Moorcroft Wilson, *Siegfried Sassoon: The Journey from the Trenches* (London: Duckworth, 2003), 140–41.

61. Robert Nichols to Henry Head, April 6, 1930, NP.

62. Ibid.

63. Robert Nichols to Henry Head, April 13, 1930, NP.

64. Robert Nichols to Henry Head, January 14, 1931, NP.

65. Ibid.

66. Robert Nichols to Henry Head, September 17–18, 1932, NP.

67. Robert Nichols to Henry Head, February 26, 1933, NP.

68. Ruth Head to Robert Nichols, August 20, 1929, NP.

69. Nikolas Rose, *Inventing Our Selves: Psychology, Power, and Personhood* (Cambridge: Cambridge University Press, 1998).

Chapter Eight

The Encephalitis Lethargica Patient as a Window on the Soul

Paul Foley

The adoption of the neurobiological approach to psychiatric disorders was excited in 1845 by the German internist Wilhelm Griesinger (1817–68)—"We must in each case recognize that psychic disorders are disorders of the brain"[1]—and by the Austrian physician Ernst von Feuchtersleben (1806–49)—"Every psychosis is at the same time a neurosis, because without mediation of nervous activity no psychic change is manifested."[2] This physiological view dominated psychiatric thought until the end of the nineteenth century, substantially sustained by the golden age of neuroanatomy that began in the 1860s. Technical developments allowed ever finer investigation of brain structure, and it appeared to be only a matter of time before the human mind and its disorders would all be explained by functions localizable in discrete areas of brain tissue.

The optimism of biological psychiatry, however, had faded somewhat by the beginning of the twentieth century. Despite intensive efforts, neuropathology had failed to identify brain lesions in either of the two major psychiatric disorder types defined by Emil Kraepelin (1856–1926) at the end of the nineteenth century: *dementia praecox*, in 1908 rechristened *schizophrenia* by Eugen Bleuler (1857–1939), and *manic depressive psychosis*. Under the influence of new psychological models of mental disease, including Freud's psychoanalytic theory, and partly because it facilitated the emancipation long sought by many psychiatrists from their neurological and internist colleagues, such *neuroses*—brain disorders without recognized neuropathology—were largely conflated with the category of *functional disorders*, in which the psychopathology directly involved only psychic phenomena, at a dynamic level distinct from that of nervous tissue organization. In these disorders, argued many psychiatrists, *there was, in principle, no anatomical lesion to discover.*[3]

The psychological approach to brain disorders did necessarily entail a break with biological psychiatry; it simply relegated neurological considerations in psychiatry to a minor role, on the basis that where the neurological basis of a disorder was unknown or unclear, alternative research and therapeutic approaches were both appropriate and required. Bleuler, for instance, specifically asserted prior to World War I that he regarded schizophrenia as a anatomochemical disorder in which a significant brain lesion is not evident, "but its function is so disturbed that the cerebral cortex reacts in the form of schizophrenia";[4] later he described it as "a physiogenic affection, that is to say, with an organic basis, [but with] a psychogenic superstructure."[5] At the same time, however, his attempts to understand the disorder and his therapeutic model were both based upon the comparatively more accessible psychic phenomena. Even Freud commented toward the end of his life that the value of psychological therapy derived partly from the absence of alternatives:

> Here we are concerned . . . with therapy only insofar as it involves psychological means; at the moment we have no alternative. The future may teach us how to directly influence energy resources and their distribution in the psychic apparatus by means of particular chemical substances. There may even be hitherto unsuspected therapeutic possibilities.[6]

Whether the psychiatrist was more interested in the ideational content of the disordered mind (Bleuler) or in the nature of the disordered processes (Kurt Schneider), they used hypothetic constructs as tools for analysis of an intricate system. Psychological approaches that analyzed psychic activities in terms of "complexes," "reactive forms," "archetypal behavioral templates," and similar constructs did not disallow that these functional concepts described phenomena that were ultimately rooted in neurological structures. These higher-level constructs were instead employed as convenient means for decomposing psychic phenomena without requiring (impossibly) precise knowledge of their neurological basis, just as I am currently employing the user interface of a computer program to type these words without needing to concern myself with the computer code that constitutes the executive program. The constructs employed by Freud—the *Ich*, the *Über-Ich* and the *Es*—did assume a greater existential autonomy in his conceptualization of the mind, particularly following their mystification through Latinization in English translations, and their conceptual autarchy contributed to increased distance between mind and matter in psychoanalytic thought, but even here the ultimate dependence of the psyche on the brain was qualified, not repudiated.

Although many neurologists looked somewhat askance at the emergence of psychiatry as a clinical branch of brain science not based directly upon neuroanatomy and neurophysiology—in Germany the institutional separation of the two halves of brain science in which the *Nervenarzt* was expected to be competent was not completed until after World War II—the dichotomy between neurologic and functional brain disorders tended, in practical terms, to promote a division of responsibility: those who regarded themselves primarily as neurologists attended to disorders where the neuropathology was known or could be confidently inferred, while psychiatrists claimed the functional disorders as their province. Each division of brain medicine was limited in its options: a neurological diagnosis, then as now, was only final once the neuropathology had been ascertained, that is, as Stephen Casper's chapter in this volume describes, post mortem. During the patients' lifetime, the neurologist could achieve little more than to ameliorate their suffering. Psychiatry, on the other hand, could not even draw on neuropathology to verify a diagnosis, and the more severe forms of mental illness, the *psychoses*, defied all attempts at therapy apart from subjugation through sedation. The lesser mental disorders, the *neuroses*, were more amenable to therapy, but even here conditions such as hysteria could prove frustratingly intransigent. The prognosis for a patient with serious brain disease, whether neurologic or psychiatric, was not promising.

In any case, the psychological approach had gained strength in European psychiatry by 1918, and the definitive separation of psychiatry from neurology seemed imminent—to the chagrin of many neurologists who argued that it was somewhat precipitate to dissect brain function into unambiguously psychic and neurologic components. Just at this point, however, a new disorder challenged the emerging partition. *Encephalitis lethargica* (EL) was a welcome vindication for neurology: a clearly organic disorder in which it was nigh impossible to extricate the psychiatric from the neurologic components.

It also offered opportunities. The neurologist, in particular, often disparaged self-reflection as a means for learning about the disordered mind, as a faulty personality was unlikely to have access to knowledge of its own crucial defects: as one of the hallmarks of psychiatric disease is a disturbed relationship with the patient's external environment, how could it be assumed that the relationship with their own interior would be preserved? This was one of the major criticisms by neurologists of Freudian psychoanalysis, particularly as the error in the psychoanalysts' case was compounded by interpretation through the prism of a dubious and untested psycho-ideology (the proponents of which, in turn, generally regarded the results of introspection as meaningless until interpreted according to psychoanalytic principles). The neurological patient, in contrast, suffered neither the social nor the biological stigmata of disordered thought: the brain of the neurological patient was injured, not their psyche. Psychiatric symptoms might be presented by neurological patients, or, indeed, in the course of any of a number of somatic disorders, including infections, but such symptoms were regarded by psychiatrists as being fundamentally different to idiopathic psychiatric disorders, regardless of similarities in presentation. Introspection by healthy persons, on the other hand, suffered from the fact that one does not notice critical aspects of one's own psychological life until they no longer function as expected; the significance of specific functions or partial functions is most apparent when they have been compromised.

EL patients—more specifically, those in the chronic phase of the disorder—presented not only the parkinsonian and other neurological syndromes for which the disorder is now best remembered, many also suffered complex psychiatric phenomena that, had they not at some time exhibited symptoms that allowed a diagnosis of EL, would have resulted in their being classified as schizophrenic or hysteric. Indeed, debates concerning the possibility of localizing these latter disorders in the brain on the basis of the established neuropathology of EL consumed much ink and energy in the medical literature of the 1920s and 1930s, particularly in the French- and German-language journals, then the major forums for original thought in psychiatry and neurology. The surprising element for many contributors was the fact that EL largely spared the cerebral cortex—assumed by many to be home to those highest functions of the psyche formerly referred to the soul: it was a polioencephalitis superior, primarily restricted to the mesencephalon, the basement of the brain, location of the vegetative centers involved in the regulation of a palette of essential physiological functions. With few exceptions—most notably Martin Reichardt[7] and Josef Berze[8]—no one had hitherto foreseen a significant role for the brainstem in psychic processes.

The EL patient was thus of great interest for many areas of clinical and theoretical neuroscience, and the opportunities it provided researchers was recognized early. This chapter will concern itself with one particular direction: the reports by patients, especially educated patients, of their experience of EL "from within." As noted already, neurological disorders did not bear the same negative stigma as do psychiatric illnesses, so that more attention was paid by neurologists to such reports than might otherwise have been the case. Indeed, the Jena psychiatrist Rudolf Lemke (1906–57) later commented that encephalitis-associated psychosis was probably more common than the number of diagnoses indicated, simply because neurological symptoms in psychiatric patients were rarely investigated in a systematic manner.[9]

Alfred Hauptmann: Exploring EL from Within

Alfred Hauptmann (1881–1948) seized with enthusiasm the opportunity proffered by EL, publishing in 1922 the most detailed and most cited paper on EL patient self-reports: "The Deficiency of Drive—As Seen from Within (the Psychic Correlate of Akinesia)."[10] Hauptmann, son of a Silesian physician, had worked for two years in Hamburg as assistant to Max Nonne, followed by several years with Alfred Hoche in Freiburg, during which time he published a paper on the use of phenobarbital in epilepsy, regarded by some as his most important contribution to neurology. In 1926 he was appointed professor for psychiatry and neurology in Halle, where he distinguished himself with research in neurology and neuropathology until, because he was Jewish, he was dismissed from the university in 1935. Following imprisonment in Dachau (1938) he emigrated to the United States, but was unable to reestablish his career at its previous level.[11]

Hauptmann saw himself primarily as a neurologist; Stockert wrote in his obituary that Hauptmann had strongly disapproved of "over-interpreting one's findings," and that in psychiatry he had been more interested in the somatic findings than their psychological interpretation.[12] It might therefore surprise that he dedicated seventy-two journal pages to discussion of the internal experiences of his EL patients. His interest was initially engaged by the case of Gustav Sawen, a law student who had contracted EL at the age of twenty-two in 1920. At the time of Hauptmann's paper there had only been limited consideration outside France of the psychiatric aspects of EL. Hauptmann had encouraged Sawen to reflect upon his experience of his illness, as he believed that such testimony would be more valuable when delivered by a "highly intellectual" person. Not every educated patient was capable of constructive reflection, and of those who were, many tended to depression and hypochondria. Nevertheless, sufficient insight, so Hauptmann believed, was more likely to be developed in those regularly engaged in intellectual activity and accustomed to making informed judgments. The significance of the EL patient with regard to psychiatry was that the mental deficits exhibited appeared to be quite focal: that is, there was no evidence of the general disintegration of personality or loss of contact with reality that characterized schizophrenia. As a result, argued Hauptmann, the "partially mentally ill patient" could provide more valuable information than even the most empathetic clinical psychologist could hope to achieve from without.

The question he wished to first address was that of the contribution of psychic processes to *akinesia*, the pathological absence of voluntary motor activity previously described in both schizophrenia and Parkinson's disease, but which had achieved particular prominence as part of postencephalitic parkinsonism.[13] For many observers its psychiatric counterpart was expressed by the German term *Mangel an Antrieb*, a "deficiency of drive";[14] Hauptmann's specific aim was to clarify the relationship between these motor and psychic entities.

Hauptmann's expectations regarding insight were not disappointed by Sawen, except for the circumstance that in May 1921 Sawen was admitted to the Heidelberg Psychiatric Clinic—an EL patient could fall into either province of brain medicine, depending upon whom he or she first consulted, and obtain a consequently differing focus with regard to symptoms and therapy—where he came to the attention of Willi Mayer-Gross (1889–1961).

Partly influenced by the phenomenological approach to psychiatry introduced by his Heidelberg colleague Karl Jaspers (1883–1969), Mayer-Gross was also interested in patients' self-reports,[15] and so it was that he and neurologist Gabriel Steiner (1883–1965), and not Hauptmann, published and supplemented Sawen's reflections at the end of 1921.[16]

Sawen's case began remarkably, in that he suffered curious psychiatric symptoms from the beginning of his illness—*before* any motor signs or somnolence was manifest—commencing, without warning or apparent justification, with the insistent thought that he was going insane. From this point he developed a series of psychiatric symptoms that rendered his life difficult:

- His intellectual and sensory performance were largely unaffected, but were no longer linked with feelings of either pleasure or aversion. He could, for example, appreciate that a musical performance was beautiful, but without it eliciting any sense of pleasure; a full bladder would be noted and understood, but not perceived as discomfiting or requiring action.
- His accustomed fluidity of thought and movement was eroded by recurring chains of thought, compulsive phenomena (including singing), increased consciousness of both his psychological and bodily processes, an exaggerated need to consider whether a desired action or thought should be undertaken or pursued, and by bizarre forebodings.
- His ability to implement his will ultimately required him to devise curious stratagems to "trick" his mind or body to behave as required, circumventing his all-dominating psychomotor inhibition.
- The distinction in consciousness that exists between dreaming and waking was no longer unambiguous: he needed to logically analyze his situation to determine whether he was really awake.
- He was subjectively more emotional, and his *empathy* for others was increased, but his *sympathy* was diminished: that is, he was more aware of the feelings of others, but this was uncoupled from the usual affective coloring of such awareness.
- He no longer experienced hunger or tiredness; although more active in the evening than during the day, this activity was devoid of genuine enthusiasm and gratification.
- Thoughts of suicide arose, including detailed plans, not as a response to his condition, but rather because his inactive, enervated existence nagged at his conscience.

Sawen had been reduced to a supervigilant spectator, no longer a participant in even his own life. His feeling that he no longer possessed complete control of his thought processes was compounded by rapidly advancing parkinsonism, which he noted with dismay but not with the horror one might expect; in fact he was oblivious to some somatic symptoms, including the increasingly debilitating rigidity.

Mayer-Gross hesitated to overrate the value of this single account of EL, but a raft of issues raised by this case were pursued further by Hauptmann in his 1922 essay. Hauptmann incorporated extracts of varying length from twelve patient reports into a magisterial analysis of the inner life of EL patients. He was at pains to emphasize that this analysis concerned *neurological patients*, but at the same time aimed to identify and distinguish both the neurological and the psychological moments underlying their disabilities. Even those who disputed his conclusions were impressed by his scientific rigor and the clarity of expression in this paper.

Hauptmann saw no evidence in his patients for a link between their premorbid personality and their post-EL motor or psychiatric symptoms. This view clashed, for example, with those who proposed that post-EL schizophrenia-like symptoms appeared only in those with a pre-existent "schizoid personality."[17] Predisposition was a broad field in the 1920s, and Hauptmann regarded with special dismay the views expressed by some colleagues that an indecisive personality, for example, could be regarded as abnormal, let alone serve as the basis for a judgment that the brain was in some manner inferior or predisposed to psychiatric disease. The premorbid personality might shape the patient's response to EL, in the same manner that some cancer patients fight their disease until their demise, while others quickly accept the inevitable, but this was a different issue to that of the psychopathology of psychotic symptoms.

Hauptmann was particularly mindful of the role of the *will* in his patients' problems, and saw his conception of the dynamics of volition corroborated by their reports:

1. The intention or wish to think or do something is initiated by an external sensory experience, even where the initiating stimulus cannot be retrospectively identified.
2. "The will is nothing more than the state of being driven or drawn by the knowledge of an increase in pleasure, or, expressed differently, by the feeling of displeasure that arises from the need for an increase in pleasure. The action of the will is for me—when objectively viewed—in principle the same as an instinctive behavior."[18]

Hauptmann would further develop his contentious model of the will in his 1928 paper on the subcortical act. The self (*Ich*) for him is not the "director" of the mental processes associated with the will, but rather a spectator, the "resultant" of the combination of numerous interacting, calculable reflex actions, primarily "automatic processes" of the phylogenetically older basal ganglia that served the essential vegetative and animal needs of the organism. "The actions no longer appear to us to be reflex processes only because their modification through the intervention of cortical activity obscures their inevitability, and because the simultaneous phenomena of consciousness, with the appearance of a self, seem to bring about a fundamentally different kind of process. It appears that 'I' move myself, but I am in fact moved."[19]

In the 1920s this was generally regarded as an unpersuasive model of human experience (except in the Soviet Union, where reflexology would continue to exert a major role in the land of Pavlov and Lenin until well after World War II),[20] but anticipates in certain respects more recent concepts of consciousness as an emergent entity dependent upon but not predicted by the complex of processes accommodated by the brain.[21]

Hauptmann divided his patients into two broad categories. In the first group, the motivation provided by normal stimuli was insufficient to evoke action; in the second, stimuli were not capable of eliciting a normal level of response. That is, "in the one case, feeling was normal, but not sufficient to allow action; in the other, too little was felt, so that also here the action cannot proceed."[22] The EL patient thereby provided an intriguing example of how the will could not be meaningfully regarded as the keystone of consciousness, nor was it a monistic structure or function.

All patients in Hauptmann's first group reported that there had been no change in their *experience of their will*, of their *wanting*; the basis of their inactivity, their akinesia, must therefore lie elsewhere. As an example, Hauptmann cited a patient for whom an itch was as irritating as it had been before his illness, and the man *wanted* to scratch. The patient was surprised, however, to find that his hand did not move as expected in response to this wish; a great deal of concentration was now required to achieve this formerly almost automatic response, and even then the resulting movement was disjointed (636). The stimulus had been acknowledged, it was recognized as unpleasant, and an action plan devised by the self: only the implementation failed. This phenomenon was even more astounding in unilateral post-EL parkinsonians. A twenty-four-year-old patient explained that when he initiated a movement requiring both arms, only the left (not affected by parkinsonism) responded appropriately. Once again great mental effort was required to move the right arm; further, it was difficult to move the right arm in these circumstances without the left also responding. The man was adamant that his experience of will was unchanged: it was the right-side limbs that were "sick" (637). Hauptmann concluded that only the unconscious process that links the *will to move* and the *movement itself* was affected by EL. Indeed, patients recognized that the less their will was involved in an action, the more successfully it occurred (whereby the passive *occur* is deliberately chosen in place of the active *was executed*; the

German words *Ablauf* and *vor sich gehen* capture even more the idea of a process initiated by the will but then fulfilled outside of conscious control); one, for instance, had less trouble walking normally when deep in conversation with a friend (646).

It thus appeared that in these patients the *response to* or *execution of the will* was compromised, not the will itself, and that this could be overcome if the patient increased their mental or emotional involvement in the act of willing, either by placing themselves in an environment that augmented their affectivity (such as the company of friends or of strangers, the presence of danger, or even the frustration of boredom) or by intellectually building a "a wild sense of enthusiasm" (638), quasi "fake it until you make it." A sense of duty could also facilitate execution of the will; patients remarked that it was easier to respond to the demands of a third person, particularly "respect persons," with the feeling that they were "performing a favor." Hauptmann stressed, however, that this did not indicate elevated receptiveness or sensitivity for outside demands in these patients, as healthy people are often also better motivated when external exhortation is provided. Rather, the relative degree of stimulus provided by respect persons was unchanged, but sufficient to elicit the desired response (638–41).

This first group of post-EL patients shared the feature that although consciousness and will were unimpaired, the normal response to external stimuli, which Hauptmann saw as underlying all psychic and somatic action, was deficient. In other words, it was inappropriate to regard a general lack of drive or initiative as necessarily providing the psychological basis of akinesia. Rather, a "relative lack of drive," insufficient to overcome any resistance "beyond the centripetal part of the reflex loop" (636–37, 647–48, 681), was involved: that is, the transmission of the will was impeded, presumably between the thalamus and pallidum, between the affective and motor centers of the basal ganglia. Hauptmann proposed that "the provision of a *greater quantum of affect than is normally required for the execution of an action* is the essential factor here" (642). The peculiar consequences of this situation were illustrated by an akinetic woman who feared the muscular injections to which she was daily subjected, and was accordingly able to mount a well-coordinated defense when the needle was brought. This was not to say that a patient's drive could not be subsequently reduced by the repeated experience of not being able to execute a particular action as desired; this psychological response to incapacity, however, was a secondary phenomenon, and could not explain primary post-EL deficits.

Hauptmann carefully disentangled the neurologic and psychogenic components of his patients' individual conditions, even recognizing that the surprising poise with which some patients bore their burden was due less to stoic character than to ignorance of some obvious symptoms, such as rigidity or frozen demeanor. He also noted that the frozen facial expression and apparent lack of response in these patients often concealed an internal life that was as rich in intellect and emotion as prior to the illness. This had consequences for their care: Hauptmann cited the case of a woman whose medical caregivers, uninhibited by her proximity, discussed "the pointlessness of keeping her alive, the burden she represented for her community, etc.," all because they held her for an "intellectually inert creature" (654–55). One academic patient even commented that the isolation effected by reduced sensory input allowed him a greater degree of undisturbed thought, so that the composition of scientific papers had become easier. It was not that EL had altered the patient's thought processes or ability to concentrate: it had rather brought about conditions—reduced external interactions—more conducive to achieving concentration (655). And once again this must be distinguished from the long-term psychological response to EL: with the passage of time, patient complaints that their thinking had become "rusty" grew ever more frequent. Similarly, two forms of depression could be delimited, one the anticipated response to motor incapacity, the other an autonomous and "overwhelming, unjustified misery," a primary, objectless melancholia inaccessible to therapies that were not then available (658–59, 682–84).

Hauptmann's second group of patients, on the other hand, exhibited not only more advanced akinesia, but also significant impairment of affect and thought. Like Sawen, these patients described the disturbing inability to respond positively or negatively to stimuli of any sort, whether external or internal (lack of response to feelings of full bladder or hunger; lack of response to temperature despite intactness of temperature perception). In these cases, Hauptmann regarded the expression "deficiency of drive" as being appropriate. The complete dissociation of sensation and affect, which he related to the thalamus, rendered decision making close to impossible: not in the sense that one might find difficulty in choosing between two options, but rather the *absolute inability to formulate a decision or to initiate the decision-making process*, and it was this feature that these patients nominated as the worst aspect of their condition. Ultimately their burden was less oppressive than that of the first group, as their perception of their disabilities was completely devoid of emotion, and depression per se requires a functional affective life. Finally, suspicions of dementia or memory deficits in this group were often misinterpretations of the patients' absence of interest in anything, an indifference so great that the words of a conversation could literally be forgotten as quickly as they were heard (676–79).

For Hauptmann the first group presented a healthy will hindered by difficulties of execution, the second presented difficulties in the initiation or initiative per se. In practical terms, this meant that a patient from the first group, for example, readily raised a handkerchief to their nose when instructed to clean it, but the action might then break down at some point without achieving its aim; whereas it was more difficult to initiate movement in the second patient type, but, once started, it proceeded smoothly and automatically to completion.

Hauptmann epitomized his findings so:

> It is certainly possible to distinguish between disorders of volition, more objectively and less assertively expressed; disorders of affective life; and hindrance of the capacity for realization of the intact will. We have seen how misguided it is to speak of lack of drive, lack of expression, stupidity, apathy, etc., if one derives justification for the presumption of these disturbances only from the apparent manifestations of their affective and volitional life. We have seen how through the interaction and mutual influence of affective and motor components a structure with a life of its own emerges, the function of which can simulate the existence of a process, a finding which is quasi a by-product of our investigations and can possibly be fruitfully pursued even further. It is observations such as these that illustrate how, in the absence of appropriate external stimuli, the reactivity of the aforementioned apparatus, already quite limited, can be further reduced. (685)

Hauptmann recognized that the damaged brain of the EL patient (or schizophrenic) could never be repaired, but he hoped that by acknowledging the disjunction in these patients between their internal life and their interactions with their surroundings, it might be possible to devise therapeutic strategies that averted the "rusting" of the imprisoned mind.

The Moscow neurologist Alexander Geimanovich (1882–1958), who had reported the first Ukrainian EL cases in 1919, supported Hauptmann's interpretations of his patients' reports; he further argued that the lack of spontaneity in post-EL patients, in contrast to that of catatonia, was experienced as "foreign" by the patient.[23] But not everybody concurred with Hauptmann. The Austrian psychiatrists Josef Gerstmann (1887–1969) and Paul Schilder (1886–1940), for example, regarded akinesia more as a disturbance of instinctual drive—by definition not accessible to conscious introspection—as a result of which extra demands are placed upon the conscious, voluntary control of motor execution, demands that could not always be met.[24] The difference between this standpoint and that of Hauptmann is, however, not substantial, as Hauptmann also saw unconscious processes as critical in post-EL akinesia; his point had indeed been that conscious processes were fairly normal in these patients. The American pioneer psychoanalyst Smith Ely Jelliffe (1866–1945) took both Hauptmann and Schilder to task for neglecting psychoanalytic approaches to the question, thereby missing "golden opportunities for correlation."[25] Nevertheless, he acknowledged that Hauptmann's paper was "one of the most valuable in the whole series of encephalitis studies along this line," and correspondingly devoted fourteen pages to its discussion, whereby he lamented the refusal to recognize the sexual basis of many of his patients' symptoms.[26]

Gabriel Delater: A Physician with EL

Hauptmann's patients, selected for their higher intelligence, included a precision mechanic, a pastor, a businessman, and housewives. But it would naturally be of interest to learn of EL as experienced by a physician, whose medical knowledge and vocabulary might add to the precision and richness of their depiction. There is little evidence that EL preferred or spared favored particular social classes or occupations, but reports of the disorder in medical practitioners were sparse. The interpersonal transmissibility of EL was low, so that there was little increased risk for physicians who treated EL patients (the suggestion by Strauss and Wechsler in the United States that physicians were *more* frequently struck by EL was exceptional),[27] but it would nevertheless also have been undesirable to be known as an "EL-positive" physician, given the mystery surrounding the disorder.

But the earliest patient report was, in fact, the "auto-observation" published in the *Paris Médical* of October 30, 1920, by Dr. Delater, *médecin-major de 2ᵉ classe*. Apart from his military rank, Delater revealed little of his biography in this and his second paper on the subject, but sufficient to allow his identification as Gabriel Auguste Delater (1883–?), who graduated in Lyon with a doctoral dissertation on the "antiseptic properties of smoke" (1906), published a series of papers on influenza in the French army between 1918 and 1921 while working at the Paris military hospital Val-de-Grâce,[28] and co-edited a textbook of bacteriology, the *Nouveau précis de bactériologie*, in 1928; a novel that drew on his experiences in Morocco (*Bled*) appeared in 1931, a volume on his time with the French army in the first half of 1940 was published in 1946.

Delater decided that his experiences as an EL patient might be of interest, particularly as there had been few extensive reports of the psychology of EL at this time. His first symptoms had appeared three weeks after returning from Morocco (November 1919), where he had attended a "Jewish woman who slept"; there had been scattered reports of EL in Morocco at this time. After experiencing unexplained impatience and agitation for a few days, he quickly slipped into a fairly typical acute EL (ten days sleep, sialorrhea), as a result of which he was admitted to Val-de-Grâce. Like Hauptmann's patients, his consciousness was unclouded, so that he heard the first attending physician speak to his family of "dementia praecox"; upon admission to the hospital he was fully cognizant of his debility and the "numbness of my faculties that spared only my higher, perceptive consciousness, a sort of blissfully happy indifference, as I was not suffering at all."[29] The only abnormal finding of a spinal tap was increased glucose. Delater could use any muscle with only the greatest effort; spared the usual diplopia, he was nonetheless aware of his mask-like visage. His mouth was completely immobile; writing was very difficult, so that it was difficult to communicate with his doctors

(who included Charles Dopter (1873–1950), director of the contagious diseases department and laboratory of Val de Grâce, and Arnold Netter (1855–
1936), France's leading EL expert), but he did manage to convey his wish
that his sacrum be supported in bed in order to relieve his discomfort. His
sensitivity and reflexes, on the other hand, were normal. He slept a great
deal, and was surprised by his feelings when awake:

> I felt a distinct dissociation in my psyche that I must stress. I saw those who
> attended to me hurrying around; I was surprised by their concern and some-
> times, despite their discretion, by their sorrow. I was neither moved nor fright-
> ened by it, no more than to sense that I was sliding imperceptibly toward an
> extreme exhaustion: all my senses of perception preserved, but I felt no emo-
> tion, I witnessed my end as a spectator, I thought of my children who might
> be deprived of their father as though it concerned someone else, and I do not
> think that this absence of feelings was owed to a cortical deficit, but rather to
> numbness: all my faculties had faded, as had my muscle power; only my higher
> consciousness persisted when I was awake. I recognized the deranged nature
> of some ideas that resulted from concerns prior to my illness (promotion to a
> higher rank, winning the lottery, desire for an autopsy should I die), and some-
> times control was achieved only after I had repeated what I wanted to those
> around me.[30]

Three weeks into his illness, which he regarded as similar to pseudo-bul-
bar paralysis, he underwent the therapy championed by Netter but rarely
used elsewhere in EL, a turpentine-induced fixation abscess, following
which the symptoms gradually subsided. Two months after his admission to
Val-de-Grâce, the doctor was discharged as "recovered," confidently attribut-
ing his recovery to Netter's approach. The dramatic symptoms of the acute
phase had indeed passed, but eight months after the onset of EL, myoclonic
jolts in various muscle groups, marked fatigability, and increased emotional-
ity began to hamper daily life:

> This is also the peripheral transference of a state of nervous excitement that
> places me under pressure with the slightest invocation of my emotions. Then
> I have some anxiety, my throat tightens, I shake a little, I throw myself towards
> the conclusion of what I have started, my voice becomes loud and hurried, is
> frequently distorted, and I'm going so fast that sometimes I use one word in
> place of another: I gain control only when the word has already escaped my
> lips. This tension of my nervous potential is unaccompanied by any modifica-
> tion of other faculties: ideation, memory, emotions, character all appear nor-
> mal, but I feel my personality is diminished in its fight with the others.[31]

What made Delater even more interesting was that he provided a follow-
up: in 1948, he published a brief account of the succeeding years, based
upon his notes. Lumbal-sacral pain had increased since the 1920s, and

following renewed military service (the brief 1940 campaign, followed by some activity with the Résistance) he found it difficult to walk more than three hundred meters or to stand for more than fifteen minutes. Vasomotor problems, the subject of Delater's professional interest prior to World War II, became more prominent during 1943, just as the involuntary limb contractions became less troublesome; loss of use of his right side prevented writing after this time. His psychological state had not changed since 1925:

> I am no longer master of myself, I am like a machine without a brake; it is as if I am under pressure and about to burst, especially when I have to express something that interests me or moves me: then I speak volubly and cannot take the time to think, I rush feverishly to the end of what I have started, toward something indeterminate, and experience a vague anxiety that my powers might suddenly fail me, words do not come, or I confuse them, sometimes driven along by a simple consonance that does not convey any approximation of my meaning—or else I get nervous and I mumble, whereby I also thrust my head forward, I must attend closely to what I say and be careful to say it slowly when I speak.[32]

Delater disputed the standard attribution of these phenomena to the bradyphrenia (slowness of thought; often equated by French authors with the *Mangel an Antrieb*) that was characteristic of post-EL.[33] On the contrary, he discerned in himself tachyphrenia (mental *hyper*activity) and tachythymia (an extremely rare term for emotional lability), while he interpreted post-EL bradyphrenia as conceivably being a defense against this racing mind. As a result, control of the contents of his thinking was impaired, which he characterized as his psychic processes running "ahead of its center of gravity," perhaps in analogy to parkinsonian retropulsion. On the one hand, this assisted his academic output; since 1924 he had published two hundred papers and eight books (two of which won awards from the Académie de Médecine et Pharmaciens, another an award from the Association des Médecins et Pharmaciens), which, he believed, supported the idea that "genius is the product of neurosis." The psychological downside included "lack of self-confidence, subjectively and objectively decreased social standing (criticism by my superiors, expressed to others, their distrust of my habilitation, etc.)." His advancing parkinsonism also reduced the charm of accelerated thought: five afternoons had been required to bring his two-page report to paper. Although his parkinsonism was still quite mild, which he attributed to smoking and using vitamin B over the past year, his drive was very low; nevertheless, he still held hope of a complete recovery. As a final thought, he hoped to place his brain after death at the disposal of Professor Jean Lhermitte (1879–1959; a French neurologist who had written extensively on both EL and the neurological basis of psychic phenomena), "serving until the end," continuing similar notions in his first report.[34]

Delater was in some respects an atypical EL patient (the slow progress of his parkinsonism), and his judgment on the efficacy of his therapy might be questioned. The significance of his two reports lies rather in their granting a glimpse behind the mask of post-EL syndrome provided by a physician who, at the outset of his disease, was only vaguely aware of EL as a disorder, but who for more than thirty years was subjected to the frustrations and humiliations that EL brought its sufferers, and who presumably received the best treatment available. His experience also bolstered Hauptmann's contention that one needed to be cautious in attempting educe the internal life of an EL patient on the basis of their external appearance. The Dutch psychiatrist Adriaan de Wilde, writing in the 1950s, emphasized this aspect, although he believed that the post-EL patient, while presenting an appearance strongly reminiscent of catatonia, could be distinguished from schizophrenic patients through the life that was still apparent in their eyes.[35]

An anonymous American physician reported his experiences in the same year as Hauptman's paper, but in much less detail. The most striking aspect of his case were prodromal psychic phenomena for a period of two months prior to the first somatic signs, including "extraordinary sexual excitement," but mostly the tachyphrenia described by Delater: "my mind 'raced' with thoughts coming and being carried to their conclusion with such speed that the experience was extremely pleasant. These thoughts have stayed with me almost as clearly as though they were last night." Abnormal sleepiness, acute amnesia, and sexual impotence dominated both the three weeks of acute EL and the subsequent six months of convalescence; at night he was plagued by unfocused fear: "the nights were terrors for me and I was glad when the day-light returned." The author considered his recovery complete nine months into its course.[36]

The EL Patient as a Special Case

The post-EL patient was a special case who required a great deal of sensitivity with regard to treatment. Nurse Elizabeth Bixler also pleaded for recognition of the spuriousness of external appearances in EL,[37] but the reality for EL patients was in general very different, for practical reasons: the personal and financial investment required to fully accommodate their special circumstances were ultimately too high to be met, a problem recognized early.[38] The fate of the long-term EL patient was perhaps most memorably recorded by Oliver Sacks with his depressing depiction of patients at the Mount Carmel Hospital in New York;[39] descriptions from the early 1960s spoke of "geriatric wards filled with miserable patients eking out wretched existences until death granted merciful release."[40]

A different sort of patient experience was that of the first American female political journalists, Duff Gilfond (1902–98; best-known for her 1932 biography of Calvin Coolidge, *The Rise of Saint Calvin*), following her diagnosis with EL.[41] As reviewed in the current affairs weekly *Time*, her book related "with harrowing gaiety of a ten-year fight against encephalitis lethargica. . . . Her descriptions of variously officious, honest, cruel, experimental, or decent specialists and the hospital experiences she had in their charge manage to be funny in spite of everything."[42] Darkly ironic is, however, the dubiousness, at least in retrospect, of her diagnosis; probably suffering from some form of chronic headache, the diagnosis of EL appeared to be more an abrogation of responsibility on the part of her neurologist, the sixth physician on her medical odyssey, than a rigorous scientific assessment. The "Great Man," as she dubbed him, however, became the one fixed point in her search for an answer, despite fleeting dalliances with glandular, psychiatric, psychoanalytic, and other specialists, each with their very own speculative and ultimately futile approach.

An American patient account highlighted the problem of mistaken interpretation of symptoms by those around her. In her case the most troubling symptom was pathological somnolence that atypically persisted beyond the acute period: "It seemed to me that life was nothing but a command to 'wake up' when all I wanted in the world was to be left entirely alone and to be allowed to continue sleeping."[43] Nine years after the onset of the disorder her continuous drowsiness—which could unexpectedly overwhelm her in public or at home—roused suspicions among friends and employers that she was a drug addict or alcoholic, with the expected consequences for her employability. The author emphasized that her sleep was more like the half-awake state before genuine sleep, and she was often disoriented on first waking. The humiliation of her somnolent appearance was the worst consequence of her disorder, which does not appear to have involved any motor symptoms.[44]

Alterations of the Sense of "Self" in EL

The French psychiatrist Georges Petit (Asile de Bourges) published in 1923 a succinct report on the psychology of the EL patient: "there are few psychopathic syndromes, with the exception of psychasthenia, where [the patient's] awareness [of their disorder] manifests itself with such frequency and insistence as in the psychic or psycho-organic forms of epidemic encephalitis."[45] This awareness could be partial or whole, intermittent or continuous; while accepting the somatic symptoms as they arose, the patient often required time to concede the reality of the psychologic aspects. Even here, however, it was possible to maintain resigned insight throughout the evolution of the psychopathy ("I'm not myself . . . I feel I'm losing my ideas . . . My reason escapes me . . . I am no longer master of my thoughts . . . I'm going mad") (494), or that insight be diluted until after the psychiatric syndrome had fully established itself. In EL cases that ended in full recovery, consciousness of the pathological process was maintained throughout the course of the disorder, and retrospective amnesia was generally reserved for the acute, febrile stage. Petit noted, however:

> The frequent swings of consciousness and lucidity on the one hand, with incoherent confusion or automatism on the other, seem to reflect one of the most striking features of the mental state of the encephalitic: that is, the uninterrupted struggle of the coherent personality against invasion by the incessant ideo-emotional, ideo-impulsive products of morbid psychomotor automatism, continuously unleashed and ever in a state of perpetual becoming. . . . That a sick man who had devoted himself just a few minutes previously to the most deranged and most antisocial reactions, suddenly exhibits absolutely clear and certain judgment and self-criticism, constitutes one of the most peculiar phenomena, but also one of the most often observed in psycho-organic forms of epidemic encephalitis. (495)

The inconstant personality of the post-EL patient was a source of ongoing difficulties both for the sufferers themselves and for their environment, in terms of antisocial behavior ranging from importunity to criminal violence, interspersed with periods of lucid remorse of indubitable authenticity. It is also significant that even extremely deranged EL patients were sufficiently self-aware as to recognize their derangement, and to thereby suffer under this knowledge. Many sought their own incarceration: "It is necessary to admit that I had every reason to ask to come to the madmen," offered a girl in explanation (496). A review of the special needs of EL patients in the United States reported similar cases; a thirty-year-old woman requested confinement in her room to prevent harm to others:

> It's so sad to be like me. This is only the beginning, it's going to get worse. You don't understand how it is not to be yourself. I feel so vicious at times. I was always good and kind to people. There are other people in the world like me. I feel so sorry for them. I know a little girl like me, and I only pray that something will happen to her before she grows up. I want to tell you about this, because the time is coming when I won't be able to. But you're well, you can't understand! (496)

Herein lay a critical problem in the evaluating introspection of EL patients, and it largely explains the differences in opinion on this question: patients of the caliber of those assessed by Hauptmann were not only educated and introspective, but *the course and outcome of their disease were also relatively mild*. This does not reduce the value of their patient reports; at the very least they provide insights into phenomena at the initial levels of the descent into incapacity in EL. But they do seem to represent a less than typical patient collective, a problem discussed also in Howard Kushner's chapter in this volume on patients with Tourette's syndrome. It cannot be excluded, on the other hand, that it was precisely the sophisticated insight of Hauptmann's patients that slowed disease progress and ameliorated its severity, perhaps by better equipping them to adapt their minds and bodies to the inexorable changes they were undergoing.

The most comprehensive English language self-report appeared in a collection of anonymous first-person experiences of various disorders published by the *Lancet* in 1952. Composed by a physician, his seven-page account of his "creeping paralysis" was prefaced by a comment that attested to the detachment evident in many EL self-reports; despite his profession, he confessed to knowing nothing about EL apart from what he himself had experienced: "I make no enquiries, nor do I dip into periodicals and books dealing with the complaint; for it is foolish, in my estimation, to anticipate what may never happen."[46] He estimated that he contracted EL during the 1918 influenza pandemic, although he first exhibited somatic symptoms in 1924. He was forced to abandon medical practice because of memory lapses, but hypersalivation proved to be his most distressing symptom (despite serious parkinsonism). Therapy proved pointless. He nevertheless wrote:

> So here I am, at the age of 55 with difficulty in walking, talking, eating, writing, and typing, with a whole host of minor ailments; yet a happy man with dozens of compensations. How has this disease affected my character and temperament? All for the better, I think. I can bear the keenest disappointment with almost complete equanimity; . . . I am now much more sympathetic and can better understand other people's foibles, peculiarities, bothers, and ailments.
>
> My belief that man possesses a separate entity apart from his husk of a body has been greatly strengthened by my experiences. I sit, as it were, inside my carapace watching my person behaving in its vile fashion, while my being is a thing apart, held a prisoner for a time. This rather queer sensation of being outside oneself has been exaggerated by my complaint: it is most comforting, and strengthens my faith that there is not complete extinction ahead, but a better deal in a new life.[47]

Some EL patients reported even more bizarre phenomena related to their sense of self, including the feeling that particular body parts (internal or external) were no longer part of themselves, the sensitivity in which, however, was preserved. A more extreme disconnection between body and mind was described by Karl Kleist in 1934:

> She experienced states that could last hours or days during which she was "in a fog." She saw and heard everything, responded and acted, but she said: "My 'I' is not here," or expressed doubts: "Is it you, or not?" "I'm like a phantom,

a machine, an electrical man who has been charged." Sometimes experiences of duplication occurred: "I lay there with terrible pain, and next to me was another creature that was light and free and ethereal, which felt nothing, so I said to it, you could also contribute something." She heard herself speak as if from afar, her surroundings seemed distant and dead to her. . . . The fact that in encephalitis only perceptual, diencephalic disturbances of the corporeal or self-ego occur, not disturbances of cortical self-experience, is understandable given the extensive sparing of the cortex in this disease.[48]

By 1932 the complexities of post-EL conditions had been recognized, but solutions remained elusive, the lot of the post-EL patient seemed irretrievably gloomy. The Romanian neurologists Demetre Paulian and Jean Stanesco wondered whether the difficulty in defining the mental disturbances of parkinsonism had been considered by "those who have tried to investigate the psyche of these patients, *frozen in their infirmity.*"[49] It was now possible to assert what had appeared unlikely to many on both sides of clinical neuroscience in 1920:

> Without having the intention of making a separation between the cortex and mesencephalon—besides, the very narrow link between conscious psychical life and automatic life is well known—we nonetheless permit ourselves the conclusion *that the primitive origins of mental disturbances in parkinsonism are located in the lower centers of psychic activity.*[50]

The entirety of the post-EL psychiatric syndrome, according to the authors, ultimately derived from disordered emotional regulation. They cautioned against becoming bogged in the details of schizophrenia-like, hysteria-like, mania-like symptoms, and so on, as each such symptom was a relatively inconstant feature of the post-EL syndrome. More important were the consistencies:

> our patients are sad today, but tomorrow they will perhaps be joyful; they are delirious today, but tomorrow they will see the absurdity of their frenzy, the same with respect to their auditory and visual hallucinations, etc. Such phenomena make only a transient appearance in consciousness; they do not persist, because of the intellectual integrity that is almost unanimously recognized in the literature as being unharmed.[51]

But the Romanians wanted to know more, and asked their patients with an intellectual past—judges, lawyers, teachers, men of letters—"how they felt before and how they felt now, from the psychological point of view." The common response:

> Before I was in control of myself, I had a will, I did not have impulses as I do now; I now demonstrate joy and sadness like anybody else, but there is a delay in their expression as laughter or tears; I was not as irritable as I am now.[52]

In short: little evidence of intellectual decline, but rather profound impairment of volitional and emotional experiences. "Our parkinsonians present, for any initiative, a kind of *volitional stupidity* (if we might express it this way), rather than intellectual stupidity; they can work, but *they cannot want to work.*"[53] Their apparent inertia was due to the inability of the patient to make decisions: "To will, is to choose to behave." Even phenomena such as stereotypic tachyphemia were related to this lack of concentration, this lack of will: When the physician inquired as to the date, one patient responded, "It is November 10, doctor, it is 10, doctor, it is November 10, doctor, doctor," and then continued moving his lips in an inarticulate manner. This prompted the renewed inquiry: "Why are you repeating it?," to which the patient replied: "I cannot stop, doctor." This verbal automatism was the linguistic counterpart of his parkinsonian tremor: momentarily controllable, but only momentarily. This lack of control applied to every aspect of the motor or psychic behavior of the post-EL patient, "incapable of any voluntary reaction; the patients are congealed in impassive rigidity." This was not utterly irreversible in all cases: the authors cited cases of parkinsonian pianists, for instance, whose condition improved, apparently through nothing more than the exhortation to play.[54]

In his review of the Paulian and Stanesco paper, Hans Steck (1891–1980), Lausanne asylum director and author of two of the most influential papers on extrapyramidal symptoms in psychotic disease[55] and on the psychiatric aspects of extrapyramidal disorders,[56] regretted only its brevity, as publications concerning the reports of educated patients were disappointingly rare.[57] The comments of EL patients on their condition and experiences were, of course, also reported in the huge literature on the psychiatric aspects of EL that appeared during the 1920s, 1930s, and 1940s. Contrary to the views of S. L. Peng,[58] the psychiatry of EL was by no means disregarded by contemporary authors, nor was it degraded by overly reductionist approaches. While the English language literature was not as rich in this respect as that in European languages, particularly German, French, and Russian, discussions of the post-EL personality and mind could hardly have been more extensive or wide ranging, especially in the context of debates regarding the rapport between neurology and psychiatry. The undiluted voice of the EL patient with insight was, however, a rare treasure in a literature dominated by filtered excerpts of secondhand reports of their experiences.

The EL Patient as a Window on the Soul

Hauptmann introduced his 1922 paper with a confession:

> I rarely experience a more intense sense of disingenuity than when in my lectures I have to expound upon catatonic, psychomotor movement disorders to

> my students, because here I need to present doctrines concerning the genesis
> of these movement disorders and their relationship with the willpower of the
> patient, doctrines that are all too hypothetical.[59]

Hauptmann lamented the fact that catatonics and similar patients were unable to provide any usable information regarding the experience of their condition "from within." Critical analysis of contested details of psychologic processes in health and disease was thus one of the most important consequences of the EL epidemic. A common finding across the spectrum of the clinical neurosciences was that the EL patient permitted insights into the organization of the psyche that had otherwise been matters of speculation. The realization that individual components of previously described symptom groups ("disorders") could, in fact, be presented in isolation by EL patients allowed the psychiatrist access to the mechanics of these symptoms. Preservation of higher-level consciousness in EL patients enabled communication of the inner experience of particular symptoms, communication until then regarded as impossible because schizophrenic patients, as an example, retained insufficient insight to provide meaningful statements, or because the value of such statements, as products of a disturbed mind, was eroded by doubts regarding their validity. Moreover, as the psychiatrist August Bostroem (1886–1944) commented in 1924, nobody had been aware of the complexity of the nature of psychomotor symptoms such as catatonia until it was observed in nonschizophrenic EL patients.[60]

The *division of the will into cortical and subcortical components* was also facilitated by EL patients, precisely because EL patients were able to give an account of their inner view of the problem: the apparently apathetic nonresponsive exterior might reflect a breakdown in the construction of the will, the "primary insufficiency of psychic activity" that Berze (1914) also saw as the essential problem in schizophrenia, but, as Hauptmann discovered, the "willing" component of the "will" could be intact, the "doing" component, however, might no longer be capable of the realization of its plans. The monolithic nature of the will was evidently illusory, and a neurological basis for the significant role of unconscious phenomena in the elaboration of the personality established. With time neurology would become depressingly familiar with conditions of massively reduced interactivity of patients with their environment, such as the "minimal conscious state" and the "locked-in syndrome."[61] EL provided the prototype of a neurological disorder in which the visible patient did not accurately reflect the internal person or their psychological dynamics.

It is interesting in this connection that a recent report on cognitive recovery from encephalitis lethargica assessed the patient's deficits with a series of standardized neuropsychological instruments, and a rehabilitation program based upon this assessment was developed. The report, however, did not include any descriptions by patients of their internal lives, nor was volition specifically addressed by the authors.[62]

The significance of the EL patient for the clinical and theoretical neurosciences also lay in the fact that they demonstrated the intimate interconnectivity between the neurologic and psychiatric facets of the human brain, and thereby provided windows onto the psyche and its disorders that the psychiatric patients themselves could not readily afford. While practical considerations might demand that certain disorders be handled primarily by the neurologist, others by the psychiatrist, it had proved impossible to discretely demarcate "neurons" from "psychons" in the living brain:

> [The] antithesis between organic and functional disease-states still lingers at the bedside and in medical literature, though it is transparently false and has been abandoned long since by all contemplative minds.[63]

The two components of brain function were intricately interwoven with one another: as noted by Lemke in 1950,[64] the neurologic symptoms of psychiatric patients were less intensively explored than was appropriate, but the converse had also been true. The presentation of symptoms by the EL patient that until this point had been regarded as hallmarks of functional psychiatric disorders blurred the borders between psychiatry and neurology. The psychologist might protest that a neurologic disorder only mimicked certain psychiatric signs, but could not reproduce their essential nature as manifested in a psychiatric disorder; the neurologist now retorted that, until otherwise resolved, similar symptoms could be assumed to arise from similar causes and referred to specific regions of the human brain. The specialness of psychiatric symptoms as indications of purely functional disturbances was lost.

This viewpoint, however, remained highly controversial prior to World War II and for decades thereafter neuropsychiatry was eclipsed by the dominance of psychological models in psychiatric thought and clinical practice, so that neurology and psychiatry pursued completely separate paths. Ironically, this can be partly ascribed to the impassioned discussions of the similarities between EL on one side and hysteria and schizophrenia on the other (to be discussed in detail in another publication): EL was employed by proponents of psychological psychiatry to more clearly define what schizophrenia, for example, was *not*, even where this involved discarding much of what had hitherto been considered typical of the disorder, particularly its psychomotor components. An alternative to the Kraepelin-Bleuler nosology of psychiatric disease, that of the Wernicke-Kleist-Leonhard school,[65] offered a more comprehensive conceptual integration of psychomotor phenomena, but for a number of reasons, one of the most important being the demands it placed upon psychiatrists for establishing a diagnosis, it found less favor among clinical practitioners than the Kraepelin model.

Richard Hunter (National Hospital, Queen Square, London) discussed the relationship between psychiatry—"the most important branch of medicine"—and neurology in his President's Address to the History of Medicine section of the Royal Society in 1972 under the title "Psychiatry and Neurology: Psychosyndrome or Brain Disease." The paper was an entertaining discussion of the history of the interpretation of mental symptoms, with particular attention to schizophrenic symptoms observed in other, particularly extrapyramidal, disorders, both prior and subsequent to Kraepelin. His conclusion:

> The concept of psychosis or schizophrenia is a historical accident. The abnormal mental state is not the illness, nor even its essence or determinant, but an epiphenomenon. Had the epidemic of encephalitis broken out only ten years earlier, or had its manifestations in endemic form been recognized for what they were, psychiatry would look very different today.[66]

Hunter's ideas were further pursued by his student Daniel Rogers in *Motor Disorder in Psychiatry: Towards a Neurological Psychiatry*. His conclusion:

> There are not two types of psychiatric disorder, but two ways of looking at psychiatric disorder. There is not brain-based psychiatric disorder and non-brain-based disorder, but a brain-based and a non-brain-based approach to understanding psychiatric disorder. Both approaches are equally valid. The appropriate approach is the one that makes most sense of a particular disorder and leads to effective treatment.[67]

Rogers pleaded for a return to viewing motor symptoms in psychiatry and neurology as equivalent, and to viewing the brain as a unified structure in which psychic and motor functions cannot be separated, even on a cell-by-cell basis:

> There is currently a considerable research effort in both psychiatry and neurology which overlaps but paradoxically does not meet. For example, a significant divide is made between the mesolimbic and nigrostriatal dopamine projection systems from brainstem to forebrain, with the former designated as psychiatric and the latter as neurological territory. Topographical studies, however, have consistently shown that the dopamine neurons of the substantia nigra-ventral tegmental area form a single nuclear group and that these meso-telencephalic neurons should be regarded as a single system with a lateral to medial topographic arrangement in their projections to striatal and limbic cortical areas.[68]

For much of the twentieth century the psychiatric aspects of neurologic disease were underexplored; in Parkinson's disease, for example, Parkinson's original assertion that the "senses and intellects" were untouched by the disease long remained an important component of the concept.[69] Since the 1990s, however, neuropsychiatry has once more advanced its profile, yet again upon the bedrock of the application of technological advances to the understanding of the brain, including real-time brain imaging techniques. Further, the non-motor symptoms of Parkinson's disease, such as depression, daytime somnolence, and "apathy," have attracted increasing attention,[70] which is all the more appropriate when one realizes that these features of the disorder are often more detrimental to a patient's quality of life than the motor symptoms per se. For instance, the experience of living with Parkinson's disease was the subject of a phenomenological study by the psychologists Bramley and Eatough, who found that "living with Parkinson's disease has a severe impact on the individual sense of self and agency. Analysis conveys how the visible symptoms of Parkinson's disease disrupt the sense of an integrated and autonomous self."[71]

Encephalitis lethargica briefly opened a window onto the intricate interdependencies of neurological and psychological functions in the human brain, thereby providing evidence that accepted psychiatric nosologic entities should rather be regarded as syndromes, collections of symptoms associated with one another statistically, but not of necessity. These advances were facilitated in no small part by the reports provided by intelligent EL patients on their experience of their condition from behind the semblance of insensibility, reports that accordingly provided more constructive data for the fractionation and understanding of the psyche than the musings of many more philosophical interpreters of the soul.

The resurgence of biological psychiatry has not been universally greeted with enthusiasm, and the extrapolation by brain researchers of their findings to fields not traditionally within the remit of the physical sciences, such as philosophy and the freedom of will problem, have undoubtedly been perceived by many as provocations. But a return to viewing the brain as an integrated whole, rather than as the home of parallel psychic and neurologic systems, need not mean the reduction of the psyche to a soulless automaton without will; rather, it simply affords due recognition of the remarkable coalescence of vegetative, animal, and psychic functions realized by the human brain.

Notes

This paper derives from an investigation of the history of encephalitis lethargica which has been supported by the Australian Research Council (Discovery Research Grant DP0451188, and an Australian postdoctoral fellowship), the University of New South Wales, and by the National Library of Medicine (Grants for Scholarly Works in Biomedicine and Health, grant no. 1G13LM00986-01). All cited translations were prepared by the author of this paper.

1. Wilhelm Griesinger, *Die Pathologie und Therapie der psychischen Krankheiten, für Ärzte und Studirende* (Stuttgart: Adolph Krabbe, 1845), 1.

2. Ernst von Feuchtersleben, *Lehrbuch der ärztlichen Seelenkunde* (Vienna: Carl Gerold, 1845), 265.

3. The history of the drifts in meaning of the terms *neurosis, psychosis,* and *functional* cannot be discussed here; see the review by M. Dominic Beer, "The Dichotomies: Psychosis/Neurosis and Functional/Organic: A Historical Perspective," *History of Psychiatry* 7 (1996): 231–55.

4. E. Bleuler, "Die Kritiken der Schizophrenien," *Zeitschrift für die gesamte Neurologie und Psychiatrie* 22 (1914): 23.

5. Eugen Bleuler, *La schizophrénie,* Congrès des médecins aliénistes et neurologistes de France et des pays de langue française, 30ᵉ Session Genève-Lausanne, 2–7 août 1926 (Paris: Masson et Cie, 1926), 17.

6. Sigmund Freud, "Abriß der Psychoanalyse," *International Zeitschrift für Psychoanalyse und Imago* 25 (1940): 44.

7. Martin Reichardt, "Theoretisches über die Psyche," *Journal für Psychologie und Neurologie* 24 (1918): 168–84; see also M. Reichardt, "Hirnstamm und Psychiatrie," *Monatsschrift für Psychiatrie und Neurologie* 68 (Festschrift für K. Bonhoeffer) (1928): 470–506.

8. Josef Berze, *Die primäre Insuffizienz der psychischen Aktivität: Ihr Wesen, ihre Erscheinungen, und ihre Bedeutung als Grundstörung der Dementia praecox und der Hypophrenien überhaupt* (Leipzig, Vienna: Franz Deuticke, 1914); Josef Berze, "Zur Frage der Lokalisation der Vorstellungen," *Zeitschrift für die gesamte Neurologie und Psychiatrie* 44 (1919): 213–85; see also Josef Berze, "Zur Frage der Lokalisation psychischer Vorgänge," *Archiv für Psychiatrie und Nervenkrankheiten* 71 (1924): 546–80.

9. R. Lemke, "Über die symptomatische Schizophrenie," *Archiv für Psychiatrie und Nervenkrankheiten* 185 (1950): 772.

10. Hauptmann, "Der 'Mangel an Antrieb'—Von innen gesehen (Das psychische Korrelat der Akinese)," *Archiv für Psychiatrie und Nervenkrankheiten* 66 (1922): 615–86.

11. Brief biographies: von Stockert, "Alfred Hauptmann," *Archiv für Psychiatrie und Nervenkrankheiten* 180 (1948): 529–30; E. Kumbier and K. Haack, "Alfred Hauptmann (1881–1948)," *Journal of Neurology* 251 (2004): 1288–89; and U. Ehrt and M. Krasnianski, "Alfred Hauptmann (1881–1948)," *Nervenarzt* 72 (2001): 162–63.

12. von Stockert, "Alfred Hauptmann," 529.

13. Review: J. de Ajuriaguerra, "The Concept of Akinesia," *Psychological Medicine* 5 (1975): 129–37.

14. The term is usually attributed to Paul Schilder; he spoke, however, of the *"Mangel an Initiative"*: Ludwig Dimitz and Paul Schilder, "Über die psychischen Störungen bei der Encephalitis epidemica des Jahres 1920," *Zeitschrift für die gesamte Neurologie und Psychiatrie* 68 (1921): 308, 322, 330. Later in the same year the Breslau neurologist Ludwig Mann spoke of the *"Mangel an Bewegungsantrieb"*: "Über das Wesen der striären oder extrapyramidalen Bewegungsstörung (amyostatischer Symptomenkomplex)," *Zeitschrift für die gesamte Neurologie und Psychiatrie* 71 (1921): 357.

15. Cf. R. Jung, "Wilhelm Mayer-Gross, 1888–1961," *Archiv für Psychiatrie und Nervenkrankheiten* 203 (1962): 123–36.

16. W. Mayer-Gross and G. Steiner, "Encephalitis Lethargica in der Selbstbeobachtung," *Zeitschrift für die gesamte Neurologie und Psychiatrie* 73 (1921): 283–309.

17. For instance: R. Neustadt, "Zur Auffassung der Psychosen bei Metencephalitis," *Archiv für Psychiatrie und Nervenkrankheiten* 81 (1927): 99–132. See also Josef Berze, "Beiträge zur psychiatrischen Erblichkeits- und Konstitutionsforschung. II. Schizoid, Schizophrenie, Dementia praecox," *Zeitschrift für die gesamte Neurologie und Psychiatrie* 96 (1925): 603–52.

18. Hauptmann, "Der 'Mangel an Antrieb,'" 627.

19. Alfred Hauptmann, "Die subcorticale 'Handlung,'" *Journal für Psychologie und Neurologie* 37 (1928): 100.

20. See, for example, W. Bechterew, "Die Krankheiten der Persönlichkeit vom Standpunkt der Reflexologie: Zur Begründung der pathologischen Reflexologie," *Zeitschrift für die gesamte Neurologie und Psychiatrie* 80 (1923): 265–309.

21. Christian Geyer, ed., *Hirnforschung und Willensfreiheit: Zur Deutung der neuesten Experimente*, (Frankfurt am Main: Suhrkamp, 2004).

22. Hauptmann, "Der 'Mangel an Antrieb,'" 671.

23. A. I. Geĭmanovich, "Psikhoticheskoe soderzhanie epidemicheskogo encefalita," in *Infektsii i Nervnaya Sistema* (Trudy Ukrainskogo Psikhonevrologikheskogo Instituta 3), ed. A. I. Geĭmanovich (Kharkov: Vseukrainskoe Medicinskoe Izdatel'stvo "Nauchnaia Mysl," 1927). Similar in: Ludwig von Angyal, "Zur Kenntnis der postencephalitischen Antriebs- und Gedächtnisstörungen," *Zeitschrift für die gesamte Neurologie und Psychiatrie* 122 (1929): 187–203.

24. Josef Gerstmann and Paul Schilder, "Studien über Bewegungsstörungen. VI. Mitt. Unterbrechung von Bewegungsfolgen (Bewegungslücken), nebst Bemerkungen über Mangel an Antrieb," *Zeitschrift für die gesamte Neurologie und Psychiatrie* 85 (1923): 39–42.

25. Smith Ely Jelliffe, "The Mental Pictures in Schizophrenia and in Epidemic Encephalitis: Their Alliances, Differences, and a Point of View," *American Journal of Psychiatry* 83 (1927): 432.

26. Jelliffe, "Mental Pictures in Schizophrenia," 432–45.

27. Israel Strauss and Israel S. Wechsler, "Epidemic Encephalitis (Encephalitis Lethargica)," *International Journal of Public Health* 2 (1921): 449–64.

28. Delater, "La grippe dans la nation armée de 1918 à 1921," *Revue d'Hygiène et de Police Sanitaire* 45 (1923): 406–26; 523–38; 619–34.

29. Delater, "Auto-observation d'encéphalite léthargique," *Paris Médical* 10 (1920): 316.

30. Ibid., 317.

31. Ibid., 318.

32. G. Delater, "Suite sur trente ans et fin d'une auto-observation d'encéphalite léthargique," *Paris Médical* 38 (1948): 230.

33. Cf. F. Naville, "Études sur les complications et les séquelles mentales de l'encéphalite épidémique: La bradyphrénie," *L'Encéphale* 17 (1922): 369–75, 423–36.

34. Delater, "Suite sur trente ans," 229–30.

35. Jacob Adriaan De Wilde, *Over Organische Defectpsychosen: Een Klinisch-Psychiatrisch Onderzoek naar het Voorkomen van Gevolgtoestanden van Encephalitis Lethargica* (Amsterdam: Van Gorcum & Co./Dr. H. J. Prakke and H. M. G. Prakke, 1959), 170.

36. Anonymous, "Epidemic (Lethargic) Encephalitis: A Personal Experience," *Journal of the American Medical Association* 78 (1922): 407–9.

37. Elizabeth S. Bixler, "The Nurse and Neurological Problems," *American Journal of Nursing* 35 (1935): 425–30.

38. See, for example, W. Heinicke, "Die unzulängliche Fürsorge für chronische Encephalitiker," *Archiv für Psychiatrie und Nervenkrankheiten* 77 (1926): 701–3.

39. Oliver W. Sacks, *Awakenings* (London: Duckworth, 1973).

40. Paul Bernard Foley, *Beans, Roots, and Leaves: A History of the Chemical Therapy of Parkinsonism* (Marburg: Tectum, 2003), 611.

41. Duff Gilfond, *I Go Horizontal* (New York: Vanguard, 1940).

42. Anonymous, "Recent & Readable," *Time*, April 22, 1940; http://www.time.com/time/magazine/article/0,9171,763911,00.html (accessed July 16, 2010).

43. Eleanore Carey, "I Recover from Sleeping Sickness," *American Mercury* 32 (1934): 165.

44. Ibid., 165–69.

45. Georges Petit, "La conscience de l'état morbide dans les formes mentales ou psycho-organiques de l'encéphalite épidémique," *Journal de Psychologie Normale et Pathologique* 20 (1923): 493.

46. Anonymous, "Parkinsonism," in *Disabilities and How to Live with Them: True Stories Written by Patients or Former Patients*, ed. *The Lancet* (London: Lancet United Kingdom, 1952), 52.

47. Ibid., 55.

48. Kleist, "Leitvortrag über Gehirnpathologie und Klinik der Persönlichkeit und Körperlichkeit" (59. Wanderversammlung der südwestdeutschen Neurologen und Psychiater am 9. und 10. Juni 1934 in Baden-Baden), *Zentralblatt für die gesamte Neurologie und Psychiatrie* 75 (1935): 711.

49. Dem. Paulian and Jean Stanesco, "Contribution à l'étude des troubles mentaux dans le parkinsonisme," *Annales Médico-Psychologiques* 90, no. 1 (1932): 394; italics in original.

50. Ibid., 395; italics in original.

51. Ibid., 397.

52. Ibid., 398; italics in original.

53. Ibid.

54. Ibid., 399–400.

55. Hans Steck, "Les syndromes extrapyramidaux dans les maladies mentales," *Archives Suisses de Neurologie et de Psychiatrie* 19 (1926): 195–233; 20 (1927): 92–136.

56. Hans Steck, "Les syndromes mentaux postencéphalitiques," *Archives Suisses de Neurologie et de Psychiatrie* 27 (1931): 137–73.

57. Hans Steck, Review of Paulian and Stanesco, "Contribution à l'étude des troubles mentaux dans le parkinsonisme," *Zentralblatt für die gesamte Neurologie und Psychiatrie* 64 (1932): 542.

58. S. L. Peng, "Reductionism and Encephalitis Lethargica, 1916–1939," *New Jersey Medicine* 90 (1993): 459–62.

59. Hauptmann, "Der Mangel an Antrieb," 615.

60. A. Bostroem, "Encephalitische und katatone Motilitätsstörungen," *Klinische Wochenschrift* 3 (1924): 465. See also A. Bostroem, "Das Wesen der rigorfreien Starre," *Archiv für Psychiatrie und Nervenkrankheiten* 71 (1924): 128–43.

61. Review: Steven Laureys, Adrian M. Owen, and Nicholas D. Schiff, "Brain Function in Coma, Vegetative State, and Related Disorders," *Lancet Neurology* 3 (2004): 537–46.

62. Bonnie-Kate Dewar and Barbara A. Wilson, "Cognitive Recovery from Encephalitis Lethargica," *Brain Injury* 19 (2005): 1285–91.

63. Samuel Alexander Kinnier Wilson, *Neurology*, ed. A. Ninian Bruce, 2nd ed. (London: Butterworth & Co., 1954), 1:1915.

64. Lemke, "Über die symptomatische Schizophrenie," 772.

65. Karl Leonhard, "Hyperkinetisch-akinetisch Motilitätspsychose," in *Aufteilung der endogenen Psychosen und ihre differenzierte Ätiologie*, ed. Helmut Beckmann, 8th ed. (Stuttgart: Georg Thieme), 79–85. See also Klaus-Jürgen Neumärker, "Leonhard and the Classification of Psychomotor Psychoses in Childhood and Adolescence," *Psychopathology* 23 (1990): 243–52; Carlo Perris, "The Importance of Karl Leonhard's Classification of Endogenous Psychoses," *Psychopathology* 23 (1990): 282–90; and Gabor S. Ungvari, "The Wernicke-Kleist-Leonhard School of Psychiatry," *Biological Psychiatry* 34 (1993): 749–52.

66. Richard Hunter, "Psychiatry and Neurology: Psychosyndrome or Brain Disease," *Proceedings of the Royal Society of Medicine* 66 (1973): 364.

67. Daniel Rogers, *Motor Disorder in Psychiatry: Towards a Neurological Psychiatry* (Chichester: John Wiley & Sons, 1992), 113.

68. Rogers, *Motor Disorder in Psychiatry*, 114.

69. James Parkinson, *Essay on the Shaking Palsy* (London: Whittingham and Rowland, 1817), 1.

70. For example, Richard Levy and Virginie Czernecki, "Apathy and the Basal Ganglia," *Journal of Neurology* 253, suppl. 7 (2006): 54–61; Kathy Dujardin et al., "Characteristics of Apathy in Parkinson's Disease," *Movement Disorders* 22 (2007): 778–84; S. E. Starkstein, and A. F. G. Leentjens, "The Nosological Position of Apathy in Clinical Practice," *Journal of Neurology, Neurosurgery & Psychiatry* 79 (2008): 1088–92.

71. Natalie Bramley and Virginia Eatough, "The Experience of Living with Parkinson's Disease: An Interpretative Phenomenological Analysis Case Study," *Psychology & Health* 20 (2005): 223.

Part Five

Historians Construct the "Neurological Patient"

Chapter Nine

Neuropatients in Historyland

Roger Cooter

If the patient is the hole at the center of the history of the neurological patient, it is only in the sense of an invisible performing subject. The *concept* of the patient has never been missing. It is implicit to the history of neurology, as it is to the rest of the history of medicine. Like all concepts and categories, however, it is a shifting product of its historical times. It moves with its historiography. In illustration of this, we need look no further than the contributions to this volume by Stephen Casper and Jesse Ballenger. Like other chapters, their essays usefully draw our attention to the importance of talking about patients in the history of neurology and in the "psy" sciences more generally. They remind us that it is in these areas of professional practice above all that talking matters—the talking, that is, *of patients.* Since it is very often only through the patient's voice that expertise is constituted in the domains of neurology, psychology, and psychiatry, the subjectivity of the patient is the name of the game. If there is no verbally constituted subjectivity, then there is no game. (Or perhaps we should say *was* no game, for brain mapping appears to be taking over the process of defining the interior of the patient subject.) But what the chapters by Casper and Ballenger also reveal, at an implicit level, is the discursive nature of the concept of the patient, and how its framing is peculiar to its historical moment. Each of these chapters is a register of the historically constituted episteme of its author. It is on the nature of these registers that I would like briefly to remark—that is, to comment on the importance of talking about *the historians* of the would-be neurological patient.

Let me say first, though, that the patient in the historiography of medicine has had a hard time. Not until the mid-1970s was it even conceived as a topic for explicit discussion. It was Charles Webster in his 1976 manifesto for the new social history of medicine who declared that the resurrection of the patient "should be an essential part of our brief."[1] Hitherto, the patient was largely irrelevant. The history of medicine was not about patients but about those who treated them, along with the institutional, intellectual, economic, social, and cultural contexts in which treatment was pursued. But the topic was slow to take root outside of women's history and the history of the mad.

It was in 1985, when the social history of medicine was at its height, that Roy Porter, the doyen of the field, published his germinal paper, "The Patient's View: Doing Medical History from Below."[2] For Porter the "doing" was justified partly on the grounds that the patient had disappeared from modern medicine.[3] But this view, while sociologically robust ever since the publication in 1976 of Nicholas Jewson's "Disappearance of the Sick Man," was becoming obsolete by the time of Porter's article.[4] The sick, far from becoming silenced through modern biomedicine, were proving to be an ever more strident voice in the free-market rhetoric of the 1980s, and were being encouraged through that rhetoric.[5] At the same time, the concurrent move to the privatization of health care was allied to the *de*-professionalization of medical practitioners. Increasingly, therefore, bioethically minded health consumers, politicians, and patient activists were occupying (and voicing) the moral high ground, while the medical profession's arbitrary and autonomous authority was quieted. In the social structural story of the doctor-patient relationship, it was patients, not doctors, who were coming out on top.[6] Today, arguably, the patient is more on top than ever, or at least more pervasive in the so-called politics of life, for, according to this position, we have all become patients in the sense that we routinely self-fashion our identity though biomedical discourse. The hopes we entertain for our own health and longevity and that of our loved ones, are fully enmeshed in the language of molecular genetics and, increasingly now, the language of "the neural."[7]

Yet despite the changes that rendered Porter's paper intellectually superfluous by the time it was published, it can nevertheless be regarded as a late product of its historiographical times.[8] In its mission to recover the patient from the condescensions of medical and medicalized posterity, it was—as with Webster's original call—at one with the agenda of E. P. Thompson in his classic *The Making of the English Working Class* (1963). Of course, the historical recovery of patients was no easy matter given the shortage of records or archives specifically on or by them. Historical evidence could seldom be other than anecdotal. What is more important to note here is, first, the social structural understanding of power inherent to this historical exercise. And second, how, as history from below, the exercise was only ever cast as the other side of the same coin of the pilloried history of medicine conducted from the top down. By the very nature of the top-down/bottom-up dichotomy, the idea of a patient-orientated history of medicine could only reveal more stories about the exercise and reproduction of power in the social relations of medicine. Significantly, Porter's pleas in the mid-1980s for such histories were contained in books seeking to historicize patients *and* practitioners.[9] As germane to the present discussion is that *the category* "the patient" was left passive—as anesthetized as the human patients that Porter sought to resurrect from the past. Like the concept of the "social" in the social history of medicine (to say nothing of the concept of "history" itself),[10] Porter did not question the category of "the patient." In common with 1970s and 1980s medical sociologists,[11] he simply took the concept for granted, deploying it unproblematically. Ironically, then, Porter's more-or-less successful attempt at bringing the patient into historical view simultaneously deflected attention from both the history of the concept and the category of the patient. The patient was simply not a key word in the Raymond Williams's sense, despite that its appropriation by medicine was largely an eighteenth-century phenomenon—the chronological heartland of Porter's social history.[12]

As it happened, the celebration of the patient's arrival at the table of the history of medicine (albeit etherized in historical essentialism) was short lived. No sooner was the aspiration to attend to patients historically in vogue than it was upstaged by a fundamentally different agenda that literally dealt that aspiration a body blow: the somatic turn inspired by Foucault's biopolitically inclined project to historicize reason and examine "how men govern themselves and others by the production of truth."[13] As a part of the postmodern literary turn devoted to the analysis of discourse, the somatic turn privileged the body as a textual site for the discursive analysis of modernity.[14] In the course of this exercise virtually every foundational and essentialist notion around the body, including its biologization, was called into question. All that hitherto had seemed so solid to historians, or was assumed timeless, natural, and epistemologically autonomous, began to melt into air. The historian's *a*historical conception and deployment of "the patient" as an autonomous agent began to become apparent; denaturalized, the concept was able to be opened to historical analysis instead of being put beyond it. No longer possible to take for granted, the idea of the patient was problematized as a product of historical creation—at least in theory.

Broadly speaking the chapters by Casper and Ballenger reflect the two different spaces for imaging the patient, the one modernist and structuralist in orientation and understanding, the other postmodernist and poststructuralist. Despite varying degrees of overlap in their expression, they signify distinct tales of historiographical mediation, or two different discursive registers for the conceptualization of the neurological patient.

Casper's chapter is cast within, and contributes to, a Weberian understanding of modernity, one familiar to historians who have worked on late nineteenth and early twentieth-century medical specialization.[15] For Weber, writing in the early twentieth century, specialization was among the central characteristics of modern (rational and rationalizing) society, along with the integration of bureaucracy and other organizational and managerial systems; the standardization, centralization, and routinization of administrative action; and the employment of experts to define and order such systems. Specialization, Weber perceived, was a part of the process of differentiation within unifying, cohering, uniforming structures. Whereas traditional social systems operated through diverse forms of social interaction and bonding, modern industrial ones aspired to conformity, to standardization and to system through the imposition of bureaucratic planning and administration. Underlying this, as indicated by Weber's designation of such a society as rational, was a form of calculative and evaluative logic that both legitimized and advanced the extension of bureaucratic structures into ever-more intimate areas of social life.[16]

All this is subsumed in the historical questions that Casper poses for the development of techniques to investigate and assess the neurological patient. It is reflected, above all, in his metaphor of the calibrating tuning fork, which he deploys to explain how it was possible to objectify subjective patient narratives—to standardize, order, and classify the signs and symptoms of mental states so as to fit would-be neurological patients to the exercise of administrative rationality. The particular circumstances whereby inaccessible minds were transformed into ones accessible to medical professionals need not detain us here. It is not the facts of the story that matter, but rather the fact that the story is embedded in the metanarrative of modernity. Just as Weber's analysis of modernity sought to make unitary sense of the world and can therefore itself be regarded as a product of modernity (as, similarly, can Marx's articulation of a universal class consciousness), Casper's effort to recover the neurological patient is made through a Weberian-informed analysis. Indeed, in terms of his analytical frame, Casper is at one with his historical actors, those pre– and post–World War I practitioners who did so much to make up the neurological patient.

But just as a Weberian-premised reading of the making of neurology produces or implies a certain form of historicized neurological patient, so too does a non-Weberian reading. Ballenger's chapter well reflects the latter, although no more *explicitly* postmodern or poststructuralist than Casper's is explicitly Weberian. Telltale, above all, is its attention to narrativity, or rather, to the technologies of narrativity, or more precisely to the technologies of narrativity among the sufferers of Alzheimer's disease. More or less, this is equivalent to Casper's interest in the technologies of objectivity, but it is inspired by, and directed to, a different end: the exposure of plural subjectivities. The underlying logic is not modernist unificatory, but rather postmodern fragmentary, and it is to difference, not sameness, that attention is directed. Linked to this, perhaps, is Ballenger's use of the word "sufferers" instead of (medicalized) patients. Beyond the politics of political correctness, this suggests intellectual distance from the crude reifications and understandings of power inherent to the discussion of doctor-patient relations in the older structuralist sociological paradigm.[17] Again, there is no need here to go into the chapter itself—not even so as to illuminate the residues or impurities of modernist thinking within it.[18]

My point is simply that any representation of a neurological patient drawn by a historian is necessarily embedded in the dominant discourse of the historian's time, which is mediated in the prevailing historiography. It may even be that the dominant discourse at any moment in time determines the shape of the practice and theory of neurological science: as phrenology and cerebral localization in the nineteenth century mediated an idealized social order, so today it is fashionable in cognitive neurological research to posit a poststructuralist brain in which thought is conceived as the outcome of disorderly impulses that trigger avalanches of neural activity.[19] Be that as it may, there is no way in which historians can stand objectively outside that which they seek to describe or analyze. As historiographers have long appreciated, historians always stand inside the present that shapes their interests and methodologies (although none has yet taken this further to understand the present, and the presents of the past, as epistemically loaded in terms of the unstated values and virtues that historians of different epochs unwittingly bring to their task and regulate it).[20] At the very least, history writing *is* its historiography, to paraphrase E. H. Carr.[21] Hence, the historian is always an actor or participant in what he or she seeks to describe, albeit usually an unwitting actor.[22] And thus between the would-be neurological patient (as represented by the historian) and the would-be observer historian (whose self is believed to be apart from what is described) the boundary is less clear cut than we might at first imagine. Try as we might to recover the experience of the neurological patient, we remain locked in our own discursive experience and epistemic virtues, which together serve to bind the subject "the patient" to the representations we make up for them.[23] The realist dream of recovering "the patient" is impossible, for nothing is ever outside its made-up historical representation. At most, we can only recover the circumstances around "the patient" that make it up at any point in history, including the humanistic and scientistic circumstances that shape the discourse of historians. Perhaps, therefore, a final thought should be given to the discourse that now drives the desire to historically recover the neurological patient. Possibly it is still the Websterian and Porteresque agenda of arguing for egalitarian social relations. But it might also be the neurological one that, by reductively turning mind into body, now increasingly turns personhood into brainhood? If so, there is some urgency in getting on with the job, for as neurohistory now tempts historians to biological toolkits and hence to new means to essentialist history and *a*historicized patients within it,[24] so the compulsion to historical thought itself as a handmaiden to humanity may soon succumb to material neurological reduction, as moral thought now does in neuroethics.[25] Against all this we can rally, as I have suggested elsewhere, although the hourglass is fast running low.[26]

Notes

1. "Abstract of Presidential Address [by Charles Webster], delivered at the 1976 Conference of the Society for the Social History of Medicine," *Society for the Social History of Medicine Bulletin* 19 (1976): 3.

2. Roy Porter, "The Patient's View: Doing Medical History from Below," *Theory and Society* 14 (1985): 175–98.

3. This was made explicit in Roy Porter and Dorothy Porter, *Patient's Progress: Doctors and Doctoring in Eighteenth-Century England* (Stanford: Stanford University Press, 1989).

4. Nicholas Jewson, "The Disappearance of the Sick Man from Medical Cosmology, 1770–1870," *Sociology* 10 (1976): 225–44.

5. Lilian Furst, *Between Doctors and Patients: The Changing Balance of Power* (Charlottesville: University of Virginia Press, 1998).

6. A reflection of this might be read into the fact that the first monograph on the history of the patient only appeared in 2003: Michael Stolberg, *Homo Patiens: Krankheits- und Körpererfahrung in der Frühen Neuzeit* (Köln: Böhlau, 2003).

7. Nikolas Rose, *The Politics of Life Itself: Biomedicine, Power, and Subjectivity in the Twenty-First Century* (Princeton: Princeton University Press, 2007). On the cerebral subject and the neural turn in contemporary culture, see the special issue of the *History of the Human Sciences* 23 (2010); and Max Stadler, "The Neuroromance of Cerebal History," in S. Choudhury and J. Slaby, eds., *Critical Neuroscience: Between Lifeworld and Laboratory* (Oxford: Oxford University Press, forthcoming).

8. Porter's motives were political not intellectual; he does not appear to have been seeking to save "the reality" of the patient from its disappearance in Foucauldian discourse analysis (see below). Although he did not register it himself (and doubtless would have disputed the fact), his work on consumerism in the eighteenth century was perfectly suited to the individualist consumerist psychology and ideology extolled by Margaret Thatcher.

9. "We have histories of diseases but not of health, biographies of doctors but not of the sick." Roy Porter, *Patients and Practitioners: Lay Perceptions of Medicine in Pre-Industrial Society* (Cambridge: Cambridge University Press, 1985), 1–2.

10. See Roger Cooter, "After Death/After-Life: The Social History of Medicine in Post-Postmodernity," *Social History of Medicine* 20 (2007): 441–64.

11. See, for example, the work on patients and doctor-patient relations by the medical sociologist David Armstrong, *Political Anatomy of the Body* (Cambridge: Cambridge University Press, 1983), 72. Armstrong talks much about patients, but he does not interrogate the category. He shows, for example, how psychiatric patients came to be constituted not according to external criteria, as they formerly had, but rather by becoming their own referent in terms of their past personality judged against their present one. See also Claudine Herzlich and Janine Pierret, *Illness and Self in Society*, trans. Elborg Forster (Baltimore: Johns Hopkins University Press, 1987), 217ff., who dwell on the emergence of new doctor-patient relations.

12. Christopher Lawrence, "Historical Keyword: Patient," *Lancet* 371 (2008): 21.

13. Michel Foucault, "Questions of Methods," in *The Foucault Effect: Studies in Governmentality*, ed. G. Burchell, C. Gordon, and P. Miller (Chicago: Chicago University

Press, 1991), 79. On Foucault and biopower and biopolitics, see Roger Cooter and Claudia Stein, "Cracking Biopower," *History of Human Sciences* 23 (2010): 109–28.

14. See, for example, Erin O'Connor, *Raw Material: Producing Pathology in Victorian Culture* (Durham: Duke University Press, 2000).

15. Roger Cooter, *Surgery and Society in Peace and War: Orthopaedics and the Organization of Modern Medicine, 1880–1948* (London: Macmillan, 1993). For a recent contribution and bibliography, see George Weisz, *Divide and Conquer: A Comparative History of Medical Specialization* (Oxford: Oxford University Press, 2006).

16. Max Weber, "Bureaucracy," in *From Max Weber: Essays in Sociology*, ed. H. H. Gerth and C. Wright Mills (London: Routledge, 1948), 196–244, cited in Roger Cooter and Steve Sturdy, "Introduction," in *War, Medicine, and Modernity*, ed. Roger Cooter, Steven Sturdy, and Mark Harrison (Stroud: Sutton, 1998), 1. See also Steve Sturdy and Roger Cooter, "Science, Scientific Management, and the Transformation of Medicine in Britain, c.1870–1950," *History of Science* 36 (1998): 421–66.

17. The history of the politically correct use of the word "patients" is itself not uninteresting. Gerald Kutcher in his recent study of the medically unethical American experimenter on human subjects, Eugene Saenger, notes how Saenger "coded his writing by using terms like *individuals, men,* or *humans* that could be read as meaning either 'soldiers' or 'patients,' depending on the audience. He reserved expressions like *patients* for those times when he definitely wanted to situate the study as one in cancer therapy." The medical model of the atomized patient, Kutcher notes, "provided a rationale for using the responses of the patients' organs and tissues as surrogate measures for those of soldiers' organs and tissues." *Contested Medicine: Cancer Research and the Military* (Chicago: University of Chicago Press, 2009), 105, 109. It has further been noted by David Reubi that in bioethical discourse the word "patient" can deliberately erase the person within the patient: "Ethics Governance, Modernity, and Human Beings' Capacity to Reflect and Decide: A Genealogy of Medical Research Ethics in the UK and Singapore" (PhD diss., London School of Economics, 2009), 181.

18. In this respect, it shares company with a great deal of contemporary history writing that in a perverse way justifies the discipline of history, for if the differences between today's ancients and moderns were absolute and obvious there would be little need for either historical or historiographical investigation. History is inherently messy in this respect.

19. David Robinson, "Disorderly Genius," *Nature* 27 (June 2009): 34–37. A parallel is to be found in genomics where the 1980s book of life approach (informed by dominant metaphors from information technology) surrendered to a poststructuralist view of the proteins inside the gene as plural, porous, and not at all open to simple reductions. See Adam Bencard, "Life Beyond Information—Contesting Life and the Body in History and Molecular Biology," in *Contested Categories—Life Sciences in Society*, ed. Susanne Bauer and Ayo Wahlberg (Farnham: Ashgate 2009), 135–54.

20. Recent studies by historians of science on the role of invisible but regulatory "epistemic values and virtues" in configuring natural knowledge past and present fail to seek out the role of such virtues and values in their own practice as historians. See, notably, Steven Shapin, *The Scientific Life: A Moral History of a Late Modern Vocation* (Chicago: Chicago University Press, 2008); and Lorraine Daston and Peter Galison,

Objectivity (New York: Zone, 2007), who coin and excavate the idea of "epistemic virtues" in science production.

21. See, for example, E. H. Carr, "The Historian and His Facts," in *What is History?* (London: Macmillan, 1961).

22. On the resistance of historians to reflect on the nature of their own professional practice, see Ludmilla Jordanova, *History in Practice* (London: Arnold, 2000), 203.

23. The historian's appeal to experience as uncontestable evidence is itself a cultural construct. On this, see Joan W. Scott, "The Evidence of Experience," *Critical Inquiry* 17 (Summer 1991), 773–97.

24. For stunning examples of the genre, see Daniel Lord Smail, *On Deep History and the Brain* (Berkeley: University of California Press, 2008); and Iain McGilchrist, *The Master and His Emissary: The Divided Brain and the Making of the Western World* (New Haven: Yale University Press, 2009). For a review of the former, see Stephen T. Casper in *Medical History* 53 (2009): 318–19; and of the latter, see Roger Cooter, in *Wellcome History* 43 (2010): 20. The neuro turn is widely evident in art history, linguistics, economics, and ethics, among other disciplines.

25. See Neil Levy, *Neuroethics* (Cambridge: Cambridge University Press, 2007).

26. Roger Cooter, "Re-Presenting the Future of Medicine's Past: Towards a Politics of Survival," *Medical History* 55 (2011): 289–94.

Chapter Ten

The Neurological Patient in History

A Commentary

Max Stadler

On the evening of Tuesday, December 2, 2009, at 5:05 pm, Henry Gustav Molaison, aged eighty-two, died of respiratory failure in a nursing home in Connecticut; his death almost coincided, fortuitously, with a workshop on the neurological patient in history some three days later in London, the papers of which comprise this volume. This brief commentary will offer some reflections on the workshop papers, but it begins with Mr. Molaison, known to the world only by his initials, H. M.

Not coincidentally, of course, does this commentary focus on H. M., for H. M. was a historic neurological patient: having lost his sense of the past, unable to form new memories, H. M. featured in a myriad of textbooks and scientific papers. H. M. became immortalized as a case of profound amnesia, the result of an operation to resect his medial temporal lobes in 1953—from his early childhood, H. M. had suffered from epilepsy. "He has taught us a great deal about the cognitive and neural organization of memory. We are in his debt," as one neuroscientist would write many years later, thanking H. M. for his persistent "dedication to research." "What's new with the amnesic patient H. M.?" she asked affectionately in her article of the same title.[1]

As an object of neuroscience, as a familiar, *patient* persona, H. M. enjoyed, it would seem, unusual degrees of intimacy and individuation; his obituaries, though, would strangely lack a sense of agency and self, indeed, that of a biography. Being passed through many an eminent laboratory of brain science, the neurological patient H. M. led an existence rather resembling a chronology of scientific observations: a public profile inseparable from the person who was Henry Molaison.

For us, what makes the case of this amnesic patient a useful entryway into a reflection upon the essays assembled here is the peculiar combination of anonymity and iconicity that is evinced by these two initials, and that came together in the patient life of Molaison. In other words, there seems to be something palpably distinct here about the neurological patient—only unusually palpable in the case of H. M.—that is not simply about questions of case and category, or merely about anonymity and matters of sources, access, and documentation. Certainly the essays in this volume suggest this much—that the patient, and H. M. is evidently just one incarnation, is a more complex and intriguing figure than the mere object of a science called neurology, more than the disciplined psychiatric subject of the Foucauldian kind, and more as well than the generic patient who was to be reinserted in our stories by a medical history *from below.*

As I read these essays, what renders the neurological patient distinct, then, as a subject and as a challenge to historical interrogation, are the very oscillations and interactions between what we may call the iconic on the one hand, and the anonymous on the other: two extreme ends of a spectrum, or dimensions, within which is located the neurological patient. Needless to say, there are other ways to think about this distinctness of the neurological patient, and neither do I propose these labels—iconicity and anonymity—as rigid denominators. But they usefully gesture at what are the complexities that enter into the fashioning of what seems to me—and this is the point—a peculiar form of neurological individuality. Indeed, in their different ways, it is these very complexities that the essays in this volume most forcefully bring out—from the *emblematic* patient, the term Kushner's essay turns to productive use, to the *scripted*, ritualistic enactments of patient and neurologist that Casper examines in his contribution.

Any such suggestion as to the peculiarities of the neurological patient must begin with a form of caveat. What I referred to as iconicity above, or a distinctness that the case of H. M. may serve to indicate, also brings with it the danger involved in prioritizing in our historical narratives this or that case, this or that neurological experience, this or that category of patient. We could indeed have started quite differently. Take, for instance, the elderly lady who is the protagonist of *Princess Margaret Blvd.* (2008), a film by Kazik Radwanski that is a cinematic reflection on Alzheimer's disease. One of the most moving scenes of the film finds her lost and helpless in the early hours of a winter day in the parking lot of a desolate suburban shopping mall; known not even by her initials, mumbling incoherent fragments of language to herself, remaining unheard and unnoticed, she teaches no one about the organization of anything in particular.

And there are, of course, the many other, thousands of nameless patients suffering from aphasia, Alzheimer's, Parkinson's, and other diseases—patients *infâmes*, to invoke Foucault's term for a historical problematic that is clearly not peculiar to the case at hand. It is certainly familiar from writing the history of patients generally. It is this danger of oversight and conflation that Kushner's essay is arguing so passionately, that of confusing—and here Kushner has in mind the neurologists—the emblematic and the not-so-emblematic patient, or what I referred to above as the two dimensions of iconicity and anonymity. It is to take H. M., as it were, for the neurological patient rather than the elderly lady with dementia. And to this I would add that being aware of these complexities should be a demand made at least equally upon us, the historians, and not so much the yardstick by which to judge our historical actors. An excitement with the exotic, extraordinary, or extreme may be a nosological will-o'-the-wisp; it certainly can be a historiographic one.

And yet it would be as wrong not to take very seriously at the same time what seems to be one of the defining peculiarities of the neurological patient: his or her curious individuality. It is a condition that may or may not be indicated by initials, but it is hard indeed to imagine another medical specialty that would have generated a similar amount of individuated disease as did neurology. H. M. is a case in point, but many more spring to mind: the tourettic patients Harold Kushner discusses in his essay for instance—the Marquise de Dampierre, the businessman "O.," Twitchy—and in very different ways, what might be called an emblematic population, the nervous kid and the Wandering Jew. The case of Robert Nichols's neuroasthenic self-fashioning, the subject of Stephen Jacyna's essay, can be seen as yet another variation of such individuation. And so can be seen those many iconic patients that populate neurological history at large: Siegfried Sassoon, Broca's Tan, Phineas Gage, Lou Gehrig, Sybil, and the curious patients Oliver Sacks parades in his popular writings.

As much as historians of medicine have come to appreciate that the Cambridge-educated, upper-class poet Sassoon doesn't exhaust the history and experience of shell shock, there seems to be preserved in the neurological patient a peculiar, irreducible form of individuality, or residues thereof, that our historical accounts need to reflect. It is, at any rate, in this connection—the complexities that underlie the constructions of neurological individuality—that I find these essays most revealing. Together they demonstrate how we can in our historical accounts make productive these oscillations and interactions—rather than seeing them as limiting, or indeed as two separate dimensions. Together they also suggest something of the very different shapes such processes of interaction can historically assume, and the great many factors that impinge on them. From Ballenger's account of the public constructions of Alzheimer's disease in the United States since the 1970s—a story of advocacy movements, of identity politics and being given a voice—to Gatley's close reading of a bohemian artistic couple coping with the trajectory into fatal neurological illness in the years surrounding the Great War, they reveal something of the intricacies of crafting neurological individuality.

The elderly, nameless lady with dementia mentioned above would thus be no exception. As both Ballenger and Lorch examine in their essays, juxtaposed to the emblems of neurological history stand the numberless, nameless patients whose voices and identities are neither straightforwardly their own, nor simply imposed and owned by others. Ballenger's essay has already been briefly mentioned as illustrating the complex interplay of multiple actors and agencies that can be involved in giving voice to neurological disease and constructing neurological identities, though here we are concerned less strictly perhaps with the iconic or emblematic than with those patients giving a public face to a disease. A similar historical complexity is evident in Lorch's contribution, which deals with a very different time period, context, and disease. It is a demonstration not least of the complexity of the historical circumstances that shape the emergence of a patient population and that thus shape and reshape the interlocking private and public dimensions of neurological identity.

Lorch's study, with its focus on civil law, significantly broadens our understanding of the factors at work in this context; as far as the legal relations of psychiatry and neurology are concerned, questions of criminal law and the advent of national systems of insurance are usually highlighted. Civil law courts, however, did not have to deal with the extreme fringes of society, insane murderers, and rapists. Instead, like the outpatient and specialty clinics that then were taking root in Britain and elsewhere, they began to make salient (among other things) a relatively benign and much broader population of speech-impaired idiots, who could not, or so it seemed, be perceived or conceptualized in terms of a unity of insanity. Their intellect was far less straightforwardly and completely corrupted, seemingly being able, when summoned by the law, to express themselves by alternative means. As Lorch shows, the aphasic patient, his or her capacity to deliver testimony, and thus his or her entitlement to a voice, will, and identity, was conditioned by transformations in British civil law that paralleled and interacted with the clinical definitions or perceptions of aphasia.

But beyond this narrower legal context, Lorch's paper suggests a range of further factors and complex cultural and social transformations at work in the emergence of the aphasic patient as a case of impaired self-expression. A great deal of conceptual and boundary-drawing work thus was spent in the Victorian period on categories such as "the expert," "the specialist," "scientific authority," or "laity," and these various, unstable groupings all had their stakes in the aphasic patient. (Lorch's paper moreover raises the question as to the significance of national contexts in this connection). Meanwhile, it was a sea change in literacy, mass schooling, and average education levels that implicated this nineteenth-century neurological patient who was capable of expression through media other than language.

This picture of aphasia is one of a tremendous amount of negotiation, dynamics involving law reforms, lawyers, medical experts, greedy family members, and revolutions in cultural technologies and media environments. To fully integrate such various dimensions into a history of the aphasic patient would seem to constitute a laudable project. It would mean to reconstruct the historicity and historical conditions of both aphasic iconicity *and* anonymity. And it would not least mean to restore a certain agency to the neurological patient; in this case, the historical means and spaces of expression available in the crafting of his or her identity.

Indeed, I would argue, taking seriously the patient as an agent in neurological historiography should lead to very fruitful elaboration of what philosopher of science Ian Hacking has labelled the process of "making up people."[2] We still must know much more about the historical processes through which the iconic, emblematic, the proto- or stereotypical narratives and images of the neurological patient get produced, appropriated, recycled, and mediated. In very different ways, the significance of a patient's literacy, education, and persona thus comes to the fore in the two contemporary cases discussed by Jacyna and Gatley, that of the neurasthenic Robert Nichols and that of the French expatriate painter Jacques Raverat, respectively. Having much in common in terms of class background, as well as geographically and culturally, the two cases impressively demonstrate how particular constellations of literacy, lay neurological knowledge, social setting, and available means and technologies of expression conspire in the specifics of self-fashioning in matters of neurological identity and the coping with neurological disease.

The crafted iconicity of a patient, we may say, is never a matter only of passivity, and as such is subject to historically specific means and conditions of self-expression. And both these cases also powerfully bring home the importance of nontextual, nonverbal means of expression and of personal interaction in such self-fashioning (or being self-fashioned). In doing so, both cases, moreover, point to factors involved in the "making up" of the neurological patient that move us well beyond the clinical encounter, or processes of disciplining, medicalization, and the boundaries defined through professional medical practice, legal systems, or the public domain. "Bodily performances," as Jacyna suggests, even a type of fatherly friendship, of imagined camaraderie, learnedness, and admiration were an essential component to Nichols's self-constructions and his transactions with his doctors. In Raverat's case, it was the intimacy of an early twentieth-century Bohemian marriage; pictorial, visual means of expression; and artistic sensibilities that mediated the patient's self-image.

Clearly, however, these were elite self-images; they were not available in every *case*. As such, they perhaps are more iconic to us as regards the interwar patient than they ever were at the time. This, of course, is not to say they were irrelevant, but rather that we still need to know more about the channels through which certain neurological images become self-images—how they turn iconic and make their reentry into the crafting of neurological identities.

But there is more to be gleaned from these essays than the circulation and construction of images and narratives. Elite or not, both Gatley's and Jacyna's cases plastically point us to a second, related theme that strikes me as crucial to several if not all of the present treatments of the neurological patient and his or her individuations. I want to conclude these brief comments on this other theme: it is the centrality of language, and of bodily and written expressions in the making up of these historical images of the neurological patient. Or, put negatively, it is the instructive absence in these various accounts of the very iconic organ that increasingly has come to shape our conceptions of neurological disease—the brain.

In fact, this absence may not be entirely coincidental. The living brain as a concrete, palpable site of observation and intervention, after all, is a matter of very recent history.[3] Notwithstanding the fact that the cerebral subject—as a discursive entity—has a long prehistory, predating, as Fernando Vidal recently has persuasively argued elsewhere, the recent surge of the neurosciences by decades and even centuries,[4] it was not until recently that neurological patients in fact carried around in their wallets the (self-reassuring) images of their own MRI brain scans or stuck them onto the doors of their fridges.[5] This is not a trivial point. Indeed the contingency of this latter, braincentric "neuroculture" is one of the crucial themes, I believe, that implicitly traverses these essays here.[6]

The case for the signal importance of bodily expression and performance, and of the theatrical and ritualistic in the lives of the neurological patient (as opposed to the central nervous system), is made most explicitly in Casper's contribution. Casper deals with the neurological examination as a type of scripted, enacted encounter between neurologist and patient mediated through textbooks and neurological pedagogy, thus coming to similar conclusions with Jacyna: ritual and bodily performance matters in the history of the neurological patient, and they matter, we may imagine, when aphasics appear in court or when tourettic patients violate social expectations and norms. By this, then, I do not mean the replacement of one romantic figure—or the "romance of the brain" as historian Susan Cozzens has aptly labelled it—by another romance, that of the *body*.[7] As Casper emphasizes, "In a world before high-definition X-rays, computer-aided analyses, and PET, CAT, and MRI imaging, the living body, normal and pathological, and the dead body, determined the neurologist's practices" (chap. 1). And they determined, I would add, in at times quite unromantic ways, the self-techniques, means of expressions, images, and imaginations available to the neurological patient.

As the essays in this volume reveal, the practices, means, and techniques of neurological individuation were subject to significant mutations and they often bore only little resemblance to the ones prevailing in our contemporary, imaging-technology mediated age of a braincentric neuroculture.

Historically, we have grown prone to forget that it was the body, the peripheral nervous and neuromuscular systems, the vegetative nervous system, and a great diversity of technologies of observation and means of expression—some image-based, some not—that have tended to come together in alternative forms of neurological culture: neurological knowledge and practices interacted in complex ways with the culturally and socially available resources as regards behavioral norms and means of expression, shaping what the neurological patient could be at a given time and period. And taken together, I would argue, these various contributions on the neurological patient invite us to pay detailed attention to these bodily cultures: the body in the history of neurology, that is, and to its historically specific means of expression; and to how, finally, these individual, neurological experiences and identities intermeshed with the emblematic narratives of neurology and its rituals.

It is as such, then, that the neurological patient in history points us beyond this iconic organ, the central nervous system—so central to our own images of the neurological—and asks us to look beyond neurology conceived as only a specialty and a matter of clinical research as well. In this, as these essays show—not in restoring the patients' perspective for its own sake (a quite sentimental endeavor)—resides the importance of reinserting the patient in our stories of the history of neurology: the neurological patient provides more than a merely a fruitful, additional area of inquiry in the history of neurology—it should prompt us to reconsider and revisit many of these themes that already have been worked into the historiography.

To be sure, if the history of neurology has been written for the most part as the biography of famous neurologists, professional historians have tended to intervene in relation to a number of themes that took the history of neurology in very different directions. But, they arguably also tended to reproduce this neurologists' perspective: clinical research, institutions, therapeutic regimes, language, war, even aesthetics (historians eagerly latched onto the early uses and importance of film and photography in neurology). We need, as the essays in this volume make clear, more complicated pictures of how these thematic complexes and historical circumstances became interwoven in the crafting of particular neurological identities. And by the same token, as I also have suggested, these essays should prompt us to reconsider from historical perspectives, in our present days of neuroscientific myopia, the place of the body, and of bodily expressions and performances in the history of the nervous system. In fact, as much as we still lack a deeper understanding of the historical dimensions of the neurological patient, this history remains by and large an historically uncharted terrain—in particular as far the twentieth century is concerned. In all these connections, I should think, the *Neurological Patient in History* offers a great many suggestive advances: from the neurological examination Casper discusses to the selffashionings of a Robert Nichols; performance, practices of giving voice, and techniques of the self, to employ another one of Foucault's winged phrases, thus loom large in these histories at hand. They also are central to Ballanger's contribution; and common to both the papers by Lorch and Kushner is a focus on language and written expression: the neurological patient's testimony (too much, an excess in the one case; too little or too incoherent in the other) and the textual work of the clinician, psychotherapist, or an Oliver Sacks. After all, this neurological patient is an individual one—insofar as it performs, has a body, possesses a language, writes, and sometimes is known by his or her initials.

Notes

1. Suzanne Corkin, "What's New with the Amnesic Patient H. M.?" *Nature Reviews Neuroscience* 3 (2002): 153–60; and Benedict Carey, "H. M., an Unforgettable Amnesiac, Dies at 82," *New York Times*, December 5, 2009.

2. Ian Hacking, "Making Up People," in *Reconstructing Individualism*, ed. T. C. Heller, M. Sosna, and D. E. Wellbery (Stanford: Stanford University Press, 1986), 222–36.

3. See esp. John Braslow, *Mental Ills and Bodily Cures: Psychiatric Treatment in the First Half of the Twentieth Century* (Berkeley: University of California Press, 1997); and Jack D. Pressman, *Last Resort: Psychosurgery and the Limits of Medicine* (Cambridge: Cambridge University Press, 1998).

4. Fernando Vidal, "Brainhood, Anthropological Figure of Modernity," *History of the Human Sciences* 22 (2009): 5–36.

5. Simon Cohn, "When Patients See Their Mental Illness," in *Technologized Images, Technologized Bodies: Anthropological Approaches to a New Politics of Vision*, ed. J. Edwards, P. Harvey, and P. Wade (Oxford: Berghahn, 2010).

6. "Neuroculture" is the term I picked up from a workshop titled "Neurocultures" (on February 20–22, 2009, at the Max Planck Institute for the History of Science, Berlin).

7. Susan Cozzens, "Knowledge of the Brain: The Visualizing Tools of Contemporary Historiography," in *The Historiography of Contemporary Science and Technology*, ed. T. Söderqvist (London: Routledge, 1997), 156.

Bibliography

Anon. "Epidemic (Lethargic) Encephalitis: A Personal Experience." *Journal of the American Medical Association* 78 (1922): 407–9.

Anon. "Parkinsonism." In *Disabilities and How to Live with Them: True Stories Written by Patients or Former Patients*, 52–58. London: The Lancet, 1952.

Anon. "The Pathology of Speech." *British Medical Journal* 2 (1879): 378–81.

Abel, Emily K. "Family Caregiving in the Nineteenth Century: Emily Hawley Gillespie and Sarah Gillespie, 1858–1888." *Bulletin of the History of Medicine* 68 (1994): 573–99.

———. *Hearts of Wisdom: American Women Caring for Kin, 1850–1940.* Cambridge: Harvard University Press, 2000.

Abbott, Andrew. *The System of Professions: An Essay on the Division of Expert Labor.* Chicago: University of Chicago Press, 1988.

Ackerknecht, Erwin H. *Medicine at the Paris Hospital, 1794–1848.* Baltimore: Johns Hopkins University Press, 1967.

Ajuriaguerra, Julián de. "The Concept of Akinesia." *Psychological Medicine* 5 (1975): 129–37.

Althaus, Julius. *Diseases of the Nervous System: Their Prevalence and Pathology.* London: Smith Elder, 1877.

Anderson, Warwick. *The Collectors of Lost Souls: Turning Kuru Scientists into Whitemen.* Baltimore: Johns Hopkins University Press, 2008.

Angyal, Ludwig von. "Zur Kenntnis der postencephalitischen Antriebs- und Gedächtnisstörungen." *Zeitschrift für die gesamte Neurologie und Psychiatrie* 122 (1929): 187–203.

Antonetta, Susanne. *A Mind Apart: Travels in a Neurodiverse World.* New York: Jeremy P. Tarcher, 2007.

Armstrong, David. *Political Anatomy of the Body.* Cambridge: Cambridge University Press, 1983.

Badley, John H. "Bedales School, Petersfield, England." *Elementary School Teacher* 5, no. 5 (1905): 257–66.

Ballenger, Jesse F. "Beyond the Characteristic Plaques and Tangles: Mid-Twentieth-Century U.S. Psychiatry and the Fight against Senility." In *Concepts of Alzheimer Disease: Biological, Clinical, and Cultural Perspectives*, edited by Peter J. Whitehouse, Konrad Maurer, and Jesse F. Ballenger, 83–103. Baltimore: Johns Hopkins University Press, 2000.

———. "Progress in the History of Alzheimer's Disease: The Importance of Context." *Journal of Alzheimer's Disease* 9 (2006): 1–9.

———. *Self, Senility, and Alzheimer's Disease in Modern America.* Baltimore: Johns Hopkins University Press, 2006.

Barnes, Arthur Stanley. "The Diagnostic Value of the Plantar Reflex." *Review of Neurology and Psychiatry* 2 (1904): 345–76.

Bartlett, Peter. "Legal Madness in the Nineteenth Century." *Social History of Medicine* 14 (2001): 107–31.

———. "Sense and Nonsense: Sensation, Delusion, and the Limitation of Sanity in Nineteenth-Century Law." In *Law and the Senses*, edited by L. Bendy and L. Flynn, 21–41. London: Pluto Press, 1996.

Bastian, Henry Charlton. "On the Various Forms of Loss of Speech in Cerebral Disease." *British Foreign Medico-chirurgical Review* 43 (1869): 209–36.

Bateman, Frederic. *On Aphasia, or Loss of Speech, and the Localisation of the Faculty of Articulate Language.* London: J. Churchill & Sons, 1870.

Beard, George Miller. "Legal Responsibility in Old Age: Based On Researchers into the Relation of Age to Work." In *The "Fixed Period" Controversy*, edited by Gerald Gruman, 4–31. New York: Arno Press, 1979.

Bechterew, W. "Die Krankheiten der Persönlichkeit vom Standpunkt der Reflexologie: Zur Begründung der pathologischen Reflexologie." *Zeitschrift für die gesamte Neurologie und Psychiatrie* 80 (1923): 265–309.

Beer, M. Dominic. "The Dichotomies: Psychosis/Neurosis and Functional/Organic: a Historical Perspective." *History of Psychiatry* 7 (1996): 231–55.

Beevor, Charles Edward. *Diseases of the Nervous System.* London: H. K. Lewis, 1898.

Bencard, Adam. "Life Beyond Information—Contesting Life and the Body in History and Molecular Biology." In *Contested Categories—Life Sciences in Society*, edited by Susanne Bauer and Ayo Wahlberg, 135–54. London: Ashgate, 2009.

Bennett, Maxwell Richard, and Peter Michael Stephan Hacker. *Philosophical Foundations of Neuroscience.* London: Blackwell, 2003.

Berg, Marc, and Annemarie Mol. *Differences in Medicine: Unravelling Practices, Techniques, and Bodies.* Durham: Duke University Press, 1998.

Bernat, James L. "Theresa Schiavo's Tragedy and Ours, Too." *Neurology* 71 (2008): 964–65.

Berze, Josef. "Beiträge zur psychiatrischen Erblichkeits- und Konstitutionsforschung. II. Schizoid, Schizophrenie, Dementia praecox." *Zeitschrift für die gesamte Neurologie und Psychiatrie* 96 (1925): 603–52.

———. *Die primäre Insuffizienz der psychischen Aktivität: Ihr Wesen, ihre Erscheinungen, und ihre Bedeutung als Grundstörung der Dementia praecox und der Hypophrenien überhaupt.* Leipzig: Franz Deuticke, 1914.

———. "Zur Frage der Lokalisation der Vorstellungen." *Zeitschrift für die gesamte Neurologie und Psychiatrie* 44 (1919): 213–85.

———. "Zur Frage der Lokalisation psychischer Vorgänge." *Archiv für Psychiatrie und Nervenkrankheiten* 71 (1924): 546–80.

Betzold, Michael. *Appointment with Doctor Death.* Troy, MI: Momentum Books, 1993.

Bichat, Xavier. *Physiological Researches on Life and Death.* Translated by F. Gold. London: J Mills Bristol, 1815.

Bickerstaff, Edwin R. *Neurological Examination in Clinical Practice.* Oxford: Blackwell, 1963.

Bivins, Roberta, and John V. Pickstone, eds. *Medicine, Madness, and Social History: Essays in Honour of Roy Porter.* Basingstoke: Palgrave Macmillan, 2007.

Bixler, Elizabeth S. "The Nurse and Neurological Problems." *American Journal of Nursing* 35 (1935): 425–30.

Bleuler, Eugen. "Die Kritiken der Schizophrenien." *Zeitschrift für die gesamte Neurologie und Psychiatrie* 22 (1914): 19–44.

———. *La schizophrénie*. Congrès des médecins aliénistes et neurologistes de France et des pays de langue française 30ᵉ Session Genève-Lausanne, 2–7 août 1926, Rapport de psychiatrie. Paris: Masson et Cie, 1926.

Bloss, Nick van. *Busy Body: My Life with Tourette's Syndrome*. London: Fusion Press, 2006.

Blustein, Bonnie Ellen. "New York Neurologists and the Specialization of American Medicine." *Bulletin of the History of Medicine* 53, no. 2 (1979): 170–83.

———. *Preserve Your Love for Science: Life of William Hammond, American Neurologist*. Cambridge: Cambridge University Press, 1991.

Bostroem, A. "Encephalitische und katatone Motilitätsstörungen." *Klinische Wochenschrift* 3 (1924): 465–69.

Bougousslavsky J., and F. Boller, eds. *Neurological Disorders in Famous Artists*. Basel: Karger, 2005.

Bourdieu, Pierre. *Homo Academicus*. Oxford: Polity Press, 2001.

———. *The Logic of Practice*. Cambridge: Polity Press, 2003.

Bourke, Joanna. *Dismembering the Male: Men's Bodies, Britain, and the Great War*. London: Reaktion, 1996.

———. "Effeminacy, Ethnicity, and the End of Trauma: The Sufferings of 'Shell-Shocked' Men in Great Britain and Ireland, 1914–1939." *Journal of Contemporary History* 35, no. 1 (2000): 57–69.

———. "Wartime." In *Companion to Medicine in the Twentieth Century*, edited by Roger Cooter and John Pickstone, 589–600. London: Routledge, 2003.

Brain, Walter Russell. *Diseases of the Nervous System*. Oxford: Oxford University Press, 1933.

Bramley, Natalie, and Virginia Eatough. "The Experience of Living with Parkinson's Disease: An Interpretative Phenomenological Analysis Case Study." *Psychology & Health* 20 (2005): 223–35.

Bramwell, Byron. *The Diseases of the Spinal Cord*. Edinburgh: Clay, 1895.

Bramwell, James P. "Case of Traumatic Aphasia: Recorded by the Patient with Remarks by J. P. Bramwell, M.D." *British Medical Journal* 2, nos. 180–81 (1867): 180.

Braslow, Joel. *Mental Ills and Bodily Cures: Psychiatric Treatment in the First Half of the Twentieth Century*. Berkeley: University of California Press, 1997.

Brissaud, Edouard, and Eugène Feindel. "Sur le traitement du torticolis mental et des tics similaires." *Journal de Neurologie* (1899): 141–49.

Bristowe, John Syer. "The Lumleian Lectures on the Pathological Relations of the Voice and Speech." *British Medical Journal* 1 (1879): 731–34.

Broca, Paul. *Nouvelle observation d'aphémie: Produite par une lésion de la troisième circonvolution frontale*. Paris: Victor Masson et Fils, 1861.

———. *Remarques sur le siège, le diagnostic, et la nature de l'aphémie: Extrait des Bulletins de la Société Anatomique, etc.* Paris: Moquet, 1863.

———. *Sur siège de la faculté du langage articulé avec deux observations d'aphémie (perte de la parole)*. Paris: Victor Masson et Fils, 1861.

————. *Du siège de la faculté du langage articulé dans l'hémisphère gauche du cerveau: Extrait des Bulletins de la Société d'Anthropologie, etc.* Paris: Moquet, 1865.

Brown, S. E. "Focal Dystonia in Musicians." *Western Journal of Medicine* 157, no. 6 (1992): 666.

Brumberg, Joan J. *Fasting Girls: The History of Anorexia Nervosa.* New York: Vintage, 1989.

Bruun, Ruth Dowling, and Bertel Bruun. *A Mind of Its Own: Tourette's Syndrome: A Story and a Guide.* New York: Oxford University Press, 1994.

Burnham, John C. *How the Idea of Profession Changed the Writing of Medical History.* London: Wellcome Institute for the History of Medicine, 1998.

————. *What is Medical History?* Cambridge: Polity Press, 2005.

Bury, Judson S. *Diseases of the Nervous System.* Manchester: Manchester University Press, 1912.

Butler, Robert N. *Why Survive?: Being Old in America.* New York: Harper & Row, 1975.

Buzzard, Thomas. *Clinical Lectures on Diseases of the Nervous System.* Philadelphia: P. Blakiston, 1882.

Bynum, William F., Anne Hardy, L. Stephen Jacyna, Christopher Lawrence, and E. M. (Tilli) Tansey, eds. *The Western Medical Tradition, 1800–2000.* Cambridge: Cambridge University Press, 2006.

Calhoun, Richard B. *In Search of the New Old: Redefining Old Age in America, 1945–1970.* New York: Elsevier, 1978.

Carey, Eleanore. "I Recover from Sleeping Sickness." *American Mercury Magazine* 32: 165–69.

Carr, Edward H. *What is History?* London: Macmillan, 1961.

Casper, Stephen T. "Atlantic Conjunctures in Anglo-American Neurology: Lewis H. Weed and Johns Hopkins Neurology, 1917–1942." *Bulletin of the History of Medicine* 82, no. 3 (2008): 646–71.

————. "The Idioms of Practice: British Neurology, 1880–1960." PhD diss., University College London, 2007.

————. Review of *On Deep History and the Brain,* by Daniel Lord Smail. *Medical History* 53 (2009): 318–19.

Certeau, Michel de. *The Practices of Everyday Life.* Berkley: University of California Press, 1988.

Charcot, Jean-Martin. *Lectures on the Diseases of the Nervous System.* Translated by George Sigerson. London: The New Sydenham Society, 1881.

Charlton, Anne, and William Charlton. *Putting Poetry First: A Life of Robert Nichols, 1893–1944.* Norwich: Michael Russell, 2003.

Clarke, Edwin, and L. Stephen Jacyna. *Nineteenth-Century Origins of Neuroscientific Concepts.* Berkeley: University of California Press, 1987.

Cohen, Brad, and Lisa Wyscocky. *Front of the Class: How Tourette Syndrome Made Me the Teacher I Never Had.* Acton, MA: Vander Wyk & Burnham, 2005.

Cole, Thomas R. *The Journey of Life: A Cultural History of Aging in America.* New York: Cambridge University Press, 1992.

Collier, James. "An Investigation upon the Plantar Reflex, with Reference to the Significance of Its Variations under Pathological Conditions, Including an Enquiry into the Aetiology of Acquired Pes Cavus." *Brain* 22, no. 1 (1899): 71–97.

Collingwood, Robin George. *Essays in the Philosophy of History*. Austin: University of Texas Press, 1965.

Collins, Joseph. *The Treatment of Diseases of the Nervous System: A Manual for Practitioners*. New York: William Wood, 1900.

Comings, David E. *Tourette Syndrome and Human Behavior*. Duarte, CA: Hope Press, 1990.

Cooter, Roger. "After Death/After-Life: The Social History of Medicine in Post-Postmodernity." *Social History of Medicine* 20 (2007): 441–64.

———. "Re-Presenting the Future of Medicine's Past: Towards a Politics of Survival." *Medical History* 55 (2011): 289–94.

———. "Review of *The Master and His Emissary: The Divided Brain and the Making of the Western World*, by Iain McGilchrist." *Wellcome History* 43 (2010): 20.

———. *Surgery and Society in Peace and War: Orthopaedics and the Organization of Modern Medicine, 1880–1948*. London: Macmillan, 1993.

Cooter, Roger, Mark Harrison, and Steve Sturdy, eds. *Medicine and Modern Warfare*. Amsterdam: Rodopi, 1999.

Cooter, Roger, and John Pickstone, eds. *Companion to Medicine in the Twentieth Century*. London: Routledge, 2003.

Cooter, Roger, and Steve Sturdy. "Introduction." In *War, Medicine, and Modernity*, edited by Roger Cooter, Steven Sturdy, and Mark Harrison, 1–9. Stroud: Sutton, 1998.

Como, Peter G. "Obsessive-Compulsive Disorder in Tourette's Syndrome." In *Behavioral Neurology of Movement Disorders*, edited by William J. Weiner and Anthony E. Lang, 249–61. New York: Raven Press, 1995.

Condrau, Flurin. "The Patient's View Meets the Clinical Gaze." *Social History of Medicine* 20 (2007): 525–40.

Core, Donald Elms. *The Examination of the Central Nervous System*. Edinburgh: E & S Livingstone, 1928.

Corkin, Suzanne. "What's New with the Amnesic Patient H. M.?" *Nature Reviews Neuroscience* 3 (2002): 153–60.

Couser, G. Thomas. *Recovering Bodies: Illness, Disability, and Life Writing*. Madison: University of Wisconsin Press, 1997.

Crichton-Browne, James. "Preface." *Medical Reports of the West Riding Lunatic Asylum* 1 (1871): iv.

Cruchet, Jean-René. "Le tic convulsif et son traitement gymnastique (méthode de Brissaud et méthode de Pitres)." MD Thesis. Bordeaux: G. Gounouilhou, Imprimeur de la Faculté de Médecine, Bordeaux, 1902.

Dandy, Walter E., and Robert Elman. "Studies in Experimental Epilepsy." *Bulletin of the Johns Hopkins Hospital* 36, no. 1 (1925): 40–49.

Daston, Lorraine, ed. *Things that Talk: Object Lessons from Art and Science*. New York: Zone, 2004.

Davis, P. A., and W. Suzlbach. Changes in the Electroencephalogram during Metrazol Therapy." *Transactions of the American Neurological Association* (1939): 144–49.

DeBaggio, Thomas. *Losing My Mind: An Intimate Look at Life with Alzheimer's*. New York: Free Press, 2002.

———. *When It Gets Dark: An Enlightened Reflection on Life with Alzheimer's*. New York: Free Press, 2003.

DeJong, Russell N. *The Neurological Examination: Incorporating the Fundamentals of Neuroanatomy and Neurophysiology.* 4th ed. New York: Harper & Row, 1979.

Delater, Gabriel. "Auto-observation d'encéphalite léthargique." *Paris Médical* 10 (1920): 316–19.

———. "La grippe dans la nation armée de 1918 à 1921." *Revue d'Hygiène et de Police Sanitaire 45* (1923): 406–26, 523–38, 619–34.

———. "Suite sur trente ans et fin d'une auto-observation d'encéphalite léthargique." *Paris Médical* 38 (1948): 229–30.

Denny-Brown, Derek, *Handbook of Neurological Examination and Case Recording.* Cambridge: Harvard University Press, 1957.

Dewar, Bonnie-Kate, and B. A. Wilson. "Cognitive Recovery from Encephalitis Lethargica." *Brain Injuries* 19 (2005): 1285–91.

Dickens, Charles. *Bleak House.* London: Nelson, 1853.

———. *The Personal History of David Copperfield.* London: Chapman & Hall, 1850.

Dimitz Ludwig, and Paul Schilder. "Über die psychischen Störungen bei der Encephalitis epidemica des Jahres 1920." *Zeitschrift für die gesamte Neurologie und Psychiatrie* 68 (1923): 299–340.

Doolittle, Glenn J. "Report of Results from Use of Ketogenic Diet and Ketogenic Diet with Water Restriction in a Series of Epileptics." Pts. 1 and 2. *Psychiatric Quarterly* 5, no. 1 (1931): 135–50; no. 2 (1931): 225–52.

Draaisma, Douwe. *Disturbances of the Mind.* Translated by Barbara Fasting. Cambridge: Cambridge University Press, 2009.

Drayton, W. "Pneumocranium in the Treatment of Traumatic Headaches, Dizziness, and Change of Character." *Archives of Neurology and Psychiatry* (1934): 1302–99.

Dror, Otniel E. "'Voodoo Death': Fantasy, Excitement, and the Untenable Boundaries of Biomedical Science." In *The Politics of Healing: Essays in the Twentieth-Century History of North American Alternative Medicine,* edited by Robert D. Johnston, 71–81. London: Routledge, 2004.

Duffin, Jacalyn. *History of Medicine: A Scandalously Short Introduction.* 2nd ed. Toronto: University of Toronto Press, 2010.

Dugas, Michel. "La maladie des tics: d'Itard aux neuroleptiques." *Revue Neurologique* 142 (1986): 817–23.

Dujardin Kathy, P. Sockeel, D. Devos, M. Delliaux, P. Krystkowiak, A. Destée, and L. Defebvre. "Characteristics of Apathy in Parkinson's Disease." *Movement Disorders* 22 (2007): 778–84.

Dumit, Joseph. *Picturing Personhood: Brain Scans and Biomedical Identity.* Princeton: Princeton University Press, 2003.

Eigen, Joel Peter. "Historical Developments in Psychiatric Forensic Evidence: The British Experience." *International Journal of Law and Psychiatry* 6 (1983): 423–29.

Eley, R. Cannon. "Epilepsy: The Value of Encephalography in the Selection of Children for Ketogenic Diets." *Journal of Pediatrics* 3, no. 2 (1933): 359–68.

Feiling, Anthony. *A History of Maida Vale Hospital for Nervous Diseases.* London: Butterworth, 1958.

Ferenczi, Sandor. "Psycho-Analytical Observation on Tic." *International Journal of Psycho-Analysis* 2 (1921): 1–30.

Ferguson, Alison, Linda Worrall, John McPhee, Rhonda Buskell, Elizabeth Armstrong, and Leanne Togher. "Testamentary Capacity and Aphasia: A Descriptive Case Report with Implications for Clinical Practice." *Aphasiology* 17, no. 10 (2003): 965–80.

Feuchtersleben, Ernst F. von. *Lehrbuch der ärztlichen Seelenkunde.* Vienna: Carl Gerold, 1845.

Finger, Stanley. *Origins of Neuroscience: A History of Explorations into Brain Function.* New York: Oxford University Press, 1994.

Fissell, Mary E. *Patients, Power, and the Poor in Eighteenth-Century Bristol.* Cambridge: Cambridge University Press, 1991.

Fleischner, E. C. "The Treatment of Tic in Childhood." *California State Journal of Medicine* 9 (1911): 379–82.

Fletcher, John Gould. "Woodcuts of Gwendolen Raverat." *Print Collector's Quarterly* 18 (1931): 330–50.

Foley, Paul B. *Beans, Roots, and Leaves: A History of the Chemical Therapy of Parkinsonism.* Marburg: Tectum, 2003.

Forman, Paul. "(Re)cognizing Postmodernity: Help for Historians—Of Science Especially." *Berichte zur Wissenschaftsgeschichte* 33 (2010): 157–75.

Foucault, Michel. *The Birth of the Clinic: An Archeology of Medical Perception.* Translated by A. M. Sheridan. London: Tavistock, 1973.

———. *Discipline and Punishment: The Birth of the Prison.* London: Penguin, 1991.

———. *Madness and Civilization: A History of Insanity in the Age of Reason.* New York: Vintage, 1988.

———. "Questions of Methods." In *The Foucault Effect: Studies in Governmentality,* edited by G. Burchell, C. Gordon, and P. Miller, 79. Chicago: Chicago University Press, 1991.

Frank, Arthur W. *The Wounded Storyteller: Body, Illness, and Ethics.* Chicago: University of Chicago Press, 1995.

Freud, Sigmund. "Abriß der Psychoanalyse." *Internationale Zeitschrift für Psychoanalyse und Imago* 25 (1940): 7–67.

Friedhoff, Arnold J., and Thomas N. Chase, eds., *Gilles de la Tourette Syndrome.* New York: Raven Press, 1982.

Furger, Julie Ann, and Adam Ward Seligman. *The Marriage Vow: Poetry and Reflections Celebrating the Married Life.* Mt. Shasta, CA: Echolalia Press, 1995.

Furst, Lilian. *Between Doctors and Patients: The Changing Balance of Power.* Charlottesville: University of Virginia Press, 1998.

Gairdner, William T. "Report of a Case of Aphasia." *British Medical Journal* 1 (1875): 568.

Gay, Peter. *Freud: A Life for Our Time.* New York: Norton, 1988.

Geĭmanovich, A. I. "Psikhoticheskoe soderzhanie epidemicheskogo encefalita." In *Infektsii i Nervnaya Sistema* (Trudy Ukrainskogo Psikhonevrologikheskogo Instituta 3), edited by A. I. Geĭmanovich. Kharkov: Vseukrainskoe Medicinskoe Izdatel'stvo "Nauchnaia Mysl," 1927.

Geison, Gerald. "Divided We Stand: Physiologists and Clinicians in the American Context." In *The Therapeutic Revolution: Essays in the Social History of American Medicine,* edited by M. J. Vogel and Charles Rosenberg, 115–29. Philadelphia: University of Pennsylvania Press, 1979.

————. *Michael Foster and the Cambridge School of Physiology: The Scientific Enterprise in Late Victorian Society.* Princeton: Princeton University Press, 1978.

Gerstmann, Josef, and Paul Schilder. "Studien über Bewegungsstörungen. VI. Mitt. Unterbrechung von Bewegungsfolgen (Bewegungslücken), nebst Bemerkungen über Mangel an Antrieb." *Zeitschrift für die gesamte Neurologie und Psychiatrie* 85 (1923): 32–43.

Geyer, Christian, ed. *Hirnforschung und Willensfreiheit: Zur Deutung der neuesten Experimente.* Edition Suhrkamp 2387. Frankfurt am Main: Suhrkamp, 2004.

Gijn, Jan van. "The Babinski Sign." *Practical Neurology* 2 (2002): 42–44.

————. *The Babinski Sign: A Centenary.* Utrecht: Universiteit Utrecht, 1996.

Gijswijt-Hofstra, Marijke, and Roy Porter, eds. *Cultures of Neurasthenia: From Beard to the First World War.* Amsterdam: Rodopi, 2001.

Gilfond, Duff. *I Go Horizontal.* New York: Vanguard, 1940.

Goetz, Christopher, M. Bonduelle, and Toby Gelfand. *Charcot: Constructing Neurology.* New York: Oxford University Press, 1995.

Goffman, Erving. *The Presentation of Self in Everyday Life.* New York: Anchor, 1959.

Gordon, Alfred. *Diseases of the Nervous System: For the General Practitioner and Student.* London: H. K. Lewis, 1908.

Gowers, William. *A Manual and Atlas of Medical Ophthalmoscopy.* London: J & A Churchill, 1879.

————. *A Manual of Diseases of the Nervous System.* London: J & A Churchill, 1892.

Graebner, William. *A History of Retirement: The Meaning and Function of an American Institution, 1885–1978.* New Haven: Yale University Press, 1967.

Griesinger, Wilhelm. *Die Pathologie und Therapie der psychischen Krankheiten, für Ärzte und Studirende.* Stuttgart: Adolph Krabbe, 1845.

Groopman, Jerome E. *How Doctors Think.* Boston: Houghton Mifflin, 2007.

Guilly, Paul. "Gilles de la Tourette." In *Historical Aspects of the Neurosciences,* edited by Frank Clifford Rose and William F. Bynum, 397–415. New York: Raven Press, 1982.

Guttmann, Paul. *A Handbook of Physical Diagnosis Comprising the Throat, Thorax, and Abdomen.* Translated by A. Napier. New York: William Wood, 1880.

Haber, Carol. *Beyond Sixty-Five: The Dilemma of Old Age in America's Past.* New York: Cambridge University Press, 1980.

Haber, Carol, and Brian Gratton. *Old Age and the Search for Security: An American Social History.* Bloomington: Indiana University Press, 1994.

Hammond, William A. *A Treatise on Diseases of the Nervous System.* New York: D. Appleton, 1871.

————, ed. *Military, Medical, and Surgical Essays: Prepared for the United States Sanitary Commission.* Philadelphia: J. B. Lippincott, 1864.

Handler, Lowell. *Twitch and Shout: A Tourette's Tale.* New York: Penguin, 1998.

Hardy, Anne. *Health and Medicine in Britain Since 1860.* New York: Palgrave, 2001.

————. "Poliomyelitis and the Neurologists: The View From England, 1896–1966." *Bulletin of the History of Medicine* 71 (1997): 249–72.

Harrington, Anne. *The Cure Within: A History of Mind-Body Medicine.* New York: W. W. Norton, 2008.

————. *Medicine, Mind, and the Double Brain: A Study in Nineteenth-Century Thought.* Princeton: Princeton University Press, 1987.

Harris, Wilfred. "The Diagnostic Value of the Plantar Reflex." *Review of Neurology and Psychiatry* 1 (1903): 320–28.

Hassall, Christopher. *Rupert Brooke: A Biography.* London: Faber & Faber, 1964.

Hauptmann, Alfred. "Der 'Mangel an Antrieb'—Von innen gesehen (Das psychische Korrelat der Akinese)." *Archiv für Psychiatrie und Nervenkrankheiten* 66 (1922): 615–86.

———. "Die subcorticale 'Handlung.'" *Journal für Psychologie und Neurologie (Leipzig)* 37 (1928): 86–100.

Hawkins, Anne Hunsaker. "A. R. Luria and the Art of Clinical Biography." *Literature and Medicine* 5 (1986): 1–15.

Heimanovich, Alexander. "Der psychotische Inhalt bei der epidemischen Encephalitis." *Zentralblatt für die ges Neurologie und Psychiatrie* 48 (1928): 46–47.

Heinicke, W. "Die unzulängliche Fürsorge für chronische Encephalitiker." *Archiv für Psychiatrie und Nervenkrankheiten* 77 (1926): 701–3.

Hellal, Paula, and Marjorie Perlman Lorch, "The Emergence of the Age Variable in Nineteenth-Century Neurology: Considerations of Recovery Patterns in Acquired Childhood Aphasia." In *Handbook of Clinical Neurology*, edited by S. Finger, F. Boller, and K. L. Tyler, 845–52. Edinburgh: Elsevier, 2010.

Helmholz, H. F. and H. M. Keith. "Ten Years' Experience with the Ketogenic Diet." *Archives of Neurology and Psychiatry* 29 (1933): 808–12.

Henderson, Cary S. *Partial View: An Alzheimer's Journal.* Dallas: Southern Methodist University Press, 1998.

Henderson, Lawrence J. "Physician and Patient as a Social System." *New England Journal of Medicine* 212 (1935): 819–23.

Herzlich, Claudine, and Janine Pierret. *Illness and Self in Society.* Translated by Elborg Forster. Baltimore: Johns Hopkins University Press, 1987.

Hibbitts, Bernard J. "Coming to Our Senses: Communication and Legal Expression in Performance Cultures." *Emory Law Journal* 4 (1992): 874–959.

Holdsworth, William. *Charles Dickens as a Legal Historian.* New Haven: Yale University Press, 1928.

Holmes, Gordon. "Disturbances of Vision from Cerebral Lesions, with Special Reference to the Cortical Representations of the Macula." *Brain* 46 (1917): 34–73.

———. *Introduction to Clinical Neurology.* Edinburgh: E & S Livingstone, 1946.

———. *The National Hospital, Queen Square.* Edinburgh: E & S Livingstone, 1954.

Holstein, Martha. "Aging, Culture, and the Framing of Alzheimer Disease." In *Concepts of Alzheimer Disease: Biological, Clinical, and Cultural Perspectives*, edited by Peter J. Whitehouse, Konrad Maurer, and Jesse F. Ballenger, 158–80. Baltimore: Johns Hopkins University Press, 2000.

———. "Alzheimer's Disease and Senile Dementia, 1885–1920: An Interpretive History of Disease Negotiation." *Journal of Aging Studies* 11 (1997): 1–13.

Howell, Joel D. *Technology in the Hospital: Transforming Patient Care in the Early Twentieth Century.* Baltimore: Johns Hopkins University Press, 1995.

Hughes, Susan. *What Makes Ryan Tick?: A Family's Triumph over Tourette Syndrome and Attention Deficit Hyperactivity Disorder.* Duarte, CA: Hope Press, 1996.

Huisman, Frank, and John Harley Warner, eds. *Locating Medical History: The Stories and Their Meanings.* Baltimore: Johns Hopkins University Press, 2006.

Humble, J. G., and Peter Hansell. *The Westminster Hospital, 1716–1966.* London: Pitman, 1966.

Hunter, Richard. "Psychiatry and Neurology: Psychosyndrome or Brain Disease." *Proceedings of the Royal Society of Medicine* 66 (1973): 359–64.

Illich, Ivan. *Limits to Medicine: Medical Nemesis, the Expropriate of Health.* London: Marion Boyars, 2000.

Israël, Lucien. *Le juif-errant à la Salpêtrière.* Paris: Collection Grands Textes, Nouvelle Objet, 1993.

Itard, Jean M. G. "Mémoire sur quelques fonctions involontaires des appareils de la locomotion, de la préhension, et de la voix." *Archives Générales de Médecine* 8 (1825): 385–407.

Jackson, John Hughlings. "On Affections of Speech from Disease of the Brain." *Brain* 1, no. 3 (1878): 304–30.

Jacyna, L. Stephen. *Lost Words: Narratives of Language and the Brain, 1825–1926.* Princeton: Princeton University Press, 2000.

———. *Medicine and Modernism: A Biography of Sir Henry Head.* London: Pickering & Chatto, 2008.

———. "Medicine in Transformation, 1800–1849." In *The Western Medical Tradition, 1800–2000,* edited by William F. Bynum, Anne Hardy, L. Stephen Jacyna, Christopher Lawrence, and E. M. Tansey, 11–101. Cambridge: Cambridge University Press, 2006.

———. "Somatic Theories of Mind and the Interests of Medicine in Britain, 1850–1879." *Medical History* 26 (1982): 233–58.

Janet, Pierre. *Les obsessions et la psychasthénie.* 2 vols. 2nd ed. Paris: Félix Alcan, 1908.

———. *Psychological Healing: A Historical and Clinical Study.* Translated by Eden Paul and Cedar Paul. London: George Allen & Unwin, 1925.

Jelliffe, Smith Ely. "The Mental Pictures in Schizophrenia and in Epidemic Encephalitis: Their Alliances, Differences, and a Point of View." *American Journal of Psychiatry* 83 (1927): 413–65.

Jelliffe, Smith Ely, and William A. White. *Diseases of the Nervous System: A Textbook of Neurology and Psychiatry.* Philadelphia: Lea & Febiger, 1917.

Jenner, Mark S. R., and Patrick Wallis, eds. *Medicine and the Market in England and Its Colonies, c. 1450–c. 1850.* Basingstoke: Palgrave Macmillan, 2007.

Jewson, Nicholas. "The Disappearance of the Sick Man from Medical Cosmology, 1770–1870." *Sociology* 10 (1976): 225–44.

Jones, Colin, and Roy Porter, eds. *Reassessing Foucault: Power, Medicine, and the Body.* London: Routledge, 1994.

Jordanova, Ludmilla. *History in Practice.* London: Arnold, 2000.

Jung, R. "Wilhelm Mayer-Gross, 1888–1961." *Archiv für Psychiatrie und Nervenkrankheiten* 203 (1962): 123–36.

Kaplan, Louise J. *Oneness and Separateness: From Infant to Individual.* New York: Simon & Schuster, 1978.

Ketterman, J. L., and H. J. Kumin. "Dehydration in Epilepsy." *Journal of the American Medical Association* 100, no. 13 (1933): 1005–6.

Kevles, Daniel, and Gerald Geison. "The Experimental Life Sciences in the Twentieth Century." *Osiris* 10 (1995): 97–121.

Kevorkian, Jack. *Prescription Medicide: The Goodness of Planned Death.* Buffalo: Prometheus, 1991.

Keynes, Geoffrey. *Gates of Memory.* Oxford: Oxford University Press, 1981.

Klein, Melanie. "Zur Genese des Tics." *Internationale Zeitschrift für Psychoanalyse* 11 (1925): 332–49. Reprinted and translated as "Contribution to the Psychogenesis of Tics." In *Contributions to Psychoanalysis, 1921–1945,* by Melanie Klein, 117–39. London: Hogarth Press, 1968.

Kleist, Karl. "Leitvortrag über Gehirnpathologie und Klinik der Persönlichkeit und Körperlichkeit." *Zentralblatt für die gesamte Neurologie und Psychiatrie* 75 (1934): 710–13.

Koehler, Peter J., G. W. Bruyn, and John M. S. Pearce. *Neurological Eponyms.* Oxford: Oxford University Press, 2000.

Kramer, Barry. "Rare Illness Reduces Its Victims to Shouts, Grunts—and Swearing." *Wall Street Journal,* June 20, 1972, 1, 15.

Kroker, Kenton. "Epidemic Encephalitis and American Neurology, 1919–1940." *Bulletin of the History of Medicine* 78 (2004): 108–47.

Kumbier, E., and K. Haack. "Alfred Hauptmann (1881–1948)." *Journal of Neurology* 251 (2004): 1288–89.

Kuhn, Thomas S. *The Structure of Scientific Revolutions.* Chicago: University of Chicago Press, 1996.

Kushner, Howard I. *A Cursing Brain?: The Histories of Tourette Syndrome.* Cambridge: Harvard University Press, 1999.

———. "Freud and the Diagnosis of Gilles de la Tourette's Illness." *History of Psychiatry* 9 (1998): 1–25.

———. "Medical Fictions: The Case of the Cursing Marquise and the (Re)Construction of Gilles de la Tourette's Syndrome." *Bulletin of the History of Medicine* 69 (1995): 224–54.

Kutcher, Gerald. *Contested Medicine: Cancer Research and the Military.* Chicago: University of Chicago Press, 2009.

Lane, Harlan. *The Wild Boy of Aveyron.* Cambridge: Harvard University Press, 1979.

Lanska, Douglas, T. A. Chumura, and Christopher Goetz. "Part 1: The History of Nineteenth-Century Neurology and the American Neurological Association." *Annals of Neurology* 53 (2003): S2–S26.

Laslett, Peter. *A Fresh Map of Life: The Emergence of the Third Age.* Cambridge: Harvard University Press, 1991.

Laureys, S., A. M. Owen, and N. D. Schiff. "Brain Function in Coma, Vegetative State, and Related Disorders." *Lancet Neurology* 3 (2004): 537–46.

Lawrence, Christopher. "Historical Keyword: Patient." *Lancet* 371 (2008): 21.

———. "Incommunicable Knowledge: Science, Technology, and the Clinical Art in Britain, 1850–1914." *Journal of Contemporary History* 20 (1985): 503–20.

Lears, Jackson. "The Ad Man and the Grand Inquisitor: Intimacy, Publicity, and the Managed Self in America, 1880–1940." In *Constructions of the Self,* edited by George Levine, 107–41. New Brunswick: Rutgers University Press, 1992.

Lederer, Susan E. *Subjected to Science: Human Experimentation in America before the Second World War.* Baltimore: Johns Hopkins University Press, 1995.

Lees, Andrew J. "Georges Gilles de la Tourette: The Man and His Times." *Revue Neurologique* 142 (1986): 808–16.

Leese, Peter. *Shell Shock: Traumatic Neurosis and the British Soldiers of the First World War.* Basingstoke: Palgrave Macmillan, 2002.

Lemke, R. "Über die symptomatische Schizophrenie." *Archiv fur Psychiatrie und Nervenkrankheiten* 185 (1950): 756–72.

Lennox, William G. "The Campaign Against Epilepsy." *American Journal of Psychiatry* 94 (1937): 251–62.

———. "The Physiological Pathogenesis of Epilepsy." *Brain* 59 (1935): 113–21.

Lennox, William G., and Stanley Cobb. "The Relation of Certain Physiochemical Processes to Epileptiform Seizures." *American Journal of Psychiatry* 85 (1929): 834–47.

Lennox, William G., and Erna Gibbs. "The Blood Flow in the Brain and the Leg of Man, and the Changes Induced by Alteration of Blood Cases." *Journal of Clinical Investigations* 11, no. 6 (1932): 1155–77.

Lennox, William G. *Epilepsy and Related Disorders.* In collaboration with Margaret A. Lennox. 2 vols. Boston: Little, Brown, 1960.

Leonhard, Karl. "Hyperkinetisch-akinetisch Motilitätspsychose." In *Aufteilung der endogenen Psychosen und ihre differenzierte Ätiologie,* edited by Helmut Beckmann, 79–85. 8th ed. Stuttgart: Georg Thieme, 2003.

Lerch, Otto. "Convulsive Tics." *American Medicine* (1901): 694–95.

Lerner, Barron H. *When Illness Goes Public: Celebrity Patients and How We Look at Medicine.* Baltimore: Johns Hopkins University Press, 2006.

Levine, Carol, and Thomas H. Murray, eds. *The Cultures of Caregiving: Conflict and Common Ground Among Families, Health Professionals, and Policy Makers.* Baltimore: John Hopkins University Press, 2004.

Levy, Neil. *Neuroethics.* Cambridge: Cambridge University Press, 2007.

Levy, Richard, and Virginie Czernecki. "Apathy and the Basal Ganglia." *Journal of Neurology* 253, suppl. no. 7 (2006): 54–61.

Lewis, Jane. "Agents of Health Care: The Relationship between Family, Professionals, and the State in the Mixed Economy of Welfare in Twentieth-Century Britain." In *Coping With Sickness,* edited by John Woodward and Robert Jutte, 161–78. Sheffield: European Association for the History of Medicine and Health, 1995.

Linden, Maurice, and Douglas Courtney. "The Human Life Cycle and Its Interruptions: A Psychologic Hypothesis." *American Journal of Psychiatry* 109 (1953): 906–15.

Lock, Margaret. *Twice Dead: Organ Transplants and the Reinvention of Death.* Berkley: University of California Press, 2001.

Lorch, Marjorie Perlman. "The Merest Logomachy: The 1868 Norwich Discussion of Aphasia by Hughlings Jackson and Broca." *Brain* 131, no. 6 (2008): 1658–70.

———. "The Unknown Source of John Hughlings Jackson's Early Interest in Aphasia and Epilepsy." *Cognitive and Behavioral Neurology* 17, no. 3 (2004): 124–32.

Löwy, Ilana. *Preventative Strikes: Women, Precancer, and Prophylactic Surgery.* Baltimore: Johns Hopkins University Press, 2010.

Lunbeck, Elizabeth. *The Psychiatric Persuasion: Knowledge, Gender, and Power in Modern America.* Princeton: Princeton University Press, 1996.

Luria, Alexsandr R. *The Man with a Shattered World: The History of a Brain Wound.* Translated by Lynn Solotaroff. London: Cape, 1973.

Lyotard, Jean-François. *The Postmodern Condition: A Report on Knowledge.* Minneapolis: University of Minnesota Press, 1984.

Macmillan, Malcolm. "Phineas Gage: A Case for All Reasons." In *Classic Cases in Neuropsychology*, edited by Chris Code, Claus-W. Wallesch, Yves Joanette, and André Roch Lecours, 243–62. Erlbaum: Psychology Press, 1996.

Macnamara, Eric D. "Habit Spasm." *Westminster Hospital Reports* (1907): 48–58.

Mahler, Margaret Schoenberger. "A Psychoanalytic Evaluation of Tic in the Psychopathology of Children: Symptomatic and Tic Syndrome." *Psychoanalytic Study of the Child* (1949): 279–310.

Mahler, Margaret Schoenberger, ed. "Tics in Children." Special issue, *Nervous Child* 4 (1945): 306–419.

Mahler, Margaret Schoenberger, and Irma L. Gross. "Psychotherapeutic Study of a Typical Case with Tic Syndrome." *Nervous Child* 4 (1945): 359–73.

Mahler, Margaret Schoenberger, and Jean A. Luke. "Outcome of the Tic Syndrome." *Journal of Nervous and Mental Diseases* 103 (1946): 433–45.

Mahler, Margaret Schoenberger, and Leo Rangell. "A Psychosomatic Study of Maladie des Tics (Gilles de la Tourette's Syndrome)." *Psychiatric Quarterly* 17 (1943): 579–603.

Malson, Lucien. *Wolf Children (followed by The Wild Boy of Aveyron by Jean Itard).* Translated by Peter Ayrton, Joan White, and Edmund Fawcett. New York: Monthly Review Press, 1972.

Mann, Ludwig. "Über das Wesen der striären oder extrapyramidalen Bewegungsstörung (amyostatischer Symptomenkomplex)." *Zeitschrift für die gesamte Neurologie und Psychiatrie* 71 (1921): 357–67.

Marks, Harry. *The Progress of Experiment: Science and Therapeutic Reform in the United States, 1900–1990.* New York: Cambridge University Press, 1997.

Matthews, Walter B. *Practical Neurology.* Oxford: Blackwell, 1963.

Maudsley, Henry. *Responsibility in Mental Disease.* 2nd ed. London: Henry S. King, 1874.

Mayer-Gross, William, and G. Steiner. "Encephalitis Lethargica in der Selbstbeobachtung." *Zeitschrift für die gesamte Neurologie und Psychiatrie* 73 (1921): 283–309.

McCandless, Peter. "Dangerous to Themselves and Others: The Victorian Debate over the Prevention of Wrongful Confinement." *Journal of British Studies* 23, no. 1 (1983): 84–104.

McClay, Wilfred M. *The Masterless: Self and Society in Modern America.* Chapel Hill: University of North Carolina Press, 1994.

McCullough, Laurence B. "Ethical Challenges Posed by Injuries and Diseases of the Nervous System." *Medical Humanities Review* 10 (1996): 108–12.

McGilchrist, Iain. *The Master and His Emissary: The Divided Brain and the Making of the Western World.* New Haven: Yale University Press, 2009.

McGowin, Diana Friel. *Living in the Labyrinth.* Thorndike, ME: Thorndike Press, 1994.

McHenry, Lawrence. *Garrison's History of Neurology.* Springfield, IL: Charles C. Thomas, 1969.

Meige, Henry. "Étude sur cértaines névropathes voyageurs: Le juif-errant à la Salpêtrière." *Nouvelle Iconographie de la Salpêtrière* 6 (1893): 191–204, 277–91, 333–58.

———. "La genèse des tics." *Journal de Neurologie* (June 5, 1902): 201–6.

————. "Tics variables, tics d'attitude." *Société du Neurologie de Paris (Bulletins Officiels)* (1901): 249–50.

Meige, Henry, and Eduard Feindel. "L'état mental des tiqueurs." *Progrès Médical* (1900): 146–49.

————. "Sur la curabilité des tics." *Gazette des Hôpitaux* (1901): 673–77.

————. *Tics and Their Treatment, with a Preface by Professor Brissaud.* Revised and updated version of *Les tics et leur traitement* (1902). Translated and edited by S. A. Kinnier Wilson. New York: William Wood, 1907.

————. "Traitement des tics." *Presse Médicale* (March 16, 1900): 125–27.

Merritt, H. Houston, and Tracy J. Putnam. "Sodium Diphenyl Hydantoinate in the Treatment of Convulsive Disorders." *Journal of the American Medical Association* 111 (1938): 1068–73.

Metcalfe, Grant E. "Induced Hypoglycemic Shock in Crytogenic Epilepsy." *Psychiatry Quarterly* 2, no. 2 (1939): 348–56.

Micale, Mark S. "The Psychiatric Body." In *Companion to Medicine in the Twentieth Century*, edited by Roger Cooter and John Pickstone, 323–46. London: Routledge, 2003.

Micale, Mark S., and Peter Lerner, eds. *Traumatic Pasts: History, Psychiatry, and Trauma in the Modern Age, 1870–1930.* Cambridge: Cambridge University Press, 2008.

Miller, Henry. "Personal Book List: Neurology." *The Lancet* 2 (1968): 972.

————. "Textbooks for Pleasure." *Journal of the American Medical Association* 192, no. 2 (1965): 145–48.

Mitchell, Silas Weir. *Injuries of Nerves and their Consequences.* New York: Dover, 1965.

————. *Lectures on Diseases of the Nervous System: Especially in Women.* Philadelphia: Lea Brothers, 1885.

————. *The Medical Department in the Civil War.* Chicago: American Medical Association, 1914.

————. *Some Personal Recollections of the Civil War.* Philadelphia, 1905. Reprinted from Transactions of the College of Physicians of Philadelphia, 1905.

Montgomery, Kathryn. *How Doctors Think: Clinical Judgment and the Practice of Medicine.* New York: Oxford University Press, 2006.

Morgan, J. P. "The First Reported Case of Electrical Stimulation of the Human Brain." *Journal of the History of Medicine and Allied Sciences* 37 (1982): 51–64.

Mott, Francis. "Presidential Address: The Inborn Factors of Nervous and Mental Disease." *Proceedings of the Royal Society of Medicine* 5, no 2 (1911): 1–30.

Mueller, Jonathan. "Neuropsychiatry and Tourette's." In *Neurology and Psychiatry: A Meeting of the Minds*, edited by Jonathan Mueller, 156–74. Basel: Karger, 1989.

Murray, Jock T. *Multiple Sclerosis: The History of a Disease.* New York: Demos, 2004.

Nascher, Ignatz L. *Geriatrics: The Diseases of Old Age and Their Treatment.* Philadelphia: P. Blakiston, 1914.

Nattrass, Frederick John. *The Commoner Nervous Diseases.* London: Oxford University Press, 1931.

Naumburg, Margaret. "The Psychodynamics of the Art Expression of a Boy Patient with Tic Syndrome." *Nervous Child* 4 (1945): 374–409.

Naville, F. "Études sur les complications et les séquelles mentales de l'encéphalite épidémique: La bradyphrénie." *L'Encéphale* 17 (1922): 369–75, 423–36.

Neumärker, Klaus-Jürgen. "Leonhard and the Classification of Psychomotor Psychoses in Childhood and Adolescence." *Psychopathology* 23 (1990): 243–52.

Neustadt, R. "Zur Auffassung der Psychosen bei Metencephalitis." *Archiv für Psychiatrie und Nervenkrankheiten* 81 (1927): 99–132.

Newman, Lindsay, and David A. Steel. *Gwen and Jacques Raverat: Paintings & Wood-Engravings, University of Lancaster Library, 1–23 June 1989.* Exhibition Catalogue. 2nd ed. Lancaster: University of Lancaster, 1989.

Nicolson, Malcom, and George W. Lowis. "The Early History of the Multiple Sclerosis Society of Great Britain and Northern Ireland: A Socio-Historical Study of Lay/Practitioner Interaction in the Context of a Medical Charity." *Medical History* 46, no. 2 (2002): 141–74.

Oberndorf, Clarence P. "Society Proceedings: New York Neurological Society and New York Academy of Medicine, Section of Neurology and Psychiatry." *Journal of Nervous and Mental Disease* 80, no. 6 (1934): 684–706.

Oliff, A. "History and Development of Neurology as a Distinct Specialty in America." *Journal of Civil War Medicine* 3 (1999): 33–41.

O'Neill, W. "A Case of Aphasia." *British Medical Journal* 2 (1877): 386.

Oppenheim, Hermann. *Diseases of the Nervous System: A Textbook for Students and Practitioners of Medicine.* London: J. B. Lippincot, 1904.

Oppenheim, Janet. *Shattered Nerves: Doctors, Patients, and Depression in Victorian England.* Oxford: Oxford University Press, 1991.

Osborn, Thomas. "On Anti-Medicine and Clinical Reason." In *Reassessing Foucault: Power, Medicine, and the Body,* edited by Colin Jones and Roy Porter, 28–47. London: Routledge, 1994.

Osler, William. "The Fixed Period." In *Aequanimitas.* 2nd ed. London: H. K. Lewis, 1906.

Paine, Richmond S., and Thomas E. Oppe, *Neurological Examination of Children.* London: Spastics Society of Medical Education and Information Unit, 1966.

Parkinson, James. *Essay on the Shaking Palsy.* London: Whittingham and Rowland, 1817.

Paulian, Demetre, and Jean Stanesco. "Contribution à l'étude des troubles mentaux dans le parkinsonisme." *Annales Médico-Psychologiques* 90, no. 1 (1932): 392–400.

Pearce, Frank S. *A Practical Treatise on Nervous Diseases for the Medical Student and General Practitioner.* London: D. Appleton, 1904.

Peng, S. L. "Reductionism and Encephalitis Lethargica, 1916–1939." *New Jersey Medicine* 90 (1993): 459–62.

Perris, Carlo. "The Importance of Karl Leonhard's Classification of Endogenous Psychoses." *Psychopathology* 23 (1990): 282–90.

Petit, Georges. "La conscience de l'état morbide dans les formes mentales ou psycho-organiques de l'encéphalite épidémique." *Journal de Psychologie Normale et Pathologique* 20 (1923): 493–97.

Piotrowski, Zygmunt A. "Rorschach Records of Children with a Tic Syndrome." *Nervous Child* 4 (1945): 350–51.

Pollock, Lewis J., and Loyal Davis. "Studies in Decerebration. V. The Effect of Differentiation upon Decerebrate Rigidity." *American Journal of Physiology* 98 (1931): 47–49.

Porter, Roy. *The Greatest Benefit of Mankind: A Medical History of Humanity from Antiquity to the Present.* New York: HarperCollins, 1997.

———. "The Patient's View: Doing Medical History from Below." *Theory and Society* 14 (1985): 175–98.

———. *Patients and Practitioners: Lay Perceptions of Medicine In Pre-Industrial Society.* Cambridge: Cambridge University Press, 1985.

Porter, Roy, and Dorothy Porter. *Patient's Progress: Doctors and Doctoring in Eighteenth-Century England.* Stanford: Stanford University Press, 1989.

Pressman, Jack. *Last Resort: Psychosurgery and the Limits of Medicine.* Cambridge: Cambridge University Press, 1998.

———. "Psychiatry and Its Origins. *Bulletin of the History of Medicine* 71, no. 1 (1997): 129–39.

Prichard, James Cowles. *A Treatise on Insanity and Other Disorders Affecting the Mind.* London: Sherwood, Gilbert, and Piper, 1835.

Pryor, William. *Virginia Woolf and the Raverats: A Different Sort of Friendship.* Bath: Clear Books, 2003.

Purves-Stewart, James Morgan. *The Diagnosis of Nervous Diseases.* London: Edward Arnold, 1906.

Rainbow, Paul, ed. *The Foucault Reader.* New York: Pantheon, 1984.

Raverat, Gwen. *Period Piece: A Cambridge Childhood.* 4th ed. London: Faber & Faber, 1952.

Reichardt, Martin. "Hirnstamm und Psychiatrie." *Monatschrift für Psychiatrie und Neurologie* 68 (1928): 470–506.

———. "Theoretisches über die Psyche." *Journal für Psychologie und Neurologie* 24 (1918): 168–84.

Reiser, Stanley J. *Medicine and the Reign of Technology.* Cambridge: Cambridge University Press, 1981.

Report on the Assistance of Indigent Patients Suffering with Epilepsy. Ann Arbor: The Minnie Frances Kleman Memorial Fund, 1936.

Reubi, David. "Ethics Governance, Modernity, and Human Beings' Capacity to Reflect and Decide: A Genealogy of Medical Research Ethics in the United Kingdom and Singapore." PhD diss., London School of Economics, 2009.

Reverby, Susan M. *Examining Tuskegee: The Infamous Syphilis Study and Its Legacy.* Chapel Hill: University of North Carolina Press, 2009.

Reverby, Susan, and David Rosner, eds. *Health Care in America: Essays in Social History.* Philadelphia: Temple University Press, 1979.

Reynolds John R. *The Diagnosis of Diseases of the Brain, Spinal Cord, Nerves, and other Appendages.* London: John Churchill, 1855.

Risse, Guenter B. *Hospital Life in Enlightenment Scotland: Care and Teaching at the Royal Infirmary of Edinburgh.* Cambridge: Cambridge University Press, 1986.

Roazen, Paul. *Freud and His Followers.* New York: Knopf, 1974.

Robertson, Mary M. "The Gilles de la Tourette Syndrome: The Current Status." *British Journal of Psychiatry* 154 (1989): 147–69.

Robson, David. "Disorderly Genius." *New Scientist* 202, no. 2714 (2009): 34–37.

Rogers, Daniel. *Motor Disorder in Psychiatry: Towards a Neurological Psychiatry.* Chichester: John Wiley & Sons, 1992.

Rohde, Kirsten, Elaine R. Peskind, and Murray R. Raskind. "Suicide in Two Patients with Alzheimer's Disease." *Journal of the American Geriatrics Society* 43 (1995): 187–89.

Rose, Nikolas. *Inventing Our Selves: Psychology, Power, and Personhood.* Cambridge: Cambridge University Press, 1998.

Rosen, George. *The Specialization of Medicine with Particular Reference to Ophthalmology.* New York: Froben Press, 1944.

Rosenberg, Charles E. *The Care of Strangers: The Rise of America's Hospital System.* New York: Basic Books, 1987.

———. "George M. Beard and American Nervousness." In *No Other Gods: On Science and American Social Thought,* edited by Charles E. Rosenberg, 98–108. Baltimore: Johns Hopkins University Press, 1997.

Rothman, Shelia. "Family Caregiving in New England: Nineteenth-Century Community Gives Way to Twentieth-Century Institutions." In *The Cultures of Caregiving: Conflict and Common Ground Among Families, Health Professionals, and Policy Makers,* edited by C. Levine and Thomas H. Murray, 75–69. Baltimore: John Hopkins University Press, 2004.

Rothschild, David. "The Practical Value of Research in the Psychoses of Later Life." *Diseases of the Nervous System* 8 (1947): 123–28.

Rowland, Lewis P. *The Legacy of Tracy J. Putnam and H. Houston Merritt: Modern Neurology in the United States.* New York: Oxford University Press, 2009.

Russell, James S. R. "Disseminated Sclerosis." In *A System of Medicine,* edited by Thomas Clifford Allbutt, 50–94. London: Macmillan, 1899.

Sacks, Oliver W. *An Anthropologist on Mars: Seven Paradoxical Tales.* New York: Vintage Press, 1996.

———. *Awakenings.* London: Duckworth, 1973.

———. *The Man That Mistook His Wife for a Hat and Other Clinical Tales.* New York: Vintage, 1985.

———. "A Surgeon's Life." *New Yorker,* March 16, 1992, 85–94.

———. "Tics." *New York Review of Books,* January 29, 1987, 337–41.

Sandor, Paul. "Gilles de la Tourette Syndrome: The Current Status." *Journal of Psychosomatic Research* 37 (1993): 211–26.

Savill, Thomas D. *A System of Clinical Medicine Dealing with the Diagnosis, Prognosis, and Treatment of Disease for Students and Practitioners.* 3rd ed. New York: William Wood, 1912.

Scott, Joan W. "The Evidence of Experience." *Critical Inquiry* 17 (1991): 773–97.

Scripture, Edward W. "Tics and Their Treatment." *Archives of Pediatrics* 26 (1909): 10–13.

Selborne, Joanna, and Lindsay Newman. *Gwen Raverat: Wood Engraver.* London: British Library; New Castle, DE: Oak Knoll Press, 2003.

Seligman, Adam Ward. *Echolalia: An Adult's Story of Tourette Syndrome.* Duarte, CA: Hope Press, 1991.

Seligman, Adam Ward, and John S. Hilkevich, *Don't Think about Monkeys.* Foreword by Oliver Sacks. Duarte, CA: Hope Press, 1992.

Sengoopta, Chandak. "'A Mob of Incoherent Symptoms?': Neurasthenia in Medical Discourse, 1860–1920." In Gijswijt-Hofstra, *Cultures of Neurasthenia,* 97–115.

Shamdasani, Sonu. "Claire, Lise, Jean, Nadia, and Gisèle: Preliminary Notes Towards a Characterisation of Pierre Janet's Psychasthenia." In Gijswijt-Hofstra, *Cultures of Neurasthenia*, 363–85.

Shapiro, Arthur K, and Elaine S. Shapiro. *Tic Syndrome and Other Movement Disorders: A Pediatricians Guide.* Pamphlet produced for the TSA and funded by the Laura B. Vogler Foundation, Inc., Bayside, New York, 1980.

———. "Treatment of Gilles de la Tourette's Syndrome with Haloperidol." *British Journal of Psychiatry* 114 (1968): 345–50.

Shapiro, Arthur K., Elaine S. Shapiro, Gerald Young, and Todd E. Feinberg. *Gilles de la Tourette Syndrome.* New York: Raven Press, 1978.

Shapiro, Arthur K., Elaine S. Shapiro, and H. Wayne. "Treatment of Tourette's Syndrome with Haloperidol, Review of 34 Cases." *Archives of General Psychiatry* 28 (1973): 92–97.

Shapiro, Elaine S., Arthur K. Shapiro, Richard D. Sweet, and Ruth D. Bruun. "The Diagnosis, Etiology, and Treatment of Gilles de la Tourette's Syndrome." In *Mental Health in Children*, vol. 1, *Genetics, Family, and Community Studies*, edited by D. V. Siva Sankar, 167–73. Westbury, NY: PJD, 1975.

Shenk, Dena, and W. Andrew Achenbaum. *Changing Perceptions of Aging and the Aged.* New York: Springer, 1994.

Shephard, Ben. *A War of Nerves: Soldiers and Psychiatrists, 1914–1994.* London: Pimlico, 2002.

Sherman, Henry C. "Some Recent Advances in the Chemistry of Nutrition." *Journal of the American Medical Association* 97, no. 20 (1931): 1425–30.

Shorter, Edward. *Bedside Manners: The Troubled History of Doctors and Patients.* Simon & Schuster, 1985.

Showalter, Elaine. *The Female Malady: Women, Madness, and English Culture.* London: Virago Press, 1985.

Sicherman, Barbara. "The Use of a Diagnosis: Doctors, Patients, and Neurasthenia." *Journal of the History of Medicine* 32 (1977): 33–54.

Smail, Daniel Lord. *On Deep History and the Brain.* Berkeley: University of California Press, 2008.

Smith, Roger. *Being Human: Historical Knowledge and the Creation of Human Nature.* New York: Columbia University Press, 2007.

———. *History of the Human Sciences.* New York: W. W. Norton, 1997.

———. *Inhibition: History and Meaning in the Sciences of the Brain and Mind.* London: Free Association Books, 1992.

Smyth, M. "Certainty and Uncertainty Science: Marking the Boundaries of Psychology in Introductory Textbooks." *Social Studies of Science* 31 (2001): 389–416.

Spalding, Frances. *Gwen Raverat: Friends, Family, and Affections.* London: The Harvill Press, 2001.

Starobinski, Jean. "The Natural and Literary History of Bodily Sensation." In *Fragments for a History of the Human Body*, edited by Michel Feher, Ramona Naddaf, and Nadia Tazi, 2:351–405. New York: Zone, 1989.

Steck, Hans. "Review of Paulian and Stanesco, 'Contribution à l'étude des troubles mentaux dans le parkinsonisme.'" *Zentralblatt für die gesamte Neurologie und Psychiatrie* 64 (1932): 542.

———. "Les syndromes extrapyramidaux dans les maladies mentales." *Archives Suisses de Nerologie et de Psychiatrie* 19 (1926): 195–233; 20 (1927): 92–136.

———. Les syndrômes mentaux postencéphalitiques. *Archives Suisses de Nerologie et de Psychiatrie* 27 (1931): 137–73.

Steen, Reginald, and Mabel Matthews. "Encephalography." *Psychiatric Quarterly* 11, no. 1 (1937): 34–43.

Stevens, Harold. "Gilles de la Tourette and his Syndrome by Serendipity." *American Journal of Psychiatry* 128 (1971): 489–91.

Stevens, Janice R., and Paul H. Blachly. "Successful Treatment of the Maladie des Tics, Gilles de la Tourette's Syndrome." *American Journal of Diseases in Children* 112 (1966): 541–45.

Stevens, Rosemary. *Medical Practice in Modern England: The Impact of Specialization on State Medicine.* New Haven: Yale University Press, 1966.

Stockert, Franz Günther von. "Alfred Hauptmann." *Archiv für Psychiatrie und Nervenkrankheiten* 180 (1948): 529–30.

Stolberg, Michael. *Homo Patiens: Krankheits- und Körpererfahrung in der Frühen Neuzeit.* Cologne: Böhlau, 2003.

Stone, Christopher, and Becie Woll. "Dumb O Jenny and Others: Deaf People, Interpreters, and the London Courts in the Eighteenth and Nineteenth Centuries." *Sign Language Studies* 8, no. 3 (2008): 226–40.

Strauss, Israel, and Israel S. Wechsler. "Epidemic Encephalitis (Encephalitis Lethargica)." *International Journal of Public Health* 2 (1921): 449–64.

Sturdy, Steve, and Roger Cooter. "Science, Scientific Management, and the Transformation of Medicine in Britain, c.1870–1950." *History of Science* 36 (1998): 421–66.

Suckling, Cornelius William. *On the Diagnosis of Diseases of the Brain, Spinal Cord, and Nerves.* London: H. K. Lewis, 1887.

Summers, Anne. "Hidden From History?: The Home Care of the Sick in the Nineteenth Century." *History of Nursing Society Journal* 4 (1993): 227–43.

Swiderski, Richard M. *Multiple Sclerosis Through History and Human Life.* Jefferson, NC: McFarland, 1998.

Szasz, Thomas. *The Myth of Mental Illness: Foundations of a Theory of Personal Conduct.* New York: Harper & Row, 1974.

Talbot, Fritz B. "The Ketogenic Diet." *Bulletin of the New York Academy of Medicine* 4 (1928): 401–10.

Talley, Colin L. *A History of Multiple Sclerosis.* Westport, CT: Praeger, 2008.

———. "A History of Multiple Sclerosis and Medicine in the United States, 1870–1960." PhD diss., University of California, San Francisco, 1998.

Taylor, Alfred Swaine, and John James Reese. *A Manual of Medical Jurisprudence.* Philadelphia: H. C. Lea's Son, 1880.

Taylor, Jill Bolte. *My Stroke of Insight: A Brain Scientist's Personal Journey.* New York: Viking, 2008.

Thomas, Edward P. *The Making of the English Working Class.* New York: Vintage, 1966.

Tibbitts, Clark, and Henry D. Sheldon. "Introduction: A Philosophy of Aging." *Annals of the American Academy of Political and Social Science* 279 (1952): 1–10.

Tomes, Nancy. "Merchants of Health: Medicine and Consumer Culture in the United States, 1900–1940." *Journal of American History* 88 (2001): 519–47.

—————. "Patients or Health-Care Consumers?: Why the History of Contested Terms Matters." In *History and Health Policy in the United States: Putting the Past Back In*, edited by Rosemary A. Stevens, Charles E. Rosenberg, and Lawton R. Burns, 83–110. New Brunswick: Rutgers University Press, 2006.

Tourette, Georges Gilles de la. "Étude sur une affection nerveuse caractérisée par de l'incoordination motrice accompagnée d'écholalie et de coprolalie (jumping, latah, myriachit)." *Archives de Neurologie* 9 (1885): 19–42, 158–200.

—————. "La maladie des tics convulsifs." *La Semaine Médicale* 19 (1899): 153–56.

Trollope, Anthony. *Orley Farm.* London: Chapman and Hall, 1862.

Trousseau, Armand. "De l'aphasie, maladie décrite récemment sous le nom impropre d'aphémie." *Gazette des Hôpitaux Civils et Militaires* 37 (1864).

Tylor, Edward Burnett. *Early Researches into the History of Mankind and the Development of Civilization.* Boston: Estes & Lauriat, 1878.

Ungvari, Gabor S. "The Wernicke-Kleist-Leonhard School of Psychiatry." *Biological Psychiatry* 34 (1993): 749–52

Vidal, Fernando. "Brainhood, Anthropological Figure of Modernity." *History of the Human Sciences* 22 (2009): 5–36.

Waggoner, R. W. "Encephalography." *The American Journal of the Medical Sciences* 174, no. 5 (1927): 459–64.

Walshe, Francis M. R. "The Babinski Plantar Response, Its Forms, and Its Physiological and Pathological Significance." In *Further Critical Studies in Neurology.* Edinburgh: E & S Livingstone, 1965.

—————. *Critical Studies in Neurology.* Edinburgh: E & S Livingstone, 1948.

—————. *Diseases of the Nervous System Described for Practitioners and Students.* Edinburgh: E & S Livingstone, 1940.

Walton, John. *The Spice of Life: From Northumbria to World Neurology.* London: Royal Society of Medicine, 1993.

Warner, John Harley. "The Use of Patient Records by Historians: Patterns, Possibilities, and Perplexities." *Health and History* 1 (1999): 101–11.

Warner, John Harley, and Janet A Tighe, eds. *Major Problems in the History of American Medicine and Public Health: Documents and Essays.* Boston: Houghton Mifflin, 2001.

Wear, Andrew. "Medical Practice in Late Seventeenth and Early Eighteenth-Century England: Continuity and Union." In *The Medical Revolution of the Seventeenth Century*, edited by R. K. French and Andrew Wear, 294–320. Cambridge: Cambridge University Press, 1989.

—————, ed. *Medicine in Society: Historical Essays.* Cambridge: Cambridge University Press, 1992.

Weatherall, Mark W. *Gentlemen, Scientists, and Doctors: Medicine at Cambridge, 1800–1940.* Woodbridge, UK: Boydell Press, 2000.

Weir, Mitchell Silas, George R. Morehouse, and William W. Keen. *Gunshot Wounds and Other Injuries of the Nerves.* Philadelphia: J. P. Lippincott, 1864.

Weisz, George. *Divide and Conquer: A Comparative History of Medical Specialization* Oxford: Oxford University Press, 2006.

Wendell, Susan. *The Rejected Body: Feminist Philosophical Reflections on Disability.* London: Routledge, 1996.

Wexler, Alice. *The Woman Who Walked into the Sea: Huntington's and the Making of a Genetic Disease.* New Haven: Yale University Press, 2008.

Wharton, Francis, Moreton Stillé, and Alfred Stillé. *A Treatise on Medical Jurisprudence.* 2nd rev. ed. Philadelphia: Kay & Bros., 1860.

Whitehouse, Peter J. Review of *Losing My Mind: An Intimate Look at Life with Alzheimer's,*" by Thomas DeBaggio. *New England Journal of Medicine* 347 (2002): 861.

Wiebe, Robert H. *The Search for Order, 1877–1920.* New York: Hill & Wang, 1967.

Wijdicks, Eelco F. M., and Coen A. Wijdicks. "The Portrayal of Coma in Contemporary Motion Pictures." *Neurology* 66 (2006): 1300–1303.

Wilde, Jacob Adriaan de. *Over Organische Defectpsychosen: Een Klinisch-Psychiatrisch Onderzoek naar het Voorkomen van Gevolgtoestanden van Encephalitis Lethargica.* Academisch Proefschrift, Vrije Universiteit te Amsterdam. Amsterdam: Van Gorcum/Dr. H. J. Prakke and H. M. G. Prakke, 1959.

Wilks, Samuel. *Lectures on the Diseases of the Nervous System.* London: J & A Churchill, 1878.

Williams, Sir Edward Vaughan. *A Treatise on the Law of Executors and Administrators.* 7th ed., by Sir Edward Vaughan Williams and Walter V. Vaughan Williams; 6th American ed., in which the subject of wills is particularly discussed and enlarged upon, by J. C. Perkins. Philadelphia: Kay & Bros., 1877.

Williamson, Richard T. *Diseases of the Spinal Cord.* London: Hodder and Stoughton, 1908.

Wilson, David C. "The Pathology of Senility." *American Journal of Psychiatry* 111 (1955): 902–6.

Wilson, James C. "A Case of Tic Convulsif." *Archives of Pediatrics* 14 (1897): 881–87.

Wilson, Jean Moorcroft. *Siegfried Sassoon: The Journey from the Trenches.* London: Duckworth, 2003.

Wilson, Samuel Alexander Kinnier, *Neurology.* Edited by A. Ninian Bruce. 3 vols. 2nd ed. London: Williams and Wilkins, 1954–55.

Wortis, S. Bernard. "Present-Day Trends in Neuropsychiatric Research: A Round Table Discussion." *American Journal of Psychiatry* 97 (1941): 780–804.

York, George K., and David Steinberg. *An Introduction to the Life and Work of John Hughlings Jackson with a Catalogue and Raisonné of His Writings.* London: Wellcome Trust Centre for the History of Medicine, 2006.

Young, Allan. *The Harmony of Illusions: Inventing Post-Traumatic Stress Disorder.* Princeton: Princeton University Press, 1995.

Young, Robert M. *Mind, Brain, and Adaptation in the Nineteenth Century.* Oxford: Oxford University Press, 1970.

Contributors

Jesse F. Ballenger is associate professor of science, technology, and society at Pennsylvania State University. His scholarship examines the ways that medical science and practice are involved in the creation and development of categories of difference—gender, race, age, deviance—and how such categories shape knowledge, policy, and everyday experience. His published work includes *Self, Senility, and Alzheimer's Disease in Modern America: A History* (Baltimore: The Johns Hopkins University Press, 2006) and *Treating Dementia: Do We Have a Pill For It?* (Baltimore: The Johns Hopkins University Press, 2009).

Stephen T. Casper is assistant professor in humanities and social sciences at Clarkson University. His scholarship focuses on the social and cultural history of neurology and neuroscience and the global relations of science, medicine, and technology. His recent publications include articles in *Medical History, Bulletin of the History of Medicine*, and the *Journal of the History of Medicine and Allied Sciences*. He also has a book manuscript in preparation examining the emergence of clinical neurology in Britain.

Roger Cooter is a Wellcome Professorial Fellow. He specializes in the social history of ideas in science and medicine from the eighteenth to the twentieth century. He has published on the history and historiography of alternative medicine, medical ethics, medical politics, the popularization of science, phrenology, orthopedics, child health, accidents, war and medicine, food safety research, death, and disability. Coeditor and contributor to *Medicine in the Twentieth Century* (2000), he is currently working on the history of the historiography of medicine and the body; an Anglo-American history of medical ethics; and a history of biopolitics and visualization strategies in Germany and Britain, *ca.* 1880–1940. He is the coeditor of *Medical History*.

Ellen Dwyer is professor emeritus in the Department of History and professor emeritus in the Department of Criminal Justice at Indiana University, Bloomington. She has had long-standing interests in the history of social control in the United States, especially in prisons and asylums. Her current research focuses on the history of psychiatry and neurology in the United State and emphasizes the ways that race and gender shaped military neuropsychiatry during World War II.

PAUL FOLEY is lecturer in the School of Medical Sciences at the University of New South Wales, Sydney, Australia. He is currently preparing the first history of the "sleeping sickness" (encephalitis lethargica) epidemic that afflicted the world between the two world wars. About one-third of victims died during the acute phase; at least equally tragic was the fact that almost all survivors, mostly under the age of thirty, developed incurable neurological syndromes resembling Parkinson's disease. Despite the enormous acute and long-term effects of the epidemic,   its cause was never established.

KATRINA GATLEY completed her MSc in the history of science, medicine, and technology at Imperial College, London. She then began, in September 2004, a Wellcome PhD studentship at University College London. Her research explores the development of medical knowledge and therapeutic approaches through the historical case study of multiple sclerosis (MS) in Britain from the late nineteenth century to the present. Her work examines how and to what extent separate yet intertwined communities of patients, physicians, charitable single-disease groups, and healthcare companies have modulated the financing and direction of MS research programs and therapeutic practice.

L. STEPHEN JACYNA is director of the University College London Centre for the History of Medicine. His current research explores developments in neuroscientific research and the emergence of the specialty of clinical neurology upon the wider culture. In particular, he is interested in the interactions between patients and neurologists in the period following 1860, the phenomenology of neurological illness, the literary forms in which these experiences are conveyed, the use of "exemplary" patients as objects of scientific study, and the fluid boundary between "functional" and "organic" nervous disorders. His most recent monograph is *Medicine and Modernism: A Biography of Sir Henry Head* (London: Pickering & Chatto, 2008).

HOWARD I. KUSHNER is Nat C. Robertson Distinguished Professor of Science and Society at the Rollins School of Public Health at Emory University. His research interests include addiction, drug abuse prevention, mental health, and smoking prevention. He has published widely on topics related to the history of medicine, the sociology of science, public health, and medicine. He is the author of *A Cursing Brain?: The Histories of Tourette Syndrome* (Cambridge: Harvard University Press, 1999).

MARJORIE PERLMAN LORCH is professor in the Department of Applied Linguistics and Communication, Birkbeck College, University of London. Her main research interest is in how language is organized in the brain. This includes all aspects of neurogenic language and communication disorders, with a specific interest in cross-linguistic comparisons and bilingual speakers. In addition, she carries out theoretical work in neurolinguistics from a historical perspective focusing on the nineteenth-century history of ideas about language and communication. She has published widely in journals devoted to neurology, neuroscience, linguistics, the history of neuroscience, and the history of medicine.

MAX STADLER received a PhD in the history of science, technology, and medicine from The Centre for the History of Science, Technology, and Medicine at Imperial College, London in 2010. He also holds a MSc in the history of science, technology, and medicine and a BSc in cognitive science. His current project, "Human Factors," concerns a history of perception through the eyes of soldiers, factory workers, and office clerks: of the ways human perception was shaped and mediated in factories and zones of war, through man-machine interactions and by disciplines such as ergonomics, military psychology, and industrial physiology. He was a pre- and postdoctoral fellow at the Max Planck Institute for the History of Science (2009–10) and an associate researcher at the Volkswagenstiftungs project "critical neuroscience," where he continued to pursue his doctoral research interests in the history of the nervous system in the twentieth century. He has a book manuscript on the (material) history of the nervous impulse in preparation.

Index

Hammond, William, 26
Handler, Lowell, 154–56
Hannen, James, 72–73
Hardy, Frederick Daniel, 66
Hartshorne, Edward, 69
Harvard University, epilepsy research at,
45, 51, 52, 55
Hauptmann, Alfred, 187–95, 198, 203–4
Hayworth, Rita, 117–18, 121
Head, Henry, 8, 27–28; on multiple scle-
rosis, 97, 99; neurological exam of,
34; and Nichols, 167–81; Parkinson's
disease of, 167; and Riddoch, 170–71
Head, Ruth, 167, 168, 180
head trauma, 81; epilepsy from, 49, 51
heel-toe-shin text, 42n53
Henderson, Cary Smith, 123–25
Henderson, L. J., 14n1
Herzlich, Claudine, 220n11
Heseltine, Philip, 179
Hilkevich, John H., 154, 155
Hill, Leonard, 57n3
Hippocrates, 53
Hoche, Alfred, 187
Holmes, Gordon, 21, *22, 23,* 31, 34
homosexuality, 5
Horsley, Victor, 82
Hughes, Susan, 152
human experimentation, 2, 44–56, 57n8
humoral medicine, 24
Hunter, Richard, 206
hyperaesthesia, 139
hypnosis, 83, 85; Charcot on, 27; and
tics, 160n59
hypochondria, 188
hysteria, 186; and epilepsy, 49; and tics,
147

iconicity. *See* emblematic cases
"idiocy," 67–68
Illich, Ivan, 2, 3
imaging, neurological, 21, 24, 37, 228
influenza, 180, 195, 201. *See also* encephalitis lethargica
insanity, legal issues with, 63, 65, 68–69,
77
insulin therapy, 36

International League Against Epilepsy,
56
Itard, Jean Marc Gaspard, 132

Jackson, John Hughlings, 8, 27, 75,
78n9
Jacyna, L. Stephen, 225, 227–28; bio-
graphical sketch of, 254; on Henry
Head, 27, 34; on Robert Nichols,
167–81
James, William, 175
Janet, Pierre, 175–77, 180
Japan, 170
Jaspers, Karl, 189
Jelliffe, Smith Ely, 194
Jews, 27–28, 44; "wandering trait" of,
134, 225
Jewson, Nicholas, 2–4, 216
Johns Hopkins University, neurological
research at, 45
Josiah Macy Foundation, 45
Juncos, Jorge L., 157n1
Jung, Carl Gustav, 174

Kaplan, Louise J., 160n48
Kevorkian, Jack, 118–20
Keynes, Geoffrey, 82, 83, 86, 87, 89,
97–98
Keynes, John Neville, 83
Keynes, Margaret, 91
Kidd, Frank, 171
Klein, Melanie, 159n45
Kleist, Karl, 201–2, 205
Kleman Foundation, 46–49, 53, 57n12
Klugman, Maurice, 154–55
knee jerk reflex, 32
Kraepelin, Emil, 113, 184, 205, 206
Kuhn, Thomas S., 14n2, 41n36
kuru, 7
Kushner, Howard I., 13, 28, 54, 129–56,
201, 224–25, 230, 254
Kutcher, Gerald, 221n17

Laslett, Peter, 115
Lawrence, Christopher, 5
Lawrence, D. H., 178
Lederer, Susan, 44–45

262   INDEX

Printed and bound by CPI Group (UK) Ltd, Croydon, CR0 4YY

27/10/2024

14580348-0001